BABY CARE
& Child Health Problems

Author
Vikas Khatri

Editor
Seema Gupta

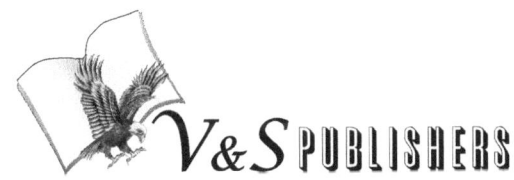

Published by:

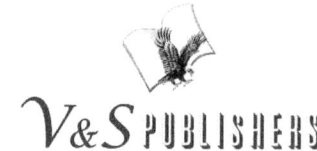

F-2/16, Ansari road, Daryaganj, New Delhi-110002
☎ 23240026, 23240027 • *Fax:* 011-23240028
Email: info@vspublishers.com • *Website:* www.vspublishers.com

Regional Office : Hyderabad
5-1-707/1, Brij Bhawan (Beside Central Bank of India Lane)
Bank Street, Koti, Hyderabad - 500 095
☎ 040-24737290
E-mail: vspublishershyd@gmail.com

Branch Office : Mumbai
Godown # 34 at The Model Co-Operative Housing, Society Ltd.,
"Sahakar Niwas", Ground Floor, Next to Sobo Central, Mumbai - 400 034
☎ 022-23510736
E-mail vspublishersmum@gmail.com

Follow us on:

All books available at **www.vspublishers.com**

© **Copyright:** *V&S* PUBLISHERS
ISBN 978-93-815887-5-8
Edition 2014

The Copyright of this book, as well as all matter contained herein (including illustrations) rests with the Publisher. No person shall copy the name of the book, its title design, matter and illustrations in any form and in any language, totally or partially or in any form. Anybody doing so shall face legal action and will be responsible for damages.

Printed at : Param Offseters Okhla New Delhi-110020

Publisher's Note

After publishing a number of books on Health and Fitness, V&S Publishers is now coming up with an exclusive and exhaustive book on ***Baby Care & Child Health Problems***. We all are aware of the fact that a baby is the most precious gift of God to a Mother. However, babies are very delicate, innocent and easily susceptible to various diseases and infections if not properly taken care of.

Therefore, a mother starts the preparations for her newborn's arrival right from the day she conceives or may be before that. She has to plan her food habits, daily routine, and take care of herself and her baby from day one till the baby is born – experiencing the pleasures and pain of the nine-month long pregnancy period.

Even after the birth of her child, she has to take the utmost care of her bundle of joy, breast-feed him/her, keep the baby clean and happy and follow the doctor's (pediatrician's) advice of vaccinating the child periodically till the age of five years. These vaccinations, medications and drops make the child immune to a number of deadly diseases like Polio, Jaundice, Hepatitis B, Chicken Pox, Measles, etc.

The book, ***Baby Care & Child Health Problems*** deals with all the above mentioned factors elaborately and systematically with special tip offs and advices from pediatricians or child specialists.

So this book can be very helpful and serve as an asset for all those mothers, who are expecting their babies to arrive soon or are busy taking care of their precious ones.

Contents

* Publisher's Note 3
* Introduction 9
* A New Life Begins 11
* Preparing for the Baby 15
* Planning a Baby Routine 17

Part I : BABY CARE   19

I. Baby Diapers 21
1. Making Cloth Diapers 21
2. Folding Cloth Diapers 22
3. Tying Cloth Diapers 24
4. Disposable Diapers 25
5. Packing a Diaper Bag 27
   FAQs 28

II. Bowel Movements and Baby's Bath 29
1. Baby Stools 29
2. Baby Toilet Training 30
3. Baby Toilet Seats 31
4. Baby Massage 32
5. Bathing Your Baby 33
6. Baby Bath Accessories 35
   FAQs 37

III. Feeding the Baby 38
1. Breast-feeding Information 38
2. Breast-feeding Positions 39
3. Breast-feeding Problems 41
4. Expressing Breast Milk 42
5. Introducing Bottle to Baby 44
6. Bottle-Feeding Tips 45
   FAQs 47

IV. Baby Sleep Patterns 48
1. Baby Sleeping Bags 48
2. Co-sleeping with Baby 49
3. Getting Baby to Sleep in Crib 50
4. Sleeping Safely 52

    5. Getting Your Baby on a Sleeping Routine 52
    6. Baby Sleep Problems 55
    7. Getting Twins to Sleep 56
    8. Positional Asphyxia in Infants 57
    FAQs 59

V. Baby Clothes 60
    1. Baby Clothing 60
    2. Buying Baby Clothes on a Budget 61
    3. Buying Clothes for the Baby Boy 63
    4. Buying Clothes for the Baby Girl 63
    5. Taking Care of Baby Clothes 65
    FAQs 66

VI. Baby Furniture and Accessories 67
    1. Baby Bedding 67
    2. Baby Carriers 69
    4. Baby Walkers 71
    5. Baby Toys 73
    6. Baby Monitors 74
    7. Baby Safe Feeder 75
    FAQs 76

VII. Premature Baby Care 77
    1. Feeding Your Premature Baby 77
    2. Premature Baby Growth Chart 79
    3. Premature Baby Health Problems 81
    4. Premature Baby Needs 82
    FAQs 84

VIII. Tips for New Mom 85
    1. Going Back to Work after Baby 85
    2. Health Tips for New Moms 86
    3. Marital Relations after Childbirth 88
    4. Travelling with a Baby 89
    FAQs 92

IX. Raising a Green Baby 93
    1. Raising Eco-Friendly Baby 93
    2. Organic Diapers 94
    3. Organic Baby Clothing 95
    FAQs 96

Part II : Child Health Problems

I. Baby Feeding 99
1. Food Guide for Babies 99
2. Feeding Problems 101
3. Transition to Bottle Feeding 104
4. Choosing Formula Milk 106
5. Guide to Choose Nipples and Bottles 107
6. Sanitising Baby Bottles 109
7. Weaning to Solid Foods 111
8. Healthy Diet for Toddlers 112
9. Feeding Schedule 114

   FAQs 115

II. Baby Hygiene 116
1. Baby Genital Care 116
2. Body Odour in Babies 117
3. Caring For Baby's Belly Button 119
4. Cleaning Baby's Eyes 121
5. Cleaning Baby's Nose 122
6. Cleaning Baby's Tongue 122
7. Cleaning Baby's Ears 123
8. Trimming Baby's Nails 124
9. Baby's Oral Hygiene 125
10. Brushing Baby's Teeth 126

    FAQs 128

III. Baby Skin Care 129
1. Baby Acne Treatment 129
2. Cradle Cap in Infants 130
3. Baby Skin Care in Winter 131
4. Baby Sun Protection 133
5. Daily Skin Care 133

   FAQs 135

IV. Common Health Problems 136
1. Body Temperature 137
2. Teething Fever 138
3. Flu 139
4. Common Cold 141
5. Asthma 142
6. Vomiting 144
7. Nappy Rash 145

8. Hypoglycemia and Colic 146
9. Irritable Bowel Syndrome 147
10. Jaundice in Newborn Babies 148
11. Anaemia 149
12. Polio 150
14. Measles 153
15. Chicken Pox 154
16. Conjunctivitis 156
17. Pneumonia 157
18. Meningitis 158
19. Hiccups in Babies 160
20. Nail-Biting in Toddlers 162
21. Restless Legs Syndrome in Babies 164
22. Shaken Baby Syndrome 165
23. Tourette Syndrome 166
24. Asperger's Syndrome 168
25. Thumb Sucking 169
26. Autism 172
27. Down Syndrome 174
28. Flat Head Syndrome 175
29. Handicaps in Children 176
30. Congenital Abnormalities 177
FAQs **178**

V. General Care **179**
1. Caring for a Sick Child 179
2. Safeguards against Accidents 180
3. Dealing with Medical Emergencies at Home 182
4. Immunization Schedule 184
Immunization Time Schedule 184
FAQs **187**

Appendix I - Average Weight and Height of Boys and Girls at Different Ages **188**

Appendix II - CDC Growth Charts **189**

Appendix III - Recipes of Common Weaning Foods **193**

Introduction

Remember that fateful day when you first held your tiny bundle of joy in your arms. Becoming a parent is the happiest day of one's life. The arrival of a new born brings delight and enthusiasm in parents' life and they look forward to see their baby grow. However, caring for your delicate baby can raise some obvious questions. A slight mishandling or carelessness can harm your baby and his/her growth and you may be left wondering where you went wrong. Apart from the regular feeding and nappy-changing, there are numerous insignificant little day-to-day jobs involved in caring for your baby the right way. Bathing and clothing him/her, breast-feeding and many such other activities require special care and attention.

Lack of proper care leaves your baby vulnerable to infections and other ailments. With low immunity, your baby is susceptible to other harmful substances in the environment. Minor skin conditions, such as heat rash, infant acne, etc may also arise as the baby's skin is thin and fragile. However, the right care can keep your baby hale and hearty, pleasant and healthy-looking and also build up his/her resistance against the above mentioned health conditions. For the lack of the right instructions' manuals, it is natural to feel baffled on how to provide the most loving and efficient care to your baby. Follow through the related chapters in this book to find the best tips and guidelines on baby care.

So help yourself and help your baby in healthy growing.

A New Life Begins

C hild care begins even before you conceive. The mother is the most important person in a child's life. If you are not ready then you will not be able to enjoy your baby nor would the baby be happy. If you are ready both physically and mentally to go through your pregnancy then the rest of the path becomes much easier. A baby is very demanding. So unless you enjoy being a mother you will find it very tough to cope with the unavoidable stress that accompanies the arrival of your little one.

Pregnancy

Pregnancy is a unique experience. You and your partner are going to become parents. Your life takes on a new dimension when you start a family. Let's have a brief idea about how pregnancy occurs. Males and females have their separate reproductive organs. The female reproductive organs include the two ovaries, fallopian tubes and the uterus. The eggs (ova) are produced in the ovaries. At the time of puberty, lots of hormonal changes take place in a girl's body. With the result, the ovaries begin to release an egg (ovum) each month. This egg travels to the uterus through fallopian tubes each month. During copulation when the sperm manages to penetrate the egg while still in the fallopian tube, fertilization occurs. If the fertilization does not occur, the egg and the tissues lining the womb are shed periodically every month. This is called menstruation. If fertilization occurs, pregnancy is established. The fertilized egg reaches the uterus and establishes itself there. New hormones are produced and new tissues are built up in the uterus to sustain the new life. A simple urine test performed six weeks after the first day of the last menstrual test may be done to confirm the pregnancy.

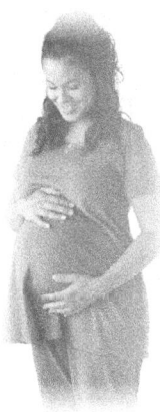

Pregnancy

Transformation

The cell formed by the union of egg and sperm is called zygote. After travelling from the fallopian tube to the womb, this cell gets attached to the lining of the uterus. With time, this zygote multiplies, matures and differentiates into various organs of the baby. The baby connects with the uterus through the placenta. Later on the placenta enlarges and is connected to the developing baby by means of the umbilical cord. The baby gets oxygen and all the nutrition from the placenta and sends its waste products to the placenta via this umbilical cord. When the baby is born, this umbilical cord is cut and clamped around two inches from the baby's end. The placenta along with the rest of the umbilical cord is expelled from the womb. The baby's umbilical cord dries up and gets shed a few days later leaving behind the belly button on baby's tummy.

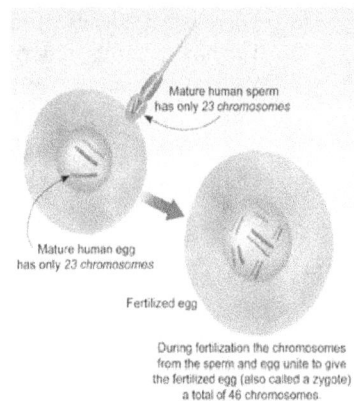

Formation of a zygote

Tests and Checkups

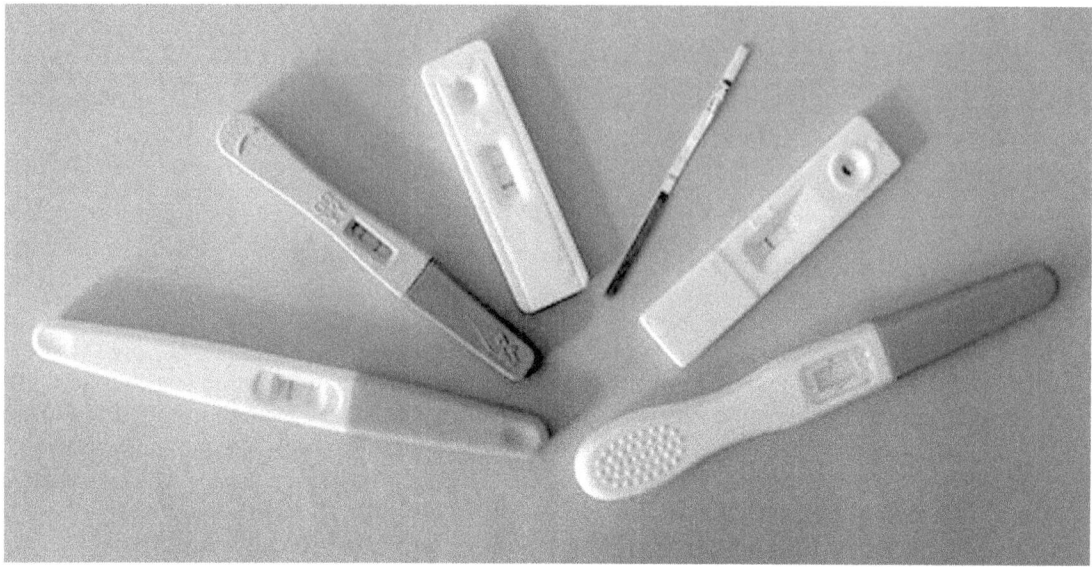

The missed periods are the first and most reliable sign for women to suspect the pregnancy. Consult your doctor as soon as possible who would confirm the pregnancy with a simple urine test.

After this, a physical examination by your doctor will be done to ensure your heart, lungs and other body systems are in perfect shape to bear the pregnancy. Throughout the pregnancy your blood pressure, heart condition and urinary status will be maintained under regular supervision for early detection of any complications. If not detected and controlled in time, they can seriously harm your baby and you.

Symptoms of Pregnancy

Here are certain features and symptoms of pregnancy which occur due to the hormonal changes and increase in the size of the womb. They are:

- The size of the breasts changes. There may be tingling and throbbing in the breasts. The veins on the surface of the breast may become more prominent. The size of the nipples increases and the surrounding area becomes darker and more prominent.
- Morning sickness in the first trimester is more common. However in some women, nausea with or without vomiting may go one further than the first trimester.
- There is a tendency of increased frequency of passing urine, especially at night.
- The bowel habits undergo change. There may be constipation.
- Your taste changes. You may develop a distaste of things which you always liked to eat and drink like tea, coffee, milk, flour, etc. There may be increased craving for things like clay, chalk or sour things.
- Some women feel emotionally drained and anxious. This occurs due to hormonal changes and it goes away on its own once the baby is born and the body reverts back to its normal form.

Development of the Baby

It is an accepted fact that the physical and mental health of the mother during pregnancy is related to the child's development, both before and after birth.

The nine months of pregnancy are divided into three parts of three months, each called trimesters.

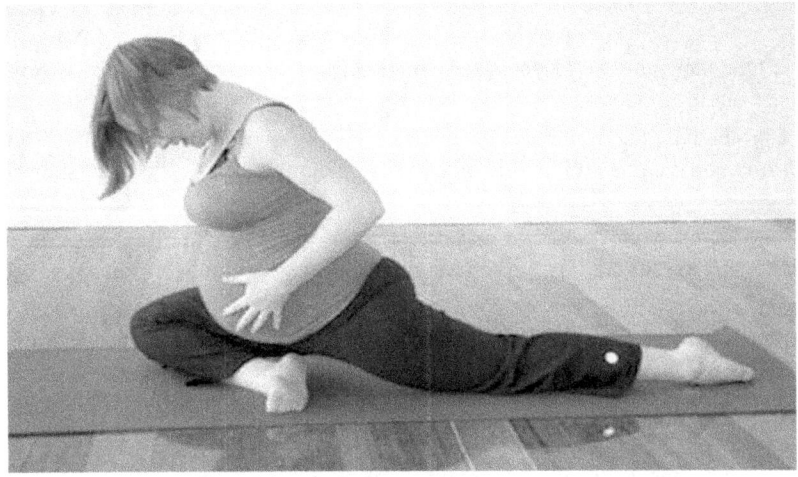
Exercising during pregnancy

- The first trimester is the most critical in terms of the formation of the baby's organs, brain, heart, kidneys, face, nose, eyes, limbs and other organs. It is during this period that most hormonal changes take place. Mild nausea and vomiting in the morning are fairly common during this trimester. To get rid of this morning sickness, avoid sudden movements and rise slowly in the morning from the lying position. It also helps to eat a dry toast or drink a cup of tea with lemon juice soon after waking up in the morning. Avoid fatty foods. Eat small but regular meals.
- During the second trimester, the pregnancy settles down and by the fifth month, you will feel the baby kicking. At first, it may not be like a pronounced kick but just a flutter or a tickle. As the months pass, you will find that the baby is more active and the frequency of movement increases.
- The third trimester is generally uneventful. Your bulge begins to show considerably. Simple yoga exercises should be done during this period for easy delivery.

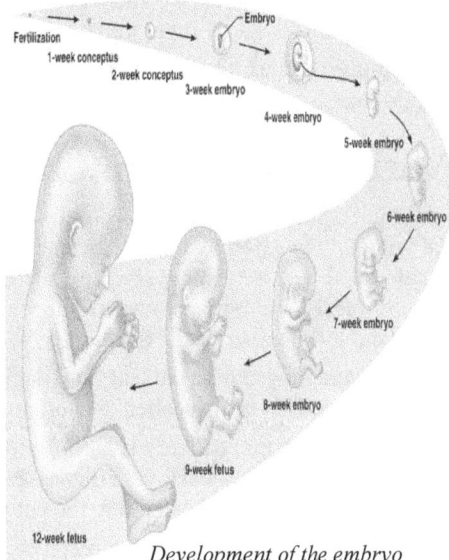
Development of the embryo

Care during Pregnancy

It is important to have regular antenatal checkups during the nine months of pregnancy.

Do not take any drugs during this period, especially during the first trimester. If it is essential then take it with the consent of your doctor because some drugs taken by you can go across the placenta to your baby. This may be harmful and damage his developing organs leading to various defects in his heart, brain, eyes, ears, etc.

Eat a healthy, nutritious diet consisting of food items of all food groups so as to provide nutrition to you as well as to the baby. Calcium, vitamin D, folic acid and iron are very important for the formation of baby's bones and teeth and to keep your haemoglobin levels high. Deficiency of folic acid in the first trimester of pregnancy is closely associated with the development of neural tube defects in the baby.

Avoid smoking and alcohol completely during pregnancy. It is also advisable to not to expose yourself to cigarette smoke released by other smokers at home or at work.

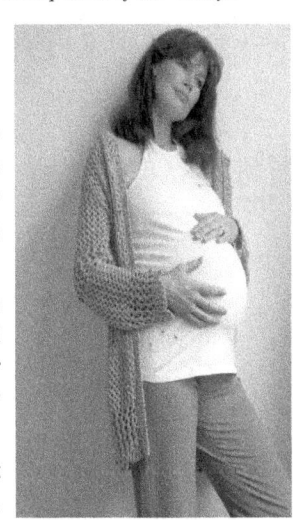

Labour

The process by which the baby and the placenta are expelled from the mother's uterus is known as labour. These symptoms indicate the onset of labour:

During pregnancy, a protective plug of mucus blocks the cervix. When the labour begins, this mucus plug loosens and is discharged through the vagina with a little blood. This phenomenon is called the 'show' and it indicates the onset of labour.

At the beginning of the labour when the cervix dilates, the amniotic sac or the water bag surrounding the baby in the womb comes down and breaks leading out a sudden gush of watery fluid coming out of the vagina.

Then regular frequent uterine contractions occur which begin as mild and brief lasting for half a minute or so. They progressively become more frequent, strong and painful lasting for a longer period.

When the onset of labour is established then the actual process of birth begins. In the first stage, the mother gets regular uterine contractions every 3 to 5 minutes and the lower portion of the uterus and the cervix dilate in order to allow easy passage for the baby.

In the second stage, strong uterine contractions begin which result in baby's head presentation. The baby's head is the first part of his body to appear and emerge out of the vagina during labour. After delivery, the baby's cord is clamped and cut. Mucus is sucked out of the baby's nose and mouth and his body is dried and he/she is wrapped in a towel.

In the third stage, which is the stage of afterbirth, the placenta and the membranes are expelled soon after the baby comes out.

Normal, Forceps or Caesarian

In normal labour, the contractions of the mother's uterus push the baby through her passage and deliver the baby out without any external aid. In case the contractions are not strong enough or the baby gets stuck in a difficult position and begins to show signs of distress, then the baby is delivered by forceps or vacuum extraction. The forceps' blades or the rubber cups of the vacuum extractor are applied to the baby's head. Then the baby is gently pulled out by an experienced doctor.

Also to avoid ragged perineal tears and damage to the mother during delivery, the doctor may make a small cut in the perineum. This is also called episiotomy. This cut is later stitched and it heals quite easily.

In cases when normal delivery is harmful to the baby or the mother, the doctor may decide to perform a caesarian operation and deliver the baby. In this case, a small cut is made in the lower abdominal wall and the uterus of the mother. After the baby is taken out, the cut parts are stitched back.

Pregnancy is not an illness. Each pregnancy is unique yet it is a perfectly normal occurrence. Regular medical advice should be taken to ensure that the pregnancy runs smoothly. There may be ups and lows in your mood, but this is not unusual. Keep your mind occupied and look after your health.

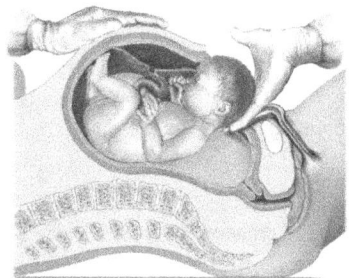 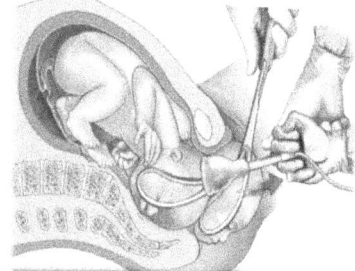

Methods of child birth

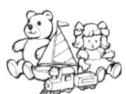

Preparing for the Baby

The arrival of the baby is the most awaited moment of your life. You would not like to spoil by having to run here and there in search of right things for the baby at the last moment. Here is a list of things which you should keep ready before the arrival of the newborn.

For the Baby

- A crib with a soft but firm baby mattress.
- Baby blankets for winter
- Pillows (optional)
- Waterproof sheeting of plastic or rubber for the crib
- Soft bed sheets and covers
- Baby clothes which are soft and comfortable
- Baby caps, socks, mittens/gloves for winter
- Soft towels
- Diapers, which are soft, such as those made from old linen in the house are very soft and should be used for the first few days as baby's skin is very delicate during this period.
- Cotton cloth pieces and wipes
- Cotton and gauze for making cotton pads
- Cotton balls for wiping baby's eyes
- Baby towels
- Mild baby soap
- Baby powder
- Baby oil
- Baby cream
- Nappy rash cream (as and when required)
- Baby bath or tub with rounded edges
- Two feeding bottles and two nipples
- A tin of milk powder
- Brushes to clean the bottles
- Bottle sterilizer

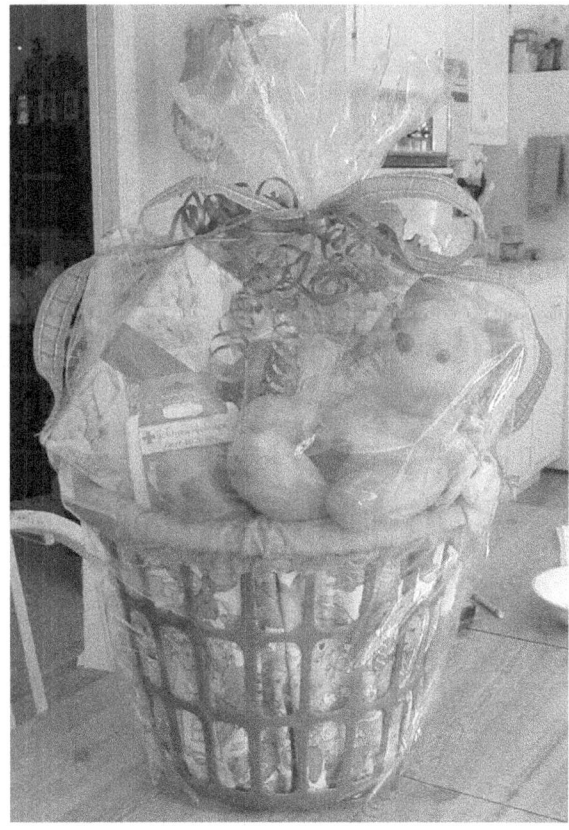

Baby accessories

For the Mother

- ❑ Maternity clothes
- ❑ Hand and body cream
- ❑ Other toiletries
- ❑ Sanitary Towels
- ❑ Breast pump (as and when required)

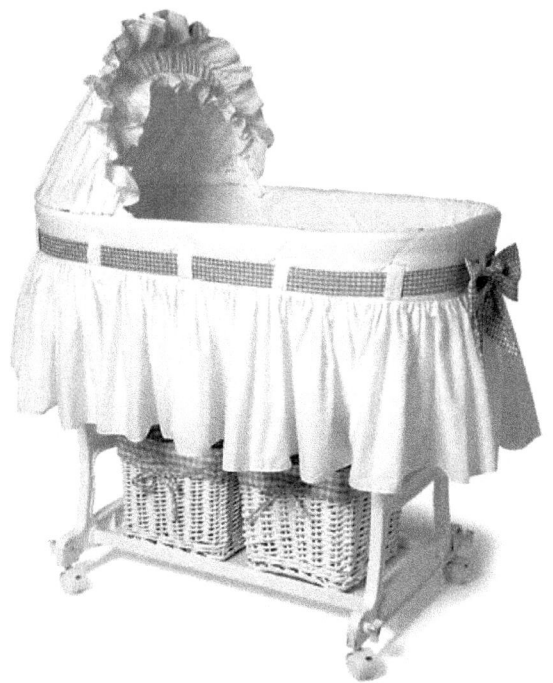
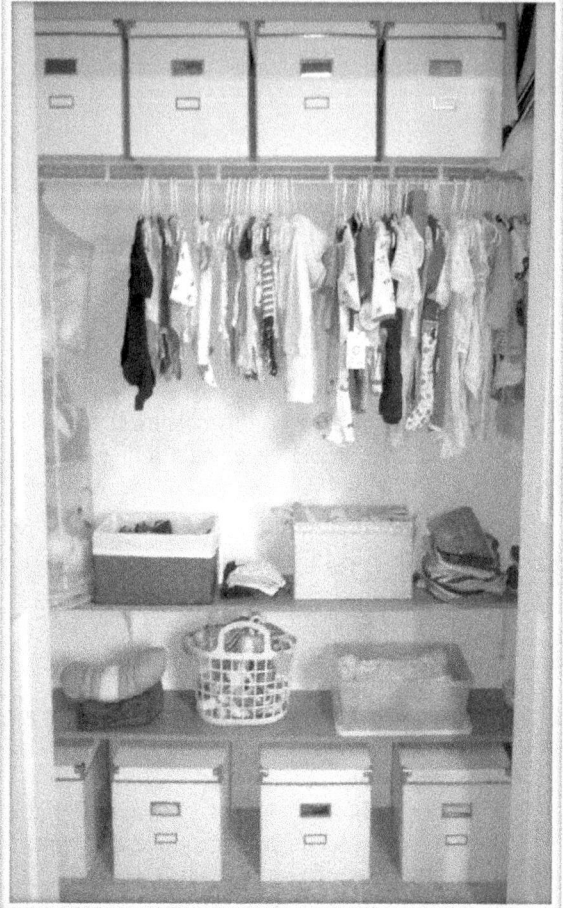
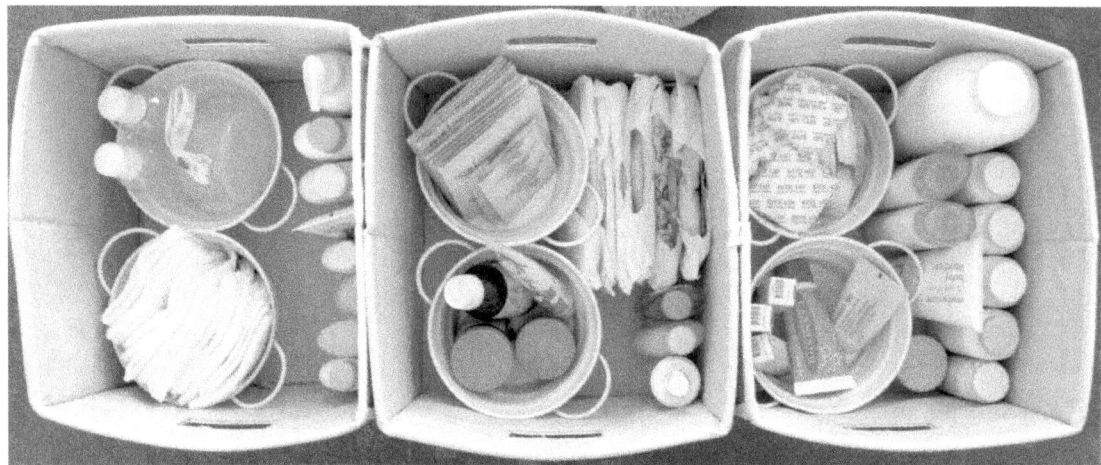

Mother and baby accessories

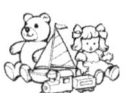

Planning a Baby Routine

The first few weeks with your baby will seem nothing more than chaotic and emotionally volatile. It will take about a month for both the mother and the baby to fit into a comfortable routine. By this time, you would have learnt how many naps he/she takes during the day and their approximate duration. You will know how often the baby needs a feed and at what intervals. You will have an idea of how many times they wake up at night. The baby will learn that you are the main caretaker and that you will feed, clean and comfort him/her when he/she cries. Depending on the way you interact and react to the baby, they will expect you to be talkative, quite, upset, calm or irritated in different situations.

Babies will also be developing their own personalities and will be learning things from you. If your behaviour is not what the baby expected in a particular situation, he/she will be upset and cry because there is a sudden unexpected change in behaviour. Babies measure their worth by the response of their caregivers. As you feed, change, bathe, clean and talk to your baby, they will look attentively at your face, observing all the changes in your expression as you speak. The first few months of a baby's life are very important from the point of view of his/her socialization. These months will form the basis for their interaction with the rest of the people. Therefore, the mother's interaction with the baby and her behaviour towards him/her assumes immense importance in the first few months.

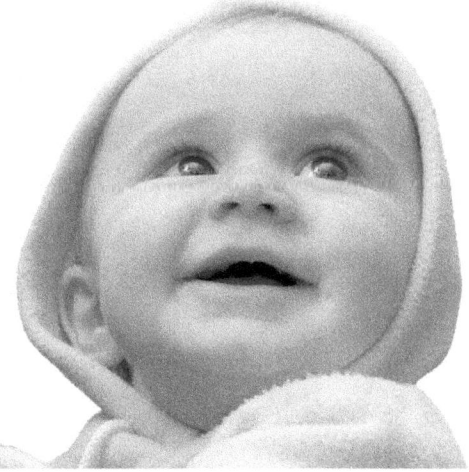

Three weeks old baby

As you have a new baby whose care will take up most of your time, it is better you make a plan and have a daily routine in place. Since you will have to take care of the baby, you may not be able to pay much attention to the rest of your family. You have an additional responsibility now that needs maximum attention and care on your part. Accept this and make changes at home to make things easier for you. Make a realistic plan that you are able to follow without much difficulty and distress. It is important to remember that you will have to plan your day around your baby. We have compiled some tips from different parents on how to manage your home and your baby in those initial days.

Tips to Plan the Baby Routine

- ❑ If you can afford it, hire someone, to help with some of the chores around the house like cleaning, ironing, shopping, etc.
- ❑ Try to keep the baby awake in the early evening time, so that he/she sleeps for a longer duration in the night. You will also be able to sleep sound if the baby doesn't wake up frequently in the night.

- ❑ You should also try to schedule the other activities of your baby, such as baths and play time along with naps and eating.
- ❑ Make sure that you stick to the same schedule during the week and on weekends. This will make it easier for the baby to fall into a set pattern.
- ❑ Take time to do something that you enjoy and that makes you happy every day. It can be talking to a friend, watching TV, or listening to music. If you are happy and relaxed, you will be able to take better care of your baby.
- ❑ On the weekends, you and your partner can take turns in looking after the baby, so that you get some time off.
- ❑ Cook your dinner early, as you will be exhausted by the evening and will have to begin cooking all over again. At least prepare most of it, so that you have very little to do later.

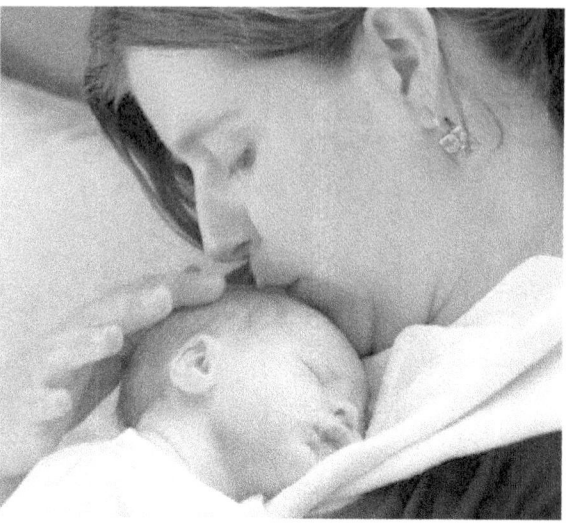

Mother putting her baby to sleep

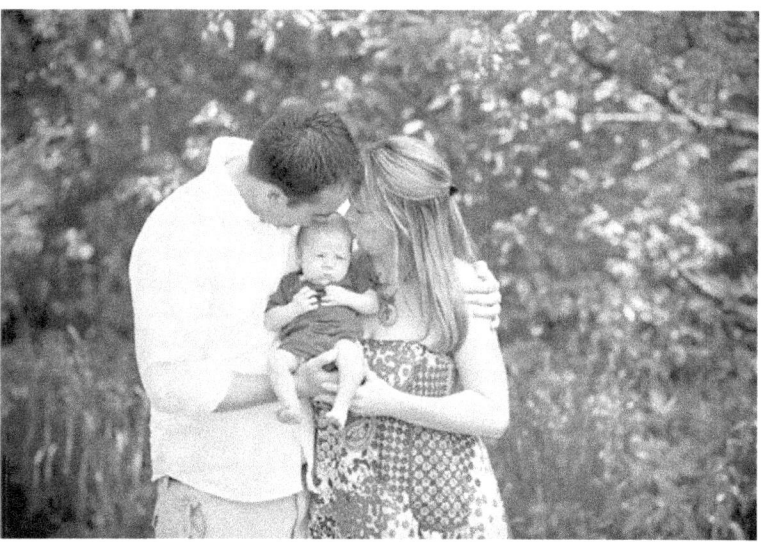

Mother, father and their child

By the age of six months, most of the babies begin to develop a rather predictable schedule for sleeping, feeding and playing. You just have to solidify those patterns by introducing your baby to a routine that is comfortable for both you and him/her. Remember, no matter how hard you work, you may not be able to do all your household chores. The important thing is not to overburden yourself, to find time for yourself and to enjoy the new baby.

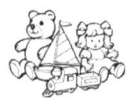

Part I
BABY CARE

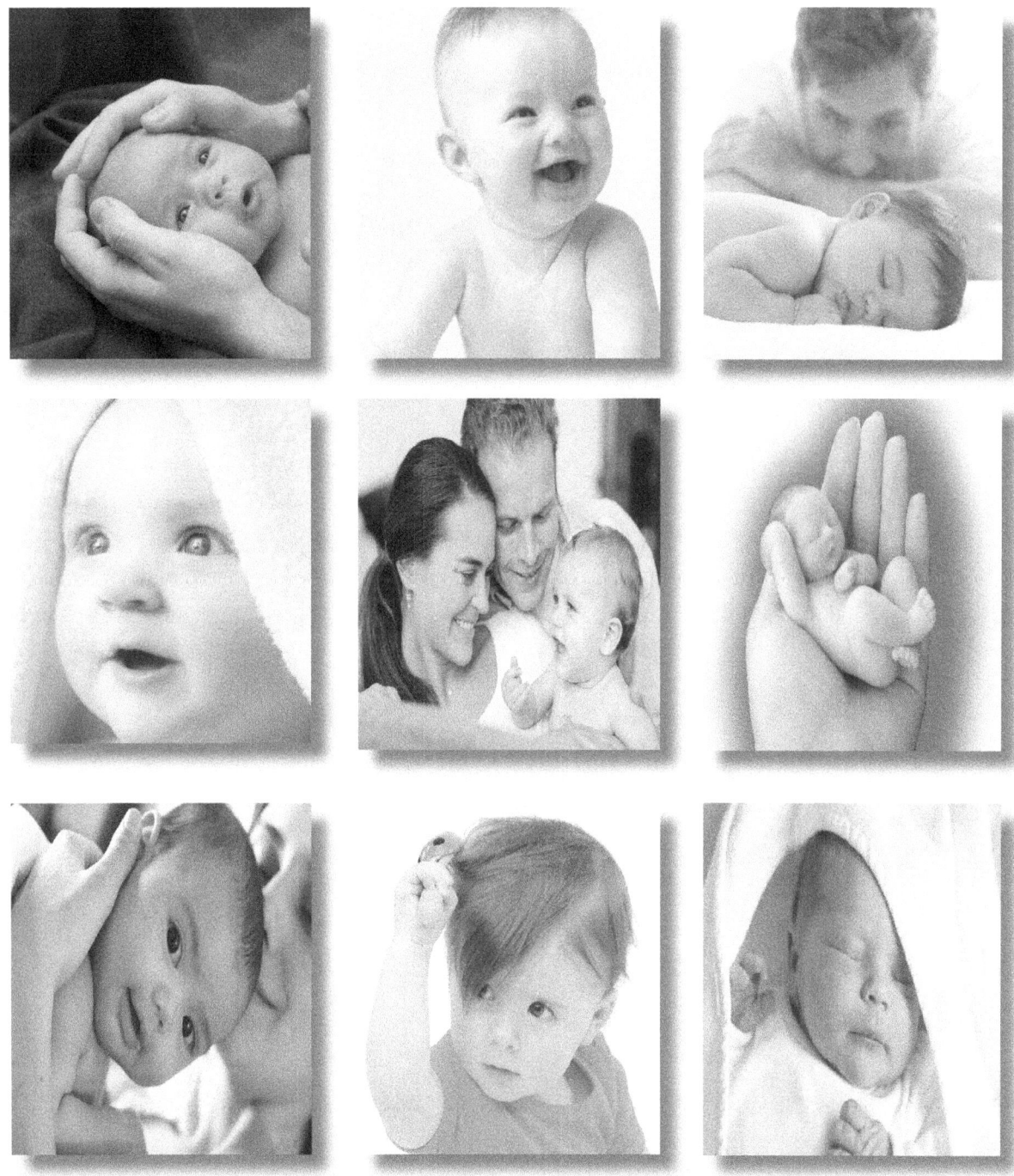

I
Baby Diapers

You have just become a parent. The excitement of labour and delivery has taken you to the next step of beginning your life with your baby. For the next few years, diapers* shall become an important part of your life. You will now wonder whether you would be using cloth or disposable diapers for your newborn. Use either of the two; your baby is sure to dirty about 10 in a day or about 70 in a week.

With the arrival of the newborn, there is a lot of joy in the air as well as lots of apprehension concerning his/her care and hygiene. For any new parent, the very thought of diapering your little one can be a scary idea. You will be amazed to see how often your baby pees and poops initially. Changing your baby after every leak is something that will command your attention most of the time. Diapers are a means to wick away wetness from your soft baby's skin, keeping him/her dry and happy. Changing your baby's diapers may seem to be a baffling chore at the start. However with a little practice, you will discover that keeping your baby dry is just a child's play. One of the important decisions that you have to make as parents is to whether put your baby on cloth diapers or disposable ones. While disposable diapers are handier and easy to use, cloth diapers are certainly the best bet. Cloth diapers are economical, environment-friendly, reusable, washable and quite easy to make.

Diapering a baby calls for some guidelines and precautions to ensure that your baby is comfortable and happy for the next few hours. If not attended well, diapers can lead to diaper rash which, when ignored, can worsen the condition. This chapter of baby care deals with the aspect of teaching new parents how to use diapers or nappies for their newborns. You will find how to make and fold cloth diapers, and pack a diaper bag. It also includes the use of disposable diapers and training a parent to tie a nappy.*

1. Making Cloth Diapers

Cloth diapers are back in vogue and are being favoured by an increasing number of parents today. Traditional cloth diapers are definitely enjoying an upper hand now, as opposed to their disposable counterparts. Apart from being economical and eco-friendly, cloth diapers are easily washable and can be reused. Also, the soft, airy feel of real cloth reduces any risk of your baby suffering painful rashes. Most parents often find it troublesome to fold a cloth diaper into a proper fit.

Choose a Style

You can begin by choosing a style for your diapers. While all-in-one (AIO) diapers are the most convenient option that comes without any pins or covers, pre-fold diapers are easy on your pockets. In case you wish to go for fitted diapers, you can sew them as per your preference.

A diaper (as known in North America) or nappy (in other countries) is a sponge-like garment worn by individuals, especially babies, who are not capable of holding their bladder or bowel movements or are unable to use the toilet.

Pick the Right Fabric

While making cloth diapers, picking the right fabric is an absolute essential. Fabrics like flannel, cotton knits, and terry make for great diapers. If you are willing for all-in-one diapers, opt for waterproof fabrics. Fleece can be used as water resistant diaper covers, as it quickly soaks away wetness from the baby's skin and keeps it dry for longer periods. It also reduces any chances of painful rashes. Terry could be used for the soaker, and a cute flannel print could be used as the external cover for your baby's diaper.

Choose a Pattern

Next step is to pick a pattern for your diapers. You can use disposable diapers for designing the pattern of your cloth diapers. Trace the outlines of the disposable diaper, carefully leaving ¼ inch for the seam. While making cloth diapers for your baby make sure that the tabs are big enough, so that they can be adjusted as the baby grows. You can also check out the various Internet websites for the pattern.

Tips to Make Cloth Diapers

- Following the pattern, cut two hourglass shaped pieces, each from the internal cloth and the external covering. Cut out a rectangular shaped cloth from the soaker and place it between the interior cloth and external covering. The soaker should run along the full length of the baby's diaper. Put the soaker on the wrong side of the interior material and sew it up.
- Now using the measuring tape, asses the girth of the baby's thigh. Cut two strips of elastic band wide enough for the comfort of your baby and stretch them to cover the whole leg opening. Now, stitch the elastic to the wrong side of the external covering along the curved side of the leg opening. Measure the baby's back and cut out half inch wide elastic piece. Stretch it, so that it covers the entire width of the diaper and then sew it to the exterior material.
- Layer the inner and the outer covering of the diaper and sew it together. Allow a small gap in the front to turn the diaper right side out.
- Using a pencil or a butter knife, mark out the seams. Fold in the seam allowance and sew it up.
- Use snaps, Velcro or other closures to secure your diaper. Velcro has a lower longevity and tends to gets frayed after repeated washes. You can use diaper pins to secure your baby's diapers.

2. Folding Cloth Diapers

Folding a cloth diaper isn't a Herculean task and all it takes is a little practice. Folding your baby's diapers can be entertaining, as it opens the space for a lot of experiments. You can fold your baby's diapers in several ways. With time, you will eventually know what works best for your baby. The key idea is to keep your baby dry and comfortable. Here are some popular ways of folding cloth diapers.

Hour-Glass Fold

- Place the diaper on a smooth surface and even out the creases.
- Position your baby on the diaper and fold in the middle of the diaper towards the center creating an hourglass shape. Draw the other half of the diaper around the front part of the baby.
- If you are using diaper covers, secure the corners with the help of a Velcro or a snap.
- In case of pull up covers, use safety pins to close the corners and then pull the cover over the diaper.
- In case you wish to go for a folded hour glass diaper, fold the diaper from one sewn corner to another and repeat the above mentioned process.

Baby Boy-friendly Folds

- Place the diaper on a smooth surface.
- Fold one-third of the cloth diaper up and then fold the edges towards the center.

- Place your baby on the diaper and pull out the remaining half of the nappy around the baby's front.
- Pull the corners of the diaper to the front and secure it with a Velcro or snap.
- This fold is particularly helpful if you are using pull up covers. In this case, you can tie the back corners to the front layer of the cloth of the front corners.

Baby Girl-friendly Folds
- Place the diaper on a smooth surface and even out all the creases.
- Fold 1/3 of the cloth down from the top and fold the bottom sides to the centre.
- Place your baby on the diaper and pull around the remaining half to the front.
- Pull the corners of the diaper to the front and secure it with a Velcro or snap.
- This fold is particularly useful if you are using pull up covers. You can fasten the front corners of the diaper to the front layers of the cloth, particularly, the back corners.

Flat-fold Diapers
- For the flat-fold diaper, you can start with folding your diaper in half.
- Fold about two-third of each side of the diaper with one side, partly covering the other to create extra absorbency in the centre.
- The flat-fold diaper is the most versatile and it can be adjusted to different sizes.

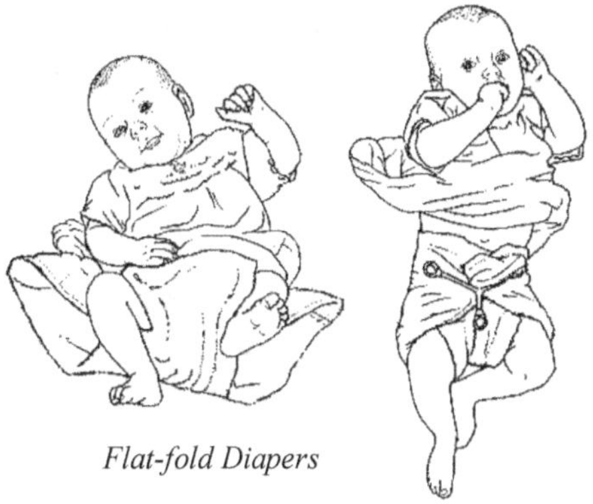

Flat-fold Diapers

Folds for Traditional Diapers

The traditional diapers are square shaped and need to be pinned up.
There are absorbent liners that can be used inside the cloth diapers, which are disposable. Cloth diapers are double lined for greater protection for night use. Diaper covers made of plastics are available to prevent leaks. They can be folded in these two styles:

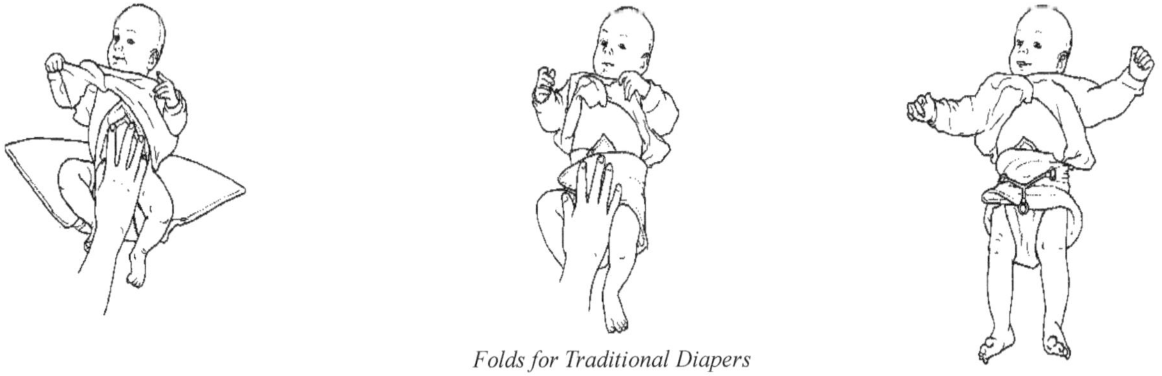

Folds for Traditional Diapers

Triangular Fold
- The square is folded into half to form a triangle.
- Place the baby gently on the triangle in such a way that his/her back is on the longest side and the opposite corner pointing to his feet.
- Bring the front part between his legs onto his stomach.
- Bring one side to overlap the middle part.
- Bring the other side to overlap the two parts. Pin them together using a safety pin.

Baby Diapers

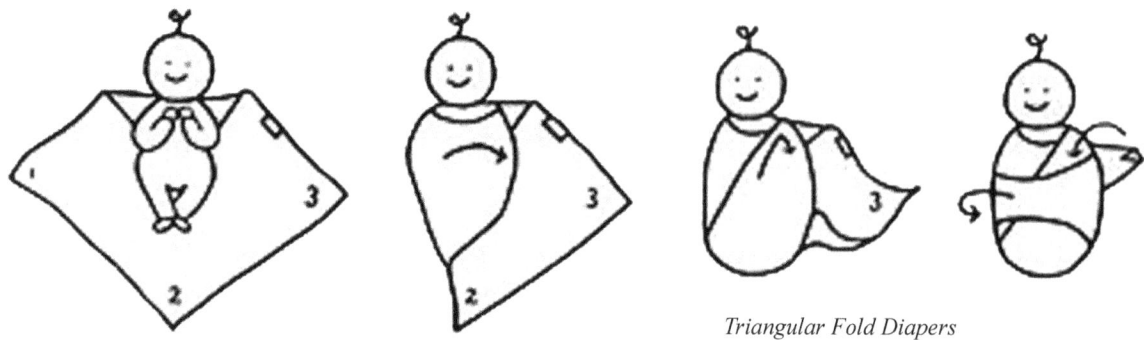

Triangular Fold Diapers

Rectangular Fold
- ❏ Fold the square into a rectangle.
- ❏ Place the baby on the rectangle.
- ❏ Bring the bottom part between his legs onto his stomach.
- ❏ Bring one side around and pin with the centre part, then bring the other side and pin again.

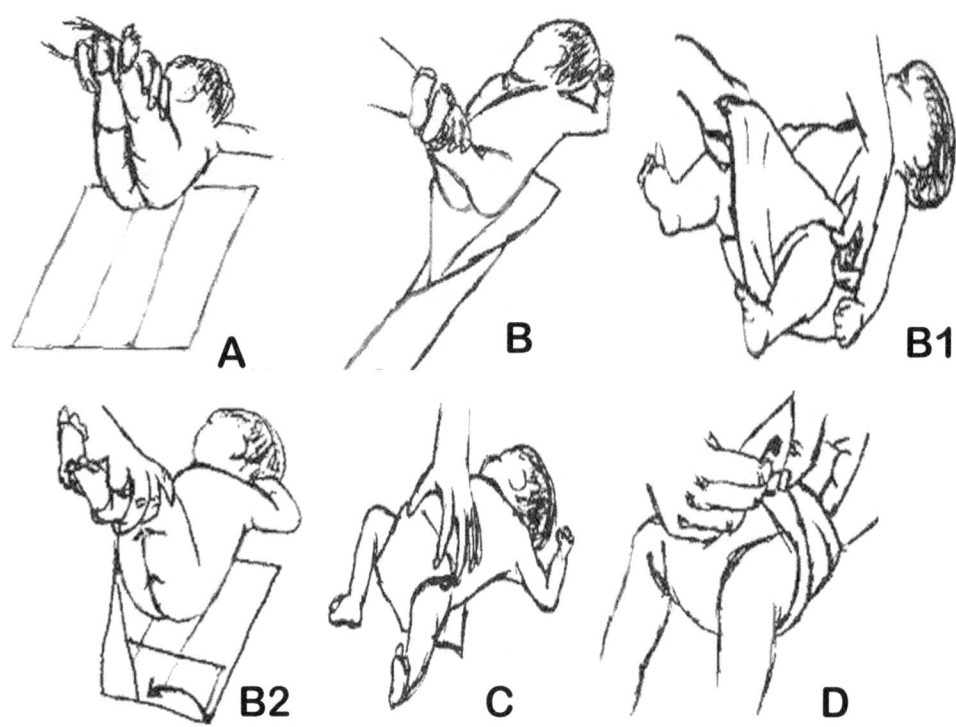

Rectangular Fold Diapers

3. Tying Cloth Diapers

Newborns and tots can make you wonder with the amount of pee and poop they generate every day. This results in lots of messy diapers. Your child needs to be kept dry all the time. On an average, a baby uses as many as 15 diapers every day. A full diaper can cause great discomfort to your little one. Your baby might catch cold, if he/she sits on a wet diaper for too long and may also develop painful skin rashes. However, going over and over that rigorous process of changing your baby's diapers can leave you high and dry at times. Most mothers often have a tough time trying to be at ease, while attending to their baby's soiled diapers.

Knowing how to tie your baby's diapers effortlessly and comfortably can ease out your endeavour and make the entire process a happy bonding time for you and your baby. Also, it can make your baby feel much more comfortable. A badly tied diaper is just the same as wearing any other uncomfortable clothing. This could badly affect your baby's sleep and could cause it to be irritable and fussy.

Tips to Tie Baby's Diapers

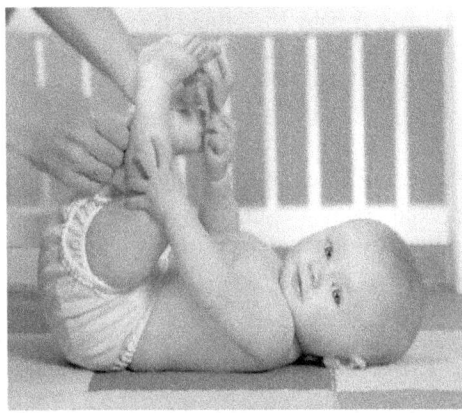
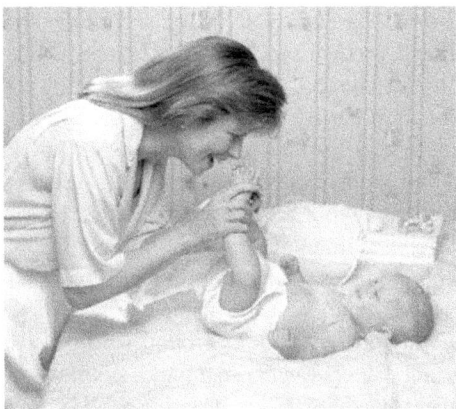

- You can place a tri-folded diaper on the wrap and then position your baby in a way that the ties are in front.
- Pad the wrap with a soaker-pad, as per your convenience.
- Fold the soaker-pad up to the baby's belly and then draw the back wings of the wrap around to the front on top of the diaper.
- Grabbing the back wings with one hand, pull the front part of the wrap with the straps up between the baby's legs and stretch it to the sides and over the diaper.
- Enclose the straps around the back and bring them to the front again and to tie them in a knot.

Tips to Use Cloth Diapers

- If the diaper requires pins, use large pins with plastic safety heads. While pinning the diaper, place your hand between the baby and the diaper. This will ensure that you do not prick the baby. Alternatively, you can use diaper tapes.
- Diapers that are wet can be put into the diaper bin. If soiled, the stools should be emptied into the toilet. You can rinse them before putting them into the diaper bin, to wash later.
- Use a solution of baking soda and water for your last rinse, as this will control odour.
- Wash diapers separately. Do not do it with the rest of your laundry.
- Use mild detergent that is recommended for baby clothing.
- Use hot water to rinse each wash.
- Wash your hands well after each diaper change to prevent germs from spreading.

4. Disposable Diapers

It's normal for parents to lose their sleep over issues relating to their child. Every parent is concerned about their baby's food, health, hygiene and even diapers. Talking of diapers, there has been a lot of discussion over disposable diapers and the traditional cloth diapers. Although it was the traditional cloth diapers that dominated the scene in the past, introduction of disposable diapers have changed the way we look at baby hygiene today. However, the opinion is divided on what is the best kind of diaper for your baby. The reason tilts from health concern to environmental issues. While traditional cloth diapers are economical and eco-friendly, disposable diapers have got an edge over being handier and easy to use. Some pediatricians do not favour using disposable diapers as they are likely to cause skin rashes, while some others are of the opinion that disposable diapers are a safe option since they wick away all moisture from the baby bottom, leaving it dry. It is sensible to change your baby's diaper frequently, if using disposable diapers. Also, keep rash creams handy and don't forget to give your baby some "open-air" time to cure any rashes caused by either kind of diapers.

Tips to Use Disposable Diapers

- Unwrap the disposable diaper and gently slip it under your baby by lifting his/her feet. Your baby's bum should rest on the top edge of the diaper, while the adhesive strips should level with your baby's belly button.
- Lift the front part of the diaper, adjusting it between your baby's legs, on top of his belly.
- Pull the adhesive strips on the rear end of the diaper to the front part and secure it comfortably. Be careful not to stick the tape to your baby's tender skin.
- If you are using disposable diapers, clean your trash regularly. This will avert growth of any harmful bacteria in your household apart from checking spread of any foul odour.
- When trashing your diaper, fold the dirty baby wipes inside the diaper. Roll it into a ball and secure it with the tapes of the dirty diaper. Put it into a cellophane grocery bag, tie it as tightly as you can and dispose it into your trash bin.
- If you notice red marks around your baby's legs and waist, opt for a loose-fitting diaper next time. Ill-fitting diapers can cause great discomfort to your baby.
- In case you notice skin rashes around your child's leg and waist, immediately shift to a different brand of diapers. Certain brands of diaper can cause skin sensitivity and allergies to your baby.
- When diapering a baby boy, position his penis downward before fastening it. This will stop leaks from seeping out over waistlines.
- If your baby's umbilical cord has not yet fallen off, be careful to fold up the waistline of your baby's diaper to prevent any kind of abrasions.
- Don't forget to wash your hands after changing your baby's diaper each time. This will prevent the spread of all kinds of harmful germs.

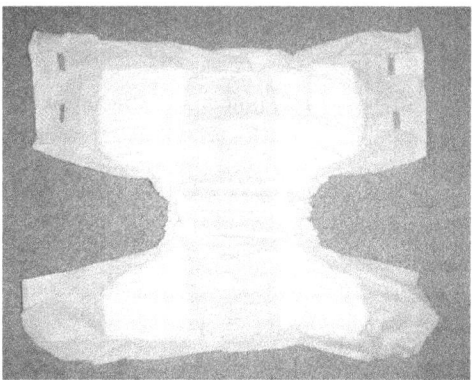
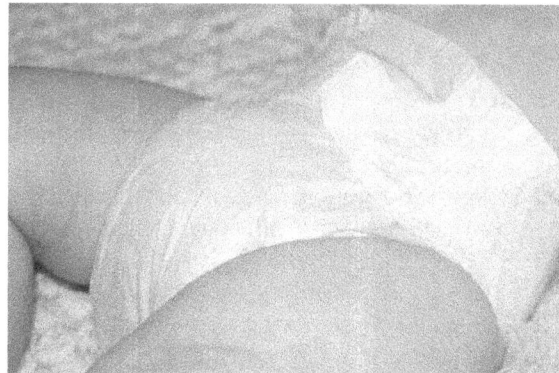

Let's Remember

- **Change diapers frequently.**
- **Look out for zinc oxide based diaper ointments to treat rashes.**
- **Don't put your baby always on diaper. Allow your baby to go without diaper for at least some part of the day.**

5. Packing a Diaper Bag

You will often see parents of little babies saddled with overstuffed diaper bags that contain almost everything, from disposable diapers to digital thermometers. When you plan to take your baby out from the comfort of your home, the focus will always be on caring for his/her little needs and having everything required, at your convenience. However, when you start deciding what assumes priority, you will be amazed at the wide range of items that you would need to choose from. At this hour, it is the diaper bag which comes to your aid. Parents are often overly careful not to exclude anything important, while packing their diaper bags. As a result, they end up cramming it with every item they come across, and then spend precious moments digging through their bag, trying to find that one small thing they need. Putting together a diaper bag requires as much careful consideration as anything else for your baby. As you get used to your child's needs, you understand that you don't really need to carry a nursery in your bag each time you go out. A little thought and smart planning is all that it takes to pack a diaper bag. Read on to know more about packing a diaper bag.

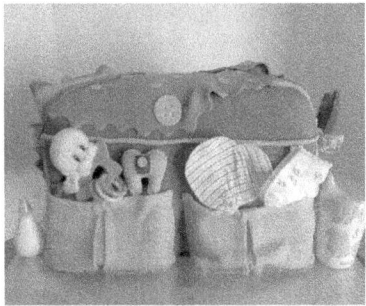

A diaper bag

Tips to Pack a Diaper Bag

- ❑ While packing diaper bags, it is essential to consider your travel time and the size of your bag first. A tote bag is just fine to cover a short outing, while you might need a large diaper bag for longer outings. You can choose from hard-sided and soft-sided bags, traditional baby bags, savvy bags, rugged-manly styles and even overnight travel cases.
- ❑ If you are planning to stay out for a short time, you can carry a bottle of milk with you. In case you wish to stay out longer, don't forget to pack in more feeding bottles. Also, do not feed your toddler with any leftover food. If you are nursing, don't forget to carry nursing pads.
- ❑ The next important thing to put into your diaper bag is diapers. Carry at least six to eight diapers for your baby, if you intend to stay out for longer hours.
- ❑ Carry anti-bacterial wipes in small containers to clean your baby's hand, face, bottom and even your own hands.
- ❑ Keep changing pads handy, in order to keep your baby from getting dirty and to wipe the dirt off your baby.
- ❑ Carry two pairs of extra clothes, bibs and socks when you are going out, just in case your little one soils his/her clothes.
- ❑ Carry a blanket to keep your baby warm.
- ❑ Using diapers for long hours can cause skin rashes. Therefore, it is important to carry a diaper cream in your bag to soothe any kind of skin irritation. This is extremely important if your baby is seated for long hours.
- ❑ Plastic bags are absolute must, in case you need to make an emergency change. Apart from holding the soiled diapers and clothes, these are extremely useful in preventing any kind of odour.
- ❑ Pack a single small toy or rattle for your child to play with, so that he/she does not get fussy while you are shopping.
- ❑ If you are planning for longer trips, don't forget to carry emergency medicines, a medicine dropper and a nasal syringe.
- ❑ Keep all the emergency contact information handy, including the contact numbers of your relatives, friends and the pediatrician.

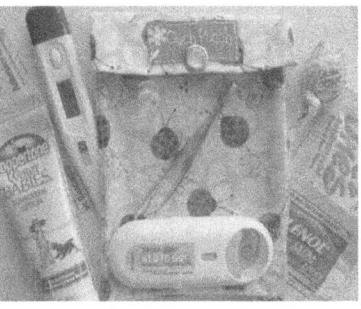

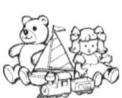

FAQs

Q-1. How can I keep my baby dry?
Ans. Prepare soft cotton pads using cotton and gauze and put them under the baby's buttocks when you are at home. As soon as they get soiled, dispose them off and use a fresh one. this way the baby will remain dry.

Q-2. What kind of diapers are the best for the baby?
Ans. Good quality disposable diapers for night and for outings are good as they save you the trouble of changing diaper number of times. But when at home or during the day, use diapers made with clean cotton cloth. These diapers are more airy and you can change them as soon as they are soiled. This way the baby remains clean at all times. This reduces the chances of your baby getting a diaper rash.

Q-3. How should I wash the cloth diapers?
Ans. To wash the cloth diapers, first clean them with soap water. Then rinse them thoroughly to wash off the soap. Wash them once more in dettol or any other anti-bacterial solution. Dry them in bright sunlight. This will disinfect the diapers completely and help in preventing rash and infection caused due to diapers.

Q-4. What should I do if the baby develops diaper rash?
Ans. If it is a mild rash, apply zinc oxide cream or a petrolatum emollient twice a day at the affected area. Keep the area dry and change the diapers frequently. In case the rash is severe and suggests fungal infection, then consult your paediatrician. Delaying this matter can cause the infection to spread to other parts of the body through blood and endanger the life of the baby.

Q-5. Is it advisable to keep my baby without diapers for some time?
Ans. During summer months, there is no harm in letting the baby go without diaper for a while as this way the skin remains dry and clean. But during the winter season, this may cause your baby to catch cold. So avoid it if possible.

Q-6. What are one-way liners?
Ans. Special one-way liners are useful since they allow urine to pass through to the towel napkin outside leaving a dry layer next to the baby's skin. These liners are now available in India in big stores.

Q-7. How are square napkins tied for girls and boys differently?
Ans. While using a square napkin, you need to place its double thickness in front for a baby boy and at the back for the baby girl.

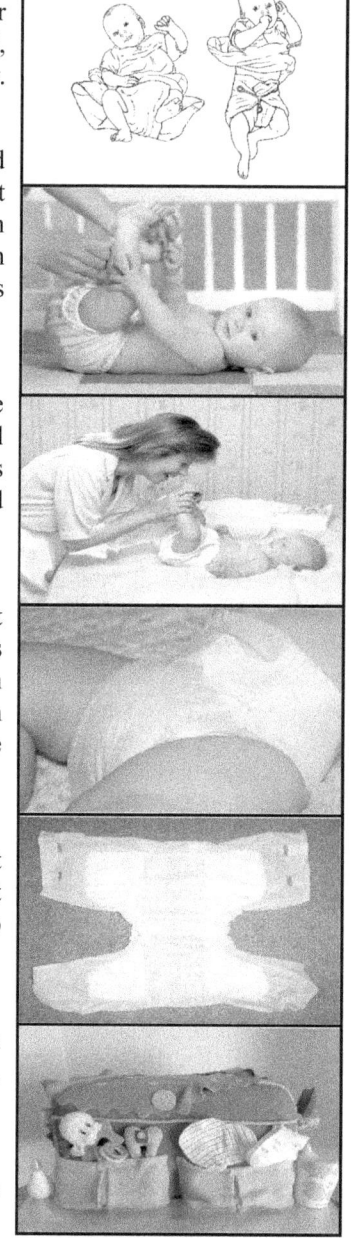

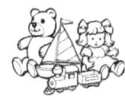

II

Bowel Movements and Baby's Bath

New mothers will learn that the two activities that take up most of their time is feeding the baby and cleaning him/her. You will have to change diapers through the day and night, at regular intervals for the first few months. There are times when you don't even have time to complete your daily household chores, since the baby is so demanding. The only way to handle this pressure is to be organised and have a system of arranging nappies, clothes, changing sheets, washing clothes. Everything required by the baby should be arranged in a systematic way, so that you can find it easily. Keeping the baby clean and dry is also important since the baby's skin is very sensitive; he/she is quite prone to develop rashes, if cleanliness and hygiene is not taken due care of. This can also make the baby irritable and cranky, which will only serve to compound your problems. To keep the baby in a cheerful and happy mood, you will have to make sure that he/she is clean and comfortable. However, the other exhausting tasks with the baby, apart from cleaning him/her, can severely test your physical stamina and mental calmness.

1. Baby Stools

The newborn baby's first nappy content is meconium, which is a greenish black substance that was in the baby's system before he/she was born. It can upset you, if you are not prepared for it. However, its presence shows that the baby's excretory system is functioning normally. The frequency or infrequency of bowel movements is an indicator of the health of the digestive system of the baby. You will have to understand the bowel movement of your baby to determine whether it is normal or a cause of concern.

Infant Bowel Movements

The frequency of stools may vary from one baby to the other. Some babies pass stools after each feed. This happens due to the gastro colic reflex, which activates the digestive system whenever the stomach is filled with more food.

Bowel Movements in Breastfed Babies

Some breastfed infants, 3-6 weeks of age, may have only one bowel movement in a few days or a complete week, which is normal. This happens as there is a very little amount of solid waste in the baby's body, which is eliminated from the child's digestive system, once in a few days. As long as the stools are soft and there are no signs indicative of constipation, the infrequency of stools is not an issue. A laxative can be given to the infant, if he/she is bothered by the long intervals between the bowel movement. The stools passed by breastfed infants are typically yellow in colour.

Bowel Movements in Formula-Fed Infants

The formula-fed infants should have, at least, one bowel movement in a day. In case, there are fewer bowel movements, the child may feel strained and uneasy because of hard stools. This may also lead to constipation. A pediatrician has to be consulted immediately in such a situation.

Bowel Movements after Four Months

As the baby begins to take solid or transition foods, the frequency of bowel movements shows an increase. The appearance and consistency of the stools will depend on the food eaten by the baby. However, the stools should appear like ordinary stools in consistency and odour. After four months, the infant may have bowel movements several times a day. Bowel movements may also be infrequent, with one stool passage in every two or three days. Some babies may also have constipation problems at this stage. Constipation caused by dehydration may result, if the baby's food contains more solids and water consumption is not adequate.

Caution

You will see that your baby's stools change a little from day to day. If there is a big change, like the stool has become very loose, very smelly, very hard or, especially, if there is mucous or blood in the stools, then you should consult your doctor immediately.

2. Baby Toilet Training

Among the innumerable things that a baby is learning, he/she must learn how to do potty in the right place meant for it. Though your baby may be too young, it has to be made a habit from an early age. Of course, toilet training for an infant differs from the toddler toilet training. The best time for early toilet training is when your child is 4-5 months old. Early toilet training depends on the understanding of the mother and child. The mother needs to understand the baby's general timing of 'pee' and also their body language. Also there are a large variety of funny toilet training seats and even toys that can be used to make the child feel curious about using them.

Tips for Baby Toilet Training

- When you have an intuition that your infant wants to do take him/her to the desired place, hold her gently and make a sound of 'pee' or 'ssss' from the mouth. After some days, your baby will be adjusted to the sound and your touch. You can choose any comfortable place.
- Pull his/her trousers up and down as children may need help with difficult clothes for some time. You can also make them wear diaper or toilet pants, while taking them to the toilet or keep them naked, if preferred.
- If after the beginning of your toilet training, your child still continues to make the diapers dirty, don't be worried. It is quite normal for the child to take around two years of time, before he/she gets adjusted to it.
- Don't pressurise the baby or don't be worried yourself in case you missed some particular timing.

Common Symptoms before Toilet

You need to understand the symptoms of your infant, after which you can confidently find out the right time to take him/her to the toilet or any other preferred place.

- The baby becomes very calm and quiet.
- He/she passes out the smelly gas.
- The body stiffens and he/she screams or become tensed up.
- The baby makes a move toward the toilet or stares at it or any such similar place.

- ❏ The baby suddenly has a look of concentration and keeps staring at some distance in vague.
- ❏ The baby makes peculiar leg movements.
- ❏ Also, there can be some changes in the behaviour of the baby. He/she can suddenly become serious.
- ❏ The baby stops playing and gives a different look.

3. Baby Toilet Seats

Toilet training can be one of the most difficult phases of parenting a newborn child. Once your kid has crossed a specific age and size, you may be interested in toilet chairs for kids, to begin the toilet training process. When it comes to buying one, you need to realise that there are a wide variety of designs available in the market, in terms of shapes, size, colour and style.

Toilet Seats for Babies

There are various types of toilet seats available in the market. Before buying a toilet seat for babies, you need to decide that whether you want the toilet seat type that sits on the floor or the one that can be attached to the toilet. Both have their advantages and disadvantages. Baby toilet seat that is attached to the floor, is easy for the child to climb and sit. However, in this case, you need to do the cleaning and also will have to train him/her separately for sitting on the bigger one later. The second option is the seat that can be attached to the general toilet. Though initially, it may pose to be a little difficult for the baby, you do not have to clean and again train the baby. Also, once the child gets a little big, you can gradually remove this extra toilet seat.

Types of Baby Toilet Seats

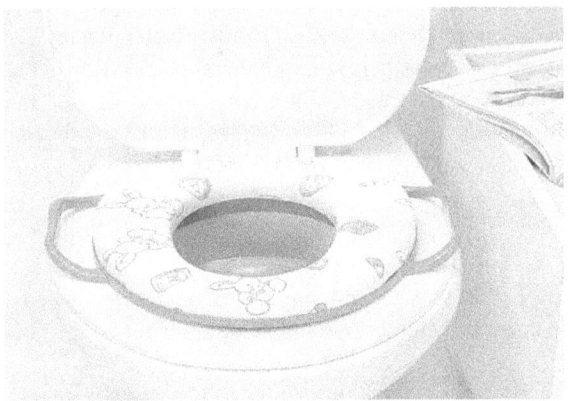
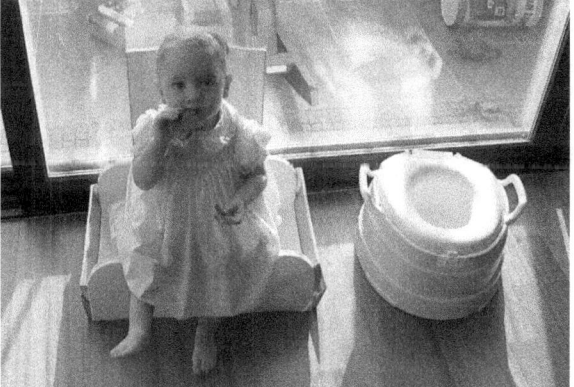
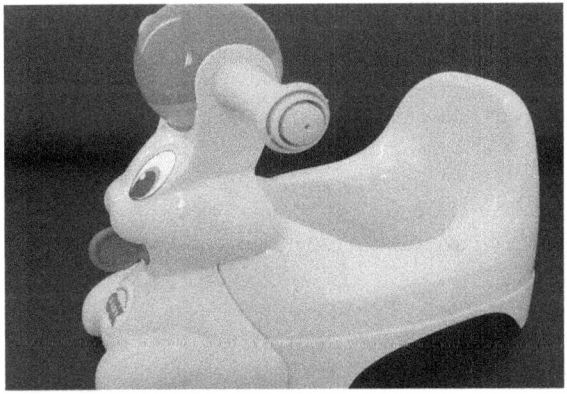
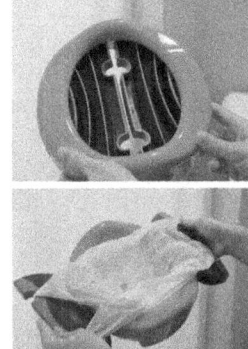
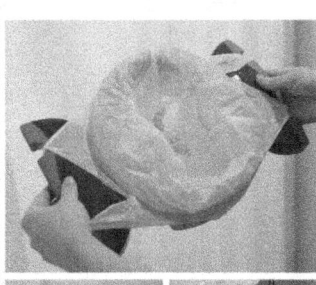
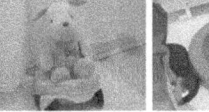

- ❑ **Moisture-Activated Seats**
  These toilet chairs have an in-built sensor to detect moisture. Once a child has finished urinating, it will begin playing a song. While some kids can be motivated to use this toilet, there may be others who get scared.
- ❑ **Decorative Toilet Seats**
  There are a number of decorative toilet chairs available to match upto the fancies of your child. You can also choose a toilet chair according to your décor or add to the fun of your child. Right from toilet chairs available in cool blue and flowery prints to ones that resemble a royal throne, the list is endless.
- ❑ **Convertible Toilet Chair**
  In such a toilet chair, the seats convert to form a stool. This can be very useful for those who have small washrooms. Convertible toilet would also encourage the child to wash his/her hands, after using the toilet. However, caution needs to be taken while converting it. Make sure the toilet chair is sturdy and stable.
- ❑ **Portable Toilet Chair**
  This is highly beneficial in case of travelling. These portable folding toilet seats for travel are compact enough to be folded easily and kept in the pouch, which is provided with the toilet seat.
- ❑ **Realistic Versions**
  It is a replica of the actual toilet chair, with the only difference being its miniature size, such type of toilet chairs are helpful for those children, who really want to use the big toilet.

4. Baby Massage

Baby massage is an ancient childcare practice that is still prevalent all over the world. Recent medical research has proven the benefits of the same. Studies have shown that premature babies when regularly massaged require minimum hospitalization. All newborns show healthy growth, more weight gain and thrive better if they are massaged well and regularly. A good oil massage soothes and calms a baby, helps him/her to relax and sleep better and makes him/her more alert during the waking hours. It is a good exercise and promotes motor activity and emotional security in a child, besides a healthy body and muscular development. It stimulates digestion and helps the baby pass gas. Here are some massage tips for infants.

Tips to Give Baby a Massage

- ❑ It is a good practice to keep all things you need ready, before you start rubbing the oil on the baby's body. This includes the baby massage oil, tissues, clean diapers and clothes. Aromatherapy oils for adults may not be suitable for the baby.
- ❑ Baby's skin is very soft and bracelet, rings and long nails might hurt your child accidentally. So, keep your fingernails short and keep aside the jewellery you wear on hands when you are massaging the baby.
- ❑ Spread a changing mat or a soft towel on a flat surface and undress the baby. Put the baby down with his or her face up.
- ❑ Rub only about half-a-teaspoon of oil at a time on your palms, so that they glide easily on the baby's body. You can apply more oil later as needed.
- ❑ Make sure that your palms are warm.
- ❑ Use smooth, gentle but firm strokes with your palm or fingers. Light circular movements on chest and stomach, stroking across the shoulders, downward movement on the arms and legs and upward movements on the back are the best.
- ❑ Do not put too much pressure on the baby's fragile body and avoid the spine area.
- ❑ Keep the baby engaged while massaging him or her by talking or singing to the infant.
- ❑ Eye contact with the baby ensures him or her of your undivided attention.

- ❑ Sudden break in contact of your hands may cause alarm to the baby. Therefore, take care to be gentle while stopping the massage.
- ❑ Do not oil baby's palms or fingers as these little ones tend to put them in their mouths or eyes often, which may cause irritation.
- ❑ Wrap the baby in a clean and warm towel after the massage and cuddle him/her.
- ❑ Do not massage the baby just before or after feeding, or when the baby is ill.
- ❑ Do not wake the baby up for a massage.
- ❑ Avoid rashes, wounds or areas where the baby has got his injections or vaccines as it may hurt.

You can continue to massage your baby till he/she is three or four years old, as the benefits of a good massage are numerous.

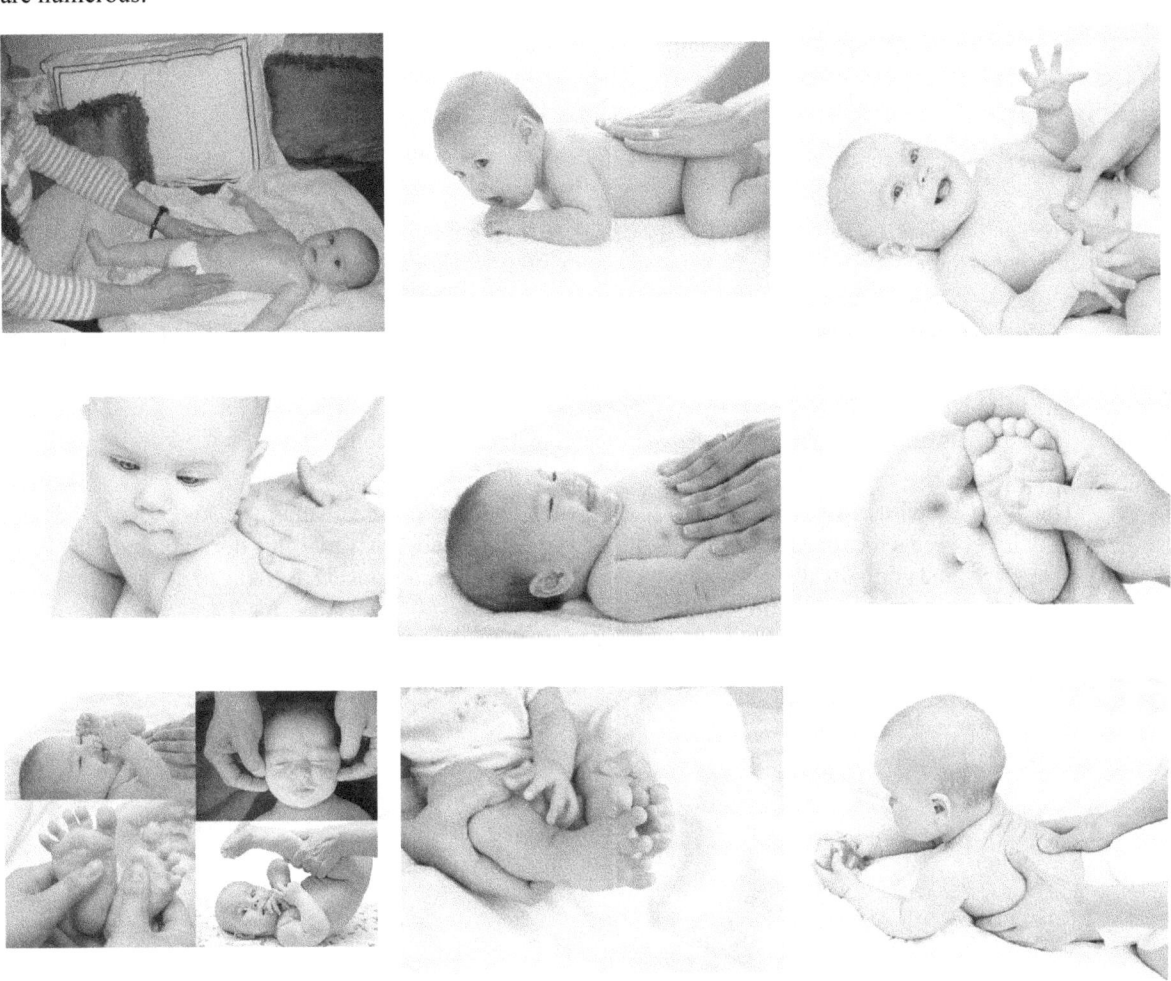

The correct way of massaging

5. Bathing Your Baby

Bathing your soft and delicate baby can be a beautiful experience for both you and the baby. It will help you a great deal to have a bath routine in place by the time your baby is a few weeks old. A calm and warm bathing environment will make the baby comfortable with the idea of bathing and he/she will be able to readily accept the new activity. Remember, some babies do not like having a bath till they are a few months old. In that case, sponge-bathing the baby may be your only option.

General Tips for Bathing

- Wrap your baby in a towel to stop him/her from waving their arms. Undress them only if you want to.
- Wipe his/her eyes with a little cotton wool that has been dipped in cooled boiled water. Begin with the inside of his eye and work outward. Wipe the other eye with another piece of cotton wool in the same way.
- Use wet cotton wool to wipe over and behind his ear. Use fresh piece of cotton wool for each ear.
- Wipe the baby's face, neck and chin with damp flannel or cotton wool.
- Pat dry with a soft towel making sure that the baby is not damp in the creases.
- Wipe dry their hands.
- Change the baby's nappy after cleaning nappy area and change into clean clothes.

Special Tips

Here are some special tips for different parts of the baby which need to be cleaned on a regular basis.

- **Hair**
  You need not wash your baby's hair every day. Just wiping it with a damp flannel cloth will remove any dirt that is there.
- **Nails**
  The easiest way to cut your baby's nails is to nibble them off. You can use a pair of scissors to cut them off, while they are asleep. The best time would be after a bath, when the nails are soft.
- **Ears and Nose**
  These organs clean themselves, so just wipe them gently with wet cotton wool.
- **Cradle Cap**
  This is a yellowish crust on the baby's scalp, which looks a little like dandruff. This occurs when the baby is between a month and six months old and almost all babies have it. This does not harm the baby in any way and normally disappears as the baby grows up. If it is noticeable, you can do the following:
- Use a baby shampoo.
- Massage one tablespoon of olive oil or almond oil into his scalp. Leave it on for an hour then wash it clean by shampooing.

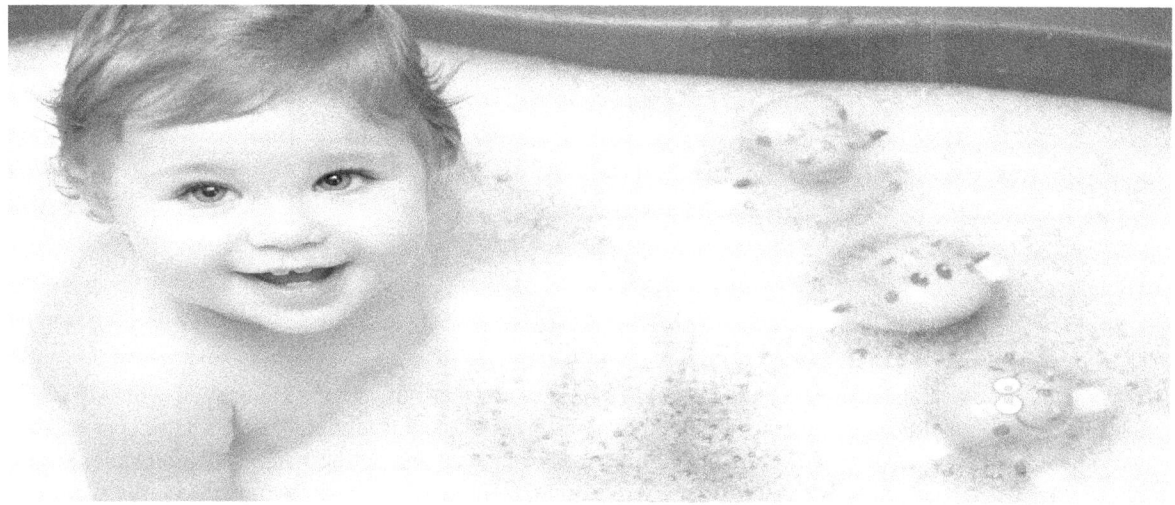

Baby in a bathtub

- ❏ Apply oil carefully to ensure that it does not enter the baby's eyes. The baby should not touch the oily scalp afterwards as it may get into his/her eyes.
- ❏ Dissolve a teaspoon of soda in 500 ml of warm water and apply on scalp with the help of cotton wool. Shampoo thoroughly. Use this regime once or twice a week.
- ❏ The flakes will become loose, if you gently comb the baby's hair.
- ❏ Never pick or scratch to loosen the flakes.
- ❏ If there are red patches on the baby's neck and behind the ears, consult a doctor immediately.

6. Baby Bath Accessories

All new parents take up the task of looking after their baby's need very seriously. They do not want to deprive their baby of even a single comfort. While giving the baby a bath, parents need to ensure that their bathroom is sufficiently equipped with the necessary baby accessories. Such accessories should not only be friendly and hygienic, but also comfortable and safe for the baby.

Bathtubs

A bathtub is one of the first things that come into mind, while furnishing a baby's bathroom. The bathtub for a baby should be comfortable, safe and fun to be in. Portable and cute bathtubs are also available in the market in different varieties. You can place them anywhere, in the bathroom or the garden, wherever you wish to bathe your baby. These portable bathtubs are convenient to use and do not cost much.

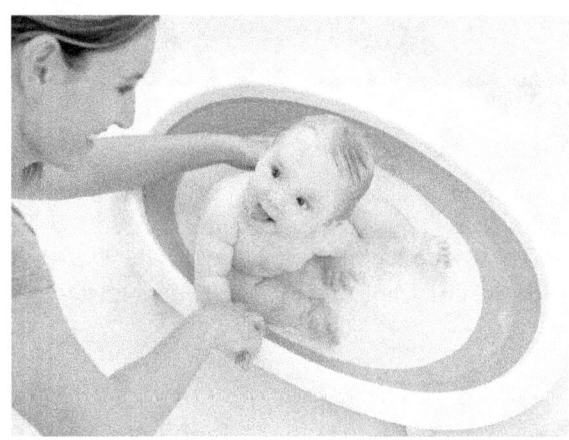

Bathing Robes

It is better to have baby-bathing robes at home. Such robes come in various designs, styles and sizes. The robe that you have chosen for your baby should be soft and fluffy, as a baby's skin is very tender and sensitive. As far as possible, you should stick to baby bathrobes made of cotton or terrycloth material. Along with being soft and comfortable, such robes easily absorb water from the baby's body and keep him/her safe and hygienic.

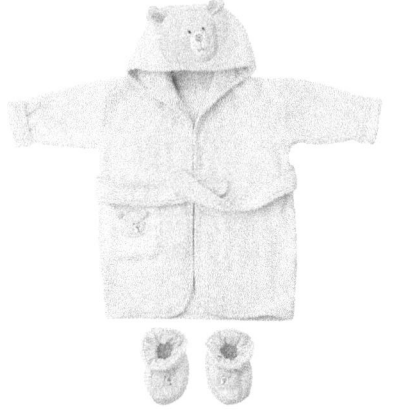
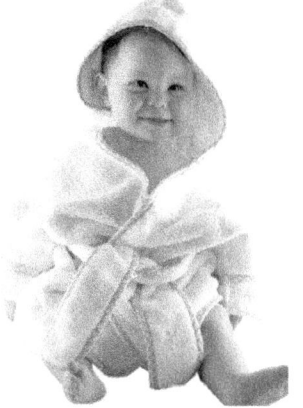

Bath Toys

Some babies do not like the idea of bathing and they make quite a protest during bath time. As a parent, it is your responsibility to make bathing experience an enjoyable one. Doing this is possible by using such bath accessories that interest a baby. Colourful bath toys serve as one of the options that can make a child happy and help him/her enjoy the bath without creating any fuss. While buying bath toys, make sure that they are cute-looking and colourful. Most importantly, they should be non-toxic, sterilised and safe for the child.

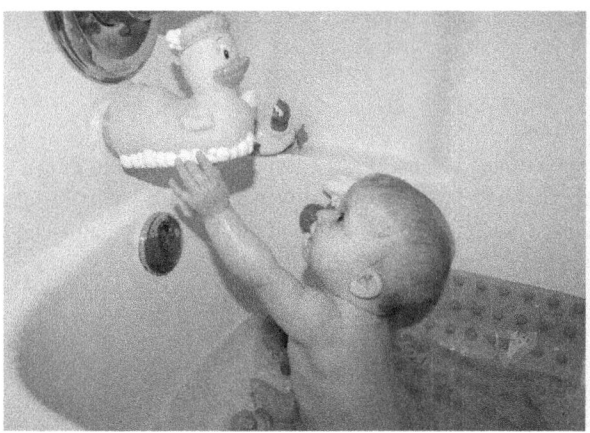
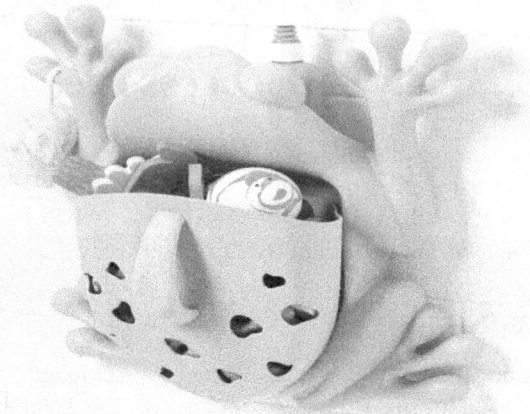

Other Accessories

Apart from the above mentioned things, there are some other accessories that will come handy while bathing a child. These include bath soap, baby shampoo, rugs, shower, curtains and hooks, soap dish, storage bin, colourful towels, tissue box cover, wall hook and wastebasket. By buying such basic bathroom accessories, you will be able to ensure that your baby has a happy, comfortable and a safe bathing experience.

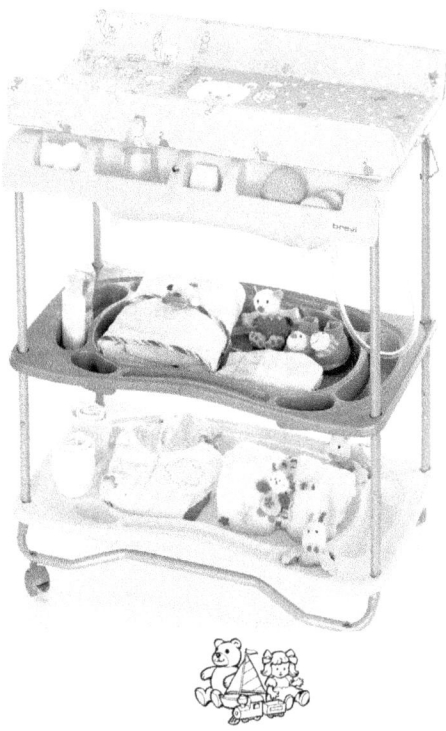

FAQs

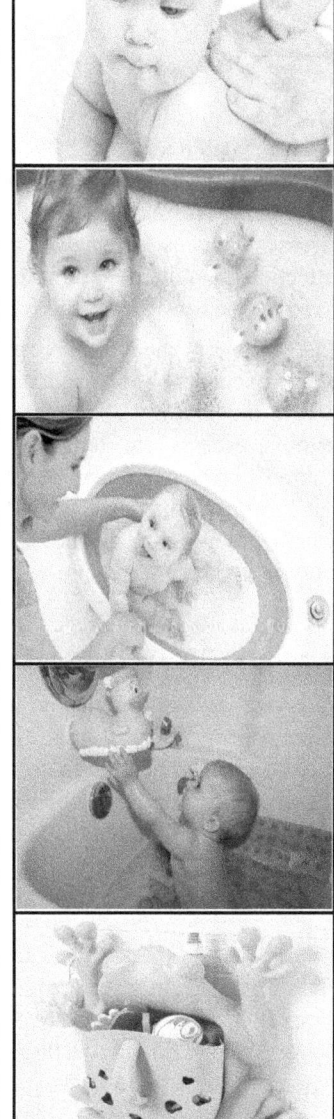

Q-1. How often should I bathe my baby?
Ans. If your baby is comfortable with it, then you should give daily bath to him/her. But if you find the baby crying during the bath or catching cold then bathing your baby on alternate days would be better. However, some sponging with warm towel and a change of clothes is important for hygiene of the baby.

Q-2. Should I clean the baby's scalp with shampoo or with soap?
Ans. Bathing the scalp once or twice a week is sufficient. To clean the scalp, use mild baby shampoo as this will not irritate the baby's eyes.

Q-3. I do not have a bath tub to bathe my baby. Can I bathe my baby without it?
Ans. In India, bathing the baby by placing him/her on the mother's outstretched feet is prevalent since old times. This is quite convenient. Just remember to take care to keep the head at a higher level than the body.

Q-4. Is it necessary to give bath to my baby with warm water even in summer season?
Ans. It is better to bathe your baby with warm water because if the water is alarmingly cold or hot then the baby does not feel comfortable in it and gets irritated.

Q-5. When my baby was born he passed a dark green and sticky stool. Was it abnormal?
Ans. The baby's first stool is called meconium. It is a thick, sticky, black-green tar-like substance which has been collecting in the intestines during the pregnancy. It is difficult to clean. But once the baby's bowels are clear of meconium, he/she begins to pass normal yellowish stools.

Q-6. Is it necessary to massage my baby?
Ans. Massaging the baby with oil is a good practice. Use coconut or olive oil for this purpose. Do the massage gently so the baby enjoys it. Make sure the oil does not go into the baby's eyes, ears, nose or mouth.

Q-7. How beneficial is the massage done with gram flour or flour dough in removing baby hair?
Ans. There is no need to apply the traditional mixture of gram flour/dough, turmeric and oil for massage. It is a myth that such a massage would remove hair from the baby's body. The hair on newborn's body would fall off anyway irrespective of whether you apply this mixture or not. It will not even prevent the baby from growing new hair on the body.

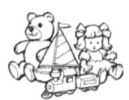

III
Feeding the Baby

Breast milk is the best food for your baby, more so, in the first six months of his/her life. Studies have proved beyond doubt that babies, who have been breastfed for the first six months of their lives, stay healthier throughout their lives. It is very important that you feed the baby the first milk your breast produces, known as colostrum. This is rich in antibodies and other substances that protect the baby from infections and illnesses. Breast-feeding is extremely healthy for your baby as it prevents many health conditions like chest infections, ear infections and diarrhoea. Protection from some diseases last long even after you have stopped breast-feeding. Feeding the baby breast milk will provide the best protection against infections.

Even mothers benefit from breast-feeding their babies. The cases of breast cancer, ovarian cancer and osteoporosis, at a later stage in life are much less among women who have breastfed their babies. A combination of breast milk and formula milk will decrease the risk of infection to a large extent. If you have a family history of diabetes, asthma, eczema, etc, formula milk can increase the risk of such diseases in the baby. In case you decide to combine breast-feeding with bottle-feeding, then the bottle-feeding should be introduced only after the baby gets used to breast-feeding. This will ensure that you have sufficient supply of breast milk. If you are unsure about whether to breast-feed or bottle-feed, it is better to start breast-feeding. Once you start bottle-feeding, it is difficult to switch to breast-feeding.

1. Breast-feeding Information

As a mother, it is your duty to take best care of your child. For the first six months, when the child is completely dependent upon breast milk, the mothers develop an emotional bond with him/her. Breast-feeding is probably the most motherly thing to do, which brings the child and the mother close to each other. So, you must cherish these moments and try to be a doting mother throughout this phase. Though initially, especially if it is your first time, breast-feeding is a little confusing and complex thing to do, with time you understand your child's habit and necessity.

The Phenomenon

Before you begin breast-feeding, you must understand how the entire phenomenon does take place. It is a very simple phenomenon, the breasts are divided into lobes and this is where the milk is produced. Individual lobes comprise 15 to 25 ducts that carry milk to the nipples and get collected at the areola before being expressed. It is when a child cries, the breasts grow hot and the blood hurries to the breasts, carrying with it sugars to the milk glands.

Getting Started

It is not easy to breast-feed as it seems. You have to take care of lots of things, so that your baby does not remain hungry. The best way to breast-feed a baby is to hold him/her close to your breast and hold your breast in a "C-hold" position, with your thumb on top and fingers beneath. You must make sure that your

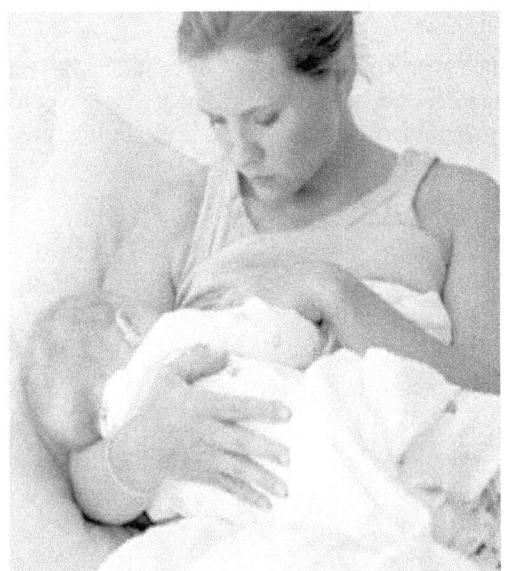
Mother feeding her baby

baby's mouth is open wide and covers your entire nipple. In case there is suction, break it by your fingers. Keep on checking for it in between. You should offer your baby both your breasts at the time of feeding.

Importance of Breast-feeding

Breast-feeding is very important for the normal mental and physical development of a newborn. The mother's milk is a complete source of all the nutrients as well as antibodies to the newborn. A breastfed baby is likely to be more strong, healthy and immune. Breast milk is easily digestible by the baby and is always available at right temperature. It also develops a sense of attachment between the mother and the baby. Apart from this, it also guards the mother against breast and ovarian cancer.

Myths about Breast-feeding

Here are some common myths about breast-feeding.

- ❑ You should not breast-feed for 24 hours after the baby receives vaccinations.
- ❑ Stop feeding completely if your nipples are cracked.
- ❑ You need not wash your nipples every time you feed.
- ❑ Those who smoke should not breast-feed at all.
- ❑ You should not breast-feed after exercising.
- ❑ Do not breast-feed if the baby has diarrhoea.

2. Breast-feeding Positions

When you are a new mother, there are a number of things that you have to learn and teach your baby. One of them is breast-feeding. Mother's milk is the only food for the newborn till the first few months. Therefore, it is important that your child learns the right breast-feeding technique as early as possible, so that he/she doesn't feel hungry after being fed, as some infants do. The mother may have to explore certain breast-feeding positions to determine the one that best suits the child. Below given are a number of positions for breast-feeding the baby.

Traditional Position

Keep a few pillows on your lap; place the baby on them, so that he/she is on the same level as your breasts. Support his/her head with your forearm in such a way that the rest of his/her body is across your stomach. You can help by cupping the baby's head in your hand (use your right hand for left breast and vice versa).

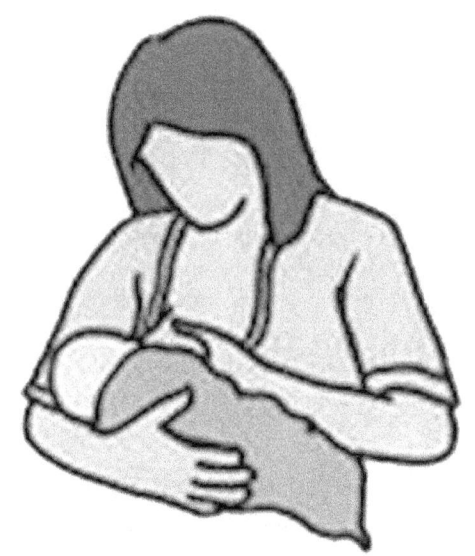
Traditional Position

Feeding the Baby

Underarm Position

Arrange a few cushions at your side and place the baby on it in such a way that his/her legs are pointing behind you. Hold your baby in such a way with your right hand that you cradle his/her head, while he/she feeds from your right breast. Women with Caesarean section use this position to avoid pressure on the scar. Twins can be breastfed together using this position.

Lying Down Position

Lie on the bed with your head resting on a pillow and place the baby close to you. The bed will give them the support they need. With your free hand bring them to your breast and support them. Keep pillows behind your back to prevent a backache.

Find a position that is comfortable for both you and your baby, so that breast-feeding is easy.

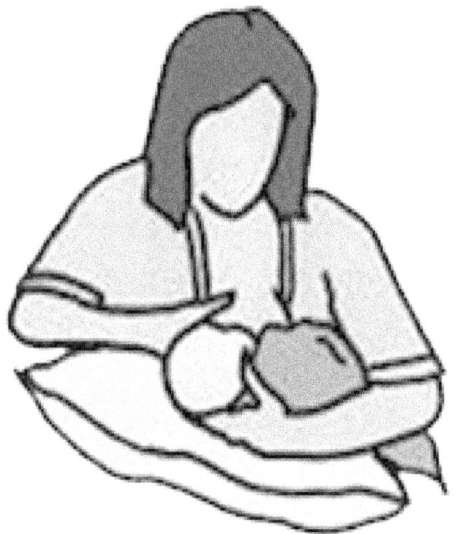
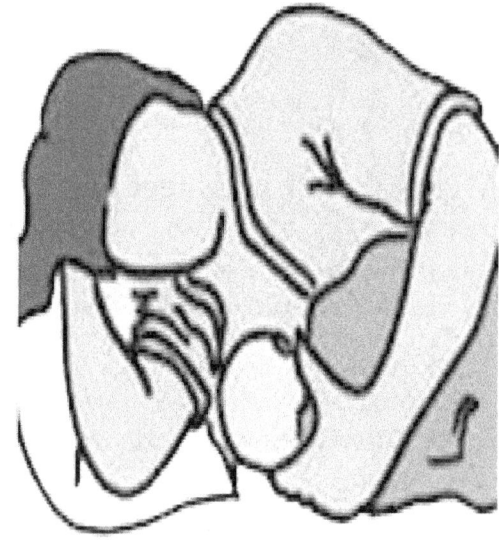

Underarm Position   *Lyingdown Position*

Beware of Things While Breast-feeding

- Baby should be tucked close to your body.
- The chin should be against your breast and stretched upward and not tucked in.
- Mouth should be open wide and their bottom lip should curl outwards.
- There should be movement of the face and jaw.
- Lower lip should take in more of the areola that the upper lip.
- The cheeks of the baby should not be sucked in.
- Lip action as if the baby is sucking a straw is a sign of wrong breast-feeding.

Beware of Sounds While Breast-feeding

- Slow and quick sounds of milk being swallowed signals that the suction is right.
- The baby should not make clicking noise.
- The baby should not smack lips.

The Feel

- ❏ You should be able to feel firmly gripped while breast-feeding.
- ❏ Letdown reflex, a tingling feeling in the breasts, usually when feeding begins as the milk flows to the baby.
- ❏ Slight pain may be felt when the baby begins to suck in the initial weeks. The pain should not last longer than the initial momentary pain.

3. Breast-feeding Problems

Both mother and baby will have to learn to master the art of breast-feeding. This will take time and what works for one pair need not necessarily work for another pair. However, breast-feeding may also pose some problems for the mother. There are some common problems associated with breast-feeding that one out of every two mothers face. While some problems disappear in due course of time, there are some that need professional help. Given below are the causes and solutions to some of the common breast-feeding problems.

Insufficient Milk Supply

The baby may want to keep feeding all the time if he/she is not positioned properly or if there is insufficient supply of milk. In the initial days, the baby may insist on feeding continuously, simply because he/she enjoys it and breast-feeding is very comforting for him/her. It could also happen if the baby is trying to increase the supply of milk. If this activity is a change from his/her normal feeding pattern, it may return to normal in a day or two. Make sure that you position the baby properly and let him/her feed on demand.

Bleeding/Sore/Cracked/Nipples

This happens because the baby is sucking your nipple and not the breast as a result of bad positioning. Dislodge the baby by inserting your finger gently into his/her mouth to break the grip. Reposition your breast, so that the breast and not just the nipple go inside the baby's mouth. Try different positions. Express milk manually and rub it on the nipples as this will help in healing. Use the less sore side to feed the baby.

Thrush that Doesn't Heal

White marks or sore nipples that don't seem to heal are known as thrush. It can appear when either you or the baby have taken a course of antibiotics or may appear without any particular reason. Both of you may have to take oral medication or use anti-fungal cream.

Flat Nipples/Lumpy, Hard and Full Breasts

Primary engorgement takes place when milk first 'fills in' on the third or fourth day. Secondary engorgement takes place when the baby reduces the number of feeds he/she takes, maybe because he/she has started sleeping for longer hours at night. If this is the case, your body will reduce the amount of milk it is producing. Feed the baby more often to reduce engorgement. If baby is unable to latch on properly, express some milk to help him/her do so. Wear warm flannel clothing to ensure milk flow or have a warm shower before feeding to ensure the same. Using chilled cabbage leaves inside your bra can reduce the swelling.

Lumps in the Breast

Free movement of milk is stopped because of a block in some duct of the breast. This can happen because you have slept in a wrong position, sat for a few hours with the seat belt across your breast or a tight bra. Massaging the area or using warm compress on the area will help the lump to dissolve. If possible, position the baby in such a way that his/her jaw is near the lump, so that he/she can feed and help in dissolving the lump. Feed from the sore side, if it doesn't work, express milk from the breast.

Inflamed, Red Areas on the Breast

Inflamed, red areas on the breast along with flu symptoms like temperature, aches with sore breast that is full; this condition is known as *Mastitis*. It is an inflammation of the breast when milk leaks into the breast tissue. Rest as much as possible, but continue to feed the baby. Use of warm and cold compress will reduce the swelling. If there is no improvement, go to your doctor, who will probably prescribe painkillers or a course of antibiotics.

Baby Refuses to be Fed from the Breast

There could be a number of reasons for this:
- A change in the taste of milk because of a change in diet or medication.
- You are using nipple cream.
- You have stopped using nipple shields.
- You are undergoing dental treatment or your periods are starting.

Breast-feeding Twins

When you have twins, the task of breast-feeding becomes a little more difficult and there is the often-asked question of about whether to feed them together or one at a time. Feeding one baby at a time improves bonding between the mother and child. However, this can be time consuming. Letting them feed together will improve your milk supply and it will be easy to remember who has had how much. If you decide to feed them together, placing one baby under each arm is the best position to use. You can also criss-cross them on your lap and feed them together. Swapping the babies between the breasts ensures equal production of milk. However, using one breast exclusively to feed one baby will customise the supply for that baby and ensure that he/she gets sufficient milk.

4. Expressing Breast Milk

There are times when you may want to express breast milk. If your breast seems too full and hurts, it would be a good idea to express the milk and store it for later use. You may want to go out and would like the person taking care of your baby to feed him/her this breast milk, instead of formula milk. Additionally, you may have to rely on milk expression techniques when you are carrying the baby out, so that you have breast milk in store for the baby. You can express milk with your hand or with a breast pump.

Hand Expression

- Take a sterile wide rimmed container to collect milk.
- Wash your hands before you begin expressing the milk.
- Close the door before you begin the process in order to avoid embarrassment for you and the intruder.
- Massage your breast gently to increase milk flow or use flannel to warm your breasts.
- Hold your breast with one hand and with the fingertips of the other, move all around the breast stroking it gently. You can use the back of your knuckles, massaging from the outer edge of the breast to the nipple.
- Once you have completely relaxed, place your hand behind the areola and start squeezing gently. You should be applying pressure on the milk sacs that are under the skin, at the edge of the areola. These sacs will feel like peas under your fingertips.
- As you squeeze in, milk will first drip out and then spurt. Move your hand all over the breast to remove milk from all the ducts.

Using Breast Pumps

There are a variety of breast pumps available today. You will have to very carefully select the pump that is best for you. If you choose the wrong one, you may harm your breast tissues. It is best to consult your doctor before buying a pump. There are two types of breast pumps:

- **Battery-operated Pumps**
  These are easy to use, but may not be very durable. These make less noise than electric pumps. Use a pump that has been designed to release suction at regular intervals to prevent excessive pressure.

- **Electric Pumps**
  There are different kinds of electric pumps available in the market. Some come with a double pumping system, which is convenient for expressing milk from both breasts at the same time. Small and light pumps are available, which can be easily carried to work and when you travel. These pumps can be recharged in your car, as they come along with adapters.

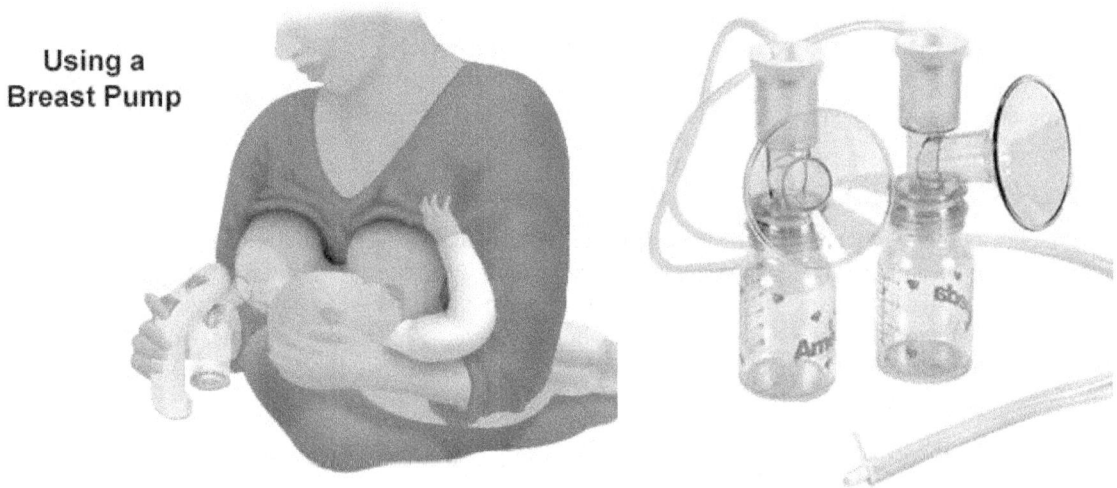

Different types of breast pumps

Storing Breast Milk

There are bags that are specially made to store expressed breast milk. You can use small disposable bottle bags or small glass or plastic bottles as well. Depending on how soon you want to use the expressed milk, you can either refrigerate or freeze it.

Tips to Store Breast Milk

- Fresh expressed milk can be stored for ten hours at room temperature. Milk brought to room temperature after refrigerating or freezing must be used within half an hour.
- Fresh expressed milk can be refrigerated for anything between five to seven days. Taste the milk to find out whether it is fresh, before giving it to your baby.
- You can store freshly expressed milk for up to six months in an average freezer, depending on the efficiency of the freezer. Make sure you store in the coldest part of the freezer and away from the door.
- Pumped milk that has been refrigerated for less than 48 hours can be frozen. If refrigerated for more than 48 hours, it should not be frozen.

- ❑ Freezing causes breast milk to expand. While filling bottles or bags, leave about one inch space from the top, so that there is place to accommodate this expansion. If you are using a disposable bag, fold the top and fasten it with a rubber band.
- ❑ Milk containers should be labelled with the time and date on which it was expressed.
- ❑ If you can express large quantities of milk, do not store it in a big bottle or bag. Use small bags or bottles. The baby will need only small quantities at a time and you can defreeze one small bag or bottle each time. Thus, wastage will be minimised.
- ❑ If you want to transport stored breast milk to use away from home, keep it cold till you use it. Use a cooler with ice or frozen packs to keep the milk cold, while transporting it.
- ❑ The oldest milk should be used first.

Defrosting Expressed Breast Milk

- ❑ To thaw breast milk, use a hot bowl of tap water or do it at room temperature. Defrost using minimum amount of heat.
- ❑ Do not microwave to defrost, as it destroys the essential vitamins and enzymes in the milk.
- ❑ Feed the baby defrosted milk, only when it has thawed completely.
- ❑ If the milk smells or tastes sour, do not use it.
- ❑ Milk that has been thawed should be kept in the refrigerator and used within 24 hours.

5. Introducing Bottle to Baby

There is no doubt about the fact that breast-feeding is better than feeding the baby formula milk. Many mothers would like to bottle-feed their babies some time later. Some babies, who have been breastfed, may take to bottle-feeding as soon as it is introduced. Babies may prefer it; especially if they are having trouble having being breastfed. But many breastfed babies refuse the bottle, when the change is introduced. Practical experience shows that this is especially true with children, when they are breastfed till an older age However, you will be introducing bottle to the baby sooner or later.

Introducing Bottle to Breastfed Baby

- ❑ You could try using different kinds of nipples. Making the teat soft by boiling it or using different types of nipples may help. Often the babies who refuse the bottle are the ones who have been breastfed for a long time.
- ❑ You should hold the baby in the same position while bottle-feeding him/her, as you do while breast-feeding him.
- ❑ You should encourage your partner or babysitter to bottle-feed the baby, as he/she will not expect to be breastfed by them and may take to bottle-feeding more easily.

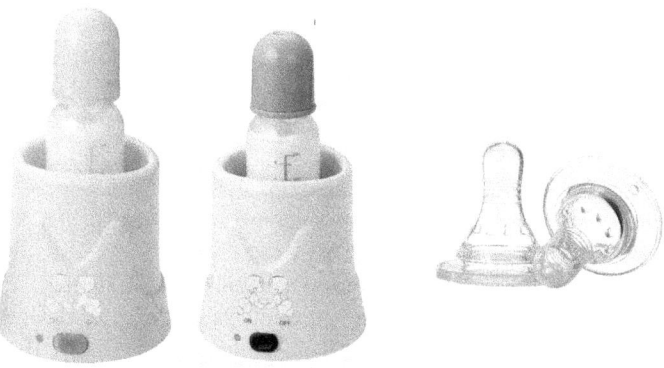

Different types of bottles and nipples

- ❏ Try changing the formula you use, as there is a chance that the baby dislikes its taste.
- ❏ Research has shown that if the bottle is introduced early, when the baby is about six weeks old, even for just one or two feeds a week, the baby is more likely to accept being bottle-fed on a regular basis.

Caution

It has been found that newborn babies, who are bottle-fed regularly, often forget how to suck milk from the breast. They may even need to relearn being breastfed. Experts are still trying to find an explanation for this behaviour. Therefore, it is best to introduce bottle-feeding only after breast-feeding is well established. If you want to avoid using a bottle, you could try spoon-feeding your baby or use cups specially made for babies. It has been found that babies, who use these cups, comfortably take to breast-feeding later on. However, it is important to learn the correct technique of using this cup from a trained person. Mothers are often concerned and wonder whether bottle-feeding will affect the health of the child. However, bottle-fed babies grow up to be just as healthy as the breastfed babies.

Breast-feeding vs Bottle-feeding

Breast-feeding does not ensure that your child will never fall ill. Although studies show that they are more resistant to common ailments as compared to formula-fed babies. Colic in babies, in both cases is more or less the same. Where sleep is concerned, it is true that formula-fed babies, sleep better and longer at night. One possible explanation is that, formula milk takes longer to digest than breast milk. Therefore, babies who are bottle-fed sleep longer between feeds. Therefore, mothers may use formula milk to ensure that babies sleep through the night. On the other hand, breast-feeding the infant during the night may be slightly inconvenient for the mother, but she doesn't need to get up and prepare bottle-milk in case the baby needs it during the night. Ultimately, it is for the mother to decide what the best option for her and her baby is.

6. Bottle-Feeding Tips

Deciding to bottle-feed your breast-feeding baby is a conscious step taken by mothers, when they want to return to their original routines. Either they want some time off from their babies, or have to return to work. It is better to think carefully about bottle-feeding because many children learn to use a cup for drinking without even going through the bottle phase. Timing plays an important role in making your baby learn to bottle-feed. If bottle-feeding is introduced too soon, then the baby may give up breast-feeding. If introduced too late, the baby may not take up the bottle and refuse to give up breast-feeding. However, not all babies need to be taught to bottle-feed, a number of them take to it without much fuss.

Bottle-Feeding an Infant

- ❏ Either use expressed breast milk or artificial milk, also called formula for bottle-feeding the infant.
- ❏ Most babies enjoy bottle-milk slightly warm. Before feeding the baby, shake the bottle and place a few drops on your inner wrist to check the temperature. Run warm tap water over the bottle, if required.
- ❏ To reduce the swallowing of air by the baby, tilt the bottle to let the milk fill the nipple and air to rise to the bottom of the bottle.
- ❏ Keep the head of the baby straight when he/she is feeding. If the head is turned sideways or backwards, the baby will not be able to swallow the milk easily.
- ❏ Switch arms while feeding the baby from the bottle. This will reduce arm fatigue and also present different views to the baby.
- ❏ Take care not to force the nipple into your baby's mouth. You should rather stimulate the baby to accept the nipple by touching his/her lips gently to the nipple.
- ❏ Look for signs indicating that the nipple hole is too large or too small. If the milk flows, instead of dripping, when the bottle is turned upside down, discard the nipple as the hole is too large. Similarly, if

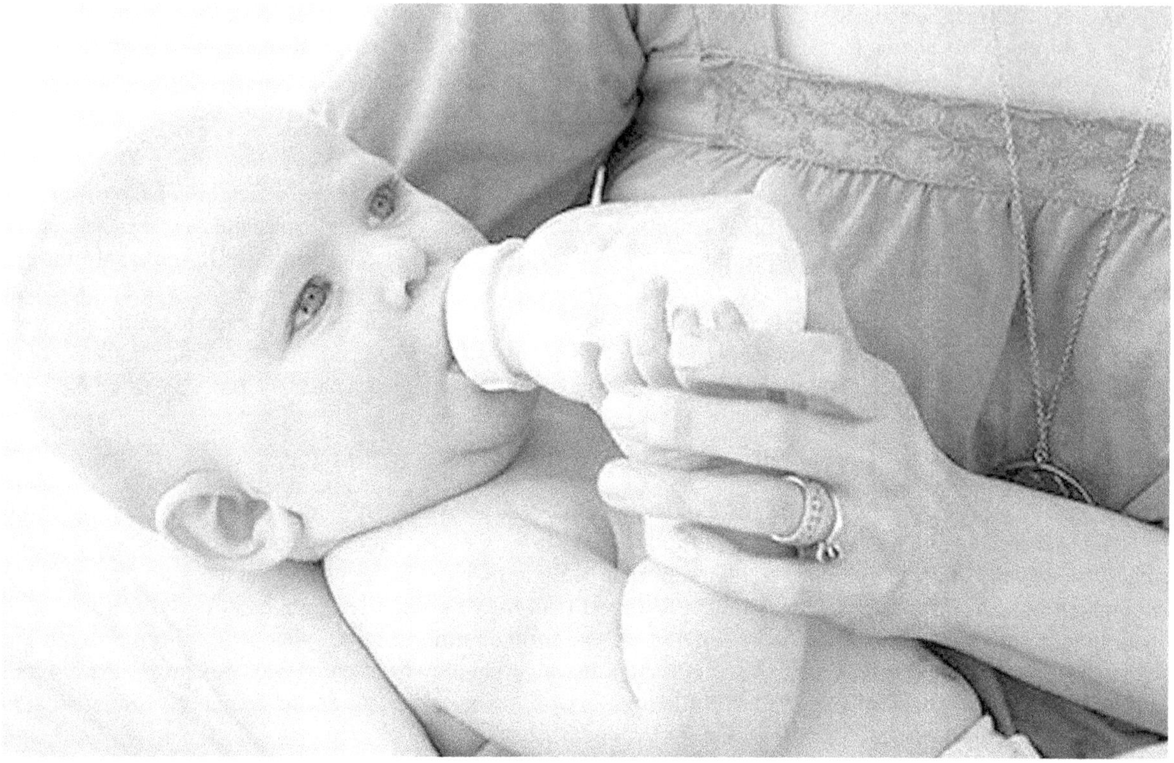

Bottle-feeding a baby

the baby tires during sucking and his/her cheeks cave in due to strong suction, the nipple hole may be too small and needs replacement.
- ❑ Always clean and sterilise the bottles by washing them properly an boiling in water, or keeping them in hot water for a while.

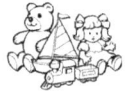

FAQs

Q-1. Is breast milk sufficient for the baby?
Ans. There is a way of knowing whether the milk is sufficient or not except to check the growth chart of the baby. You may be rest assured that your milk supply is sufficient if your baby seems satisfied after feeding for a reasonable period of time. Also if the baby is gaining weight adequately and if the baby passes urine five to six times a day, then it is an indication that your breast milk is sufficient for the baby.

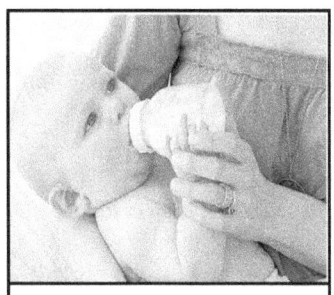

Q-2. Should I boil the stored breast milk before use?
Ans. The breast milk is sterile and needs no boiling. Boiling leads to breast milk losing its natural nutrients. The bottle of breast milk may be warmed by gradually placing it in a bowl of hot water just before feeding the baby.

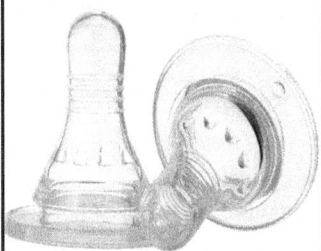

Q-3. For bottle feeding which milk is better – cow's milk or formula milk?
Ans. Cow's milk may be easily available and low on cost but there is high chance of it getting spoilt if kept for longer duration. Secondly heating and reheating of cow's milk may lead to it losing its nutritional contents considerably. Formula milk may be costly, but there is less chance of contamination if it is stored properly. Also the formula milk is fortified with many essential nutrients in such a way that it comes closest to mother's milk in terms of digestibility and nutritional value. So it is always advisable to use formula milk for the first year if you can afford it. However, if you have to use the cow's milk then always ensure that it is fresh milk and not the packaged one.

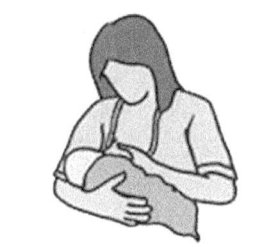

Q-4. How much milk should be given to the baby?
Ans. The quantity of milk to be given to the baby may vary. However on a general note, give around 5 to 6 ounces (1 ounce is equal to 30 ml) per kg body weight per day. If a two-month old baby weighs 5 kg then the baby requires 30 to 36 ounces of milk in a day. The baby may be fed 6 to 7 times in a day.

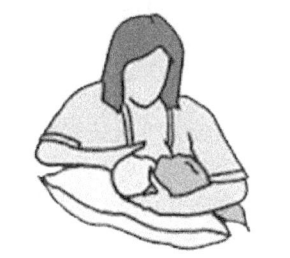

Q-5. Why do some bottle-fed babies get recurring ear infection?
Ans. The problem of ear infection is more with the bottle because when the nipple hole is too big and the baby gulps down the milk, some of it goes up into the ear via a tube connecting the ear to the area behind the nose. To stop it from recurring is by changing the nipple with a normal sized hole.

Q-6. Why do some babies bring up milk after each feed?
Ans. Most babies bring up some milk after their feeds. This milk may be small in quantity but seems quite a lot because it is mixed with saliva. This problem is more in the babies who are bottle-fed than those who are breastfed. This problem may arise due to any one of these reasons:

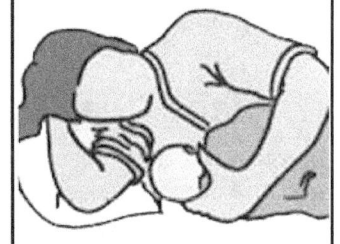

> Baby is swallowing air along with the milk. So hold the bottle properly and make sure that the nipple is always full of milk.
> After a full feed, the back of the baby is rubbed very hard. Do it gently to burp the baby.
> Baby is being pushed to take extra milk in order to finish the entire contents of the bottle. This should not be the practice. Let the baby drink as much milk as he/she can easily take.

Feeding the Baby

IV
Baby Sleep Patterns

Sleeping is an essential and important activity for your baby. In the beginning, your baby will spend the better part of the day sleeping. Growth hormones work most effectively when the baby is asleep. Initially, for the first few months, your baby will continue with his/her own sleep pattern, sleeping as and when he/she likes. As the baby grows older, he/she will slowly learn to adjust the sleep pattern to your daily routine. When the baby is about three months old, *your baby will normally sleep for 10 hours* at night on the whole, even if he/she wakes up in between. Your baby's daytime sleep can often be divided into two sessions - morning and afternoon.

Everybody has different opinion when it comes to care and upbringing of a baby, therefore sleep is no different. Even the simple task of deciding the length of a baby's nap, or how to put your baby to sleep has become complicated, because of the number of opinions you will get. As a result of the emotional involvement in caring for your baby, every small aspect becomes an issue. Most mothers are more than happy to make adjustments and will schedule their sleeping pattern to fit their baby's sleep pattern. This ensures that the mother and baby sleep together which is ideal. Sleeping together ensures strong emotional bonding between the mother and her baby. Studies have shown that babies who sleep with their mothers feel more protected.

If you feel that your baby should have a sleep pattern that is convenient for everyone at home and that does not interfere with your sleep pattern, you will have to make the baby learn a sleep pattern. One of the most common ways to make a baby sleep, is to use music, either sing to the baby or play some soothing music and before you know the baby is fast asleep. This is a method that has been tried and tested over the years and this wisdom has been passed on from generation to generation, though the type of music used may vary.

Some parents choose a particular song for each child and sing this special song day after day at the baby's bedtime. They begin this when the baby is a few days old. After some time, the baby gets conditioned and will sleep easily once you start singing the song. If you don't want your baby to get used to the habit of being rocked to sleep, you can try using a musical toy. Wind-up this toy and it will play music for a few minutes. Use this toy every time you want to make your baby sleep. Place it close to his/her cot. After sometime, the baby will get accustomed to falling asleep to the sound of the musical toy. This method will help your baby sleep comfortably even if you are away from home.

Today CDs are created with specific music, which help very young babies fall asleep. While selecting music, they use music with the same beats per minute as the heartbeat of the mother, which the baby hears while in the womb. This has a soothing effect on the young baby, helps him/her to relax and fall asleep comfortably. You can choose whatever method suits you or try all of them and decide which one works best for your baby.

1. Baby Sleeping Bags

The concept of baby sleeping bags, though considerably new in many countries, has been in vogue for quite some time. Sleeping bags are specially designed bags that are meant for the purpose of keeping a baby warm, secure and comfortable at night. When should a baby be allowed to sleep in the bags has been a subject of debate and is still controversial. While in some parts of the world, babies are made to sleep in the bags as soon as they are born, in others, they need to be a few months old to be allowed to sleep in these specially designed sleeping bags.

There are a number of reasons why parents opt for sleeping bags for their babies. It is said that the coziness of a baby sleeping bag helps reinforce the sleeping pattern of a baby and gives him/her the security needed by the baby to sleep. There are a number of things that disturb a sleeping baby - a wet nappy, hunger, pain or feeling cold. While all the other causes are grasped by parents, they hardly come to know that the baby is feeling cold. This is where baby sleeping bags come to their rescue.

Choosing the Right Sleeping Bag

- ❑ Choose your baby's sleeping bag according to the prevailing season, so that he/she stays comfortably warm. Check the TOG** of the bag carefully.
- ❑ When you are buying a new sleeping bag for your child, make sure to check that the design and weight do not add to the heating process, thereby leading to overheating.
- ❑ It is advisable to go for a sleeping bag that has deep sleeve holes, so that the air gets room to circulate throughout the bag. This will work to prevent the bag from getting overheated.
- ❑ While determining the size of your baby sleeping bag, make sure that it is small enough to prevent your baby from sliding down inside the bag. At the same time, it should be big enough to allow him/her to kick legs freely, without the risk of being uncovered.
- ❑ Never ever get a quilted sleeping bag for your baby, as it can get too hot for your baby to handle. If you feel that your baby might feel cold in it, you can always put a sheet on the sleeping bag.

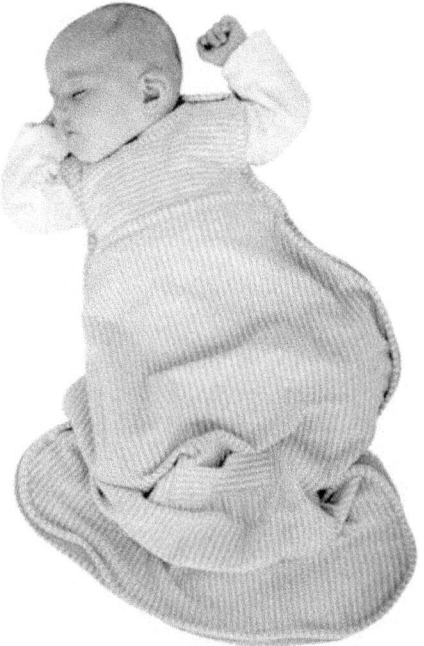

A baby in a sleeping bag

2. Co-sleeping with Baby

When we think of a young baby sleeping, the most natural assumption is that the baby will be sleeping with his mother. Babies have slept with their mothers from time immemorial. This was thought to be the best practice as constant contact between mother and baby not only gave the baby a sense of security, but also strengthened the emotional bond between the two. The increase in research and studies done on babies, in the recent times, has given rise to a debate as to whether it is better for the baby to sleep with their mother or alone in their cot. Some mothers prefer sleeping together, while others prefer to put their baby in a cot. There are some precautions which you should take while co-sleeping with your baby.

Avoid Drugs

Take care not to sleep with your baby, if you have taken any drug that may affect the pattern of your sleep. If you have consumed alcohol, avoid sleeping with the baby at all costs. Counter drugs, such as cold medicine, also dull your sense of awareness during the night and you may put your weight or roll over on the baby without realising.

**Sleeping bags are given a TOG rating according to the warmth they provide. The higher the TOG figure, the warmer will be the bag. In winter, a baby sleeping bag should have a rating of 4 TOG - 2.2 TOG. In summers, you'll need a sleeping bag with a lower TOG rating.

Make Enough Space

You need to ensure that there is enough space in the bed to accommodate you and your baby comfortably. A crowded bed is potentially unsafe for your baby. Each one on the bed should have space to move around a bit.

Use Bed Rails

You can use one or two bed rails on the bed, so that the baby doesn't roll off onto the floor. The chances of injury can also be minimised by pushing the mattress flush against a wall or placing another mattress on the floor to give support to the baby in the instance of falling.

Tie long hair

If your hair is very long, it is advisable to tie it back in order to avoid strangulation. Though such chances are very slim, it is better to tie the hair or wear a bonnet, while sleeping with the baby, as there have been instances where the babies have suffocated in sleep by getting entangled in their parent's hair.

Head and Foot Boards

Flushing the mattress against the headboard and the footboard can also ensure that the baby is not entrapped between the mattress and the bed frame. Some babies tend to wriggle themselves to the top, bottom or side of the mattresses.

Siblings and Pets

A baby should not be made to sleep next to the siblings or pets. The baby should always sleep next to the mother, so that she can breast-feed him/her during the night, if required. There is a danger that the pets or siblings may roll over the baby and injure him/her.

Bedding and Pillows

The baby should not be made to sleep with fluffy bedding, pillows or stuffed animals. In fact, babies should not even sleep close to fluffy bedding or pillows. Take care not to cover the baby's face with a blanket, unless it is extremely cold. You can cover the rest of the baby's body with a blanket, but the face should be left uncovered.

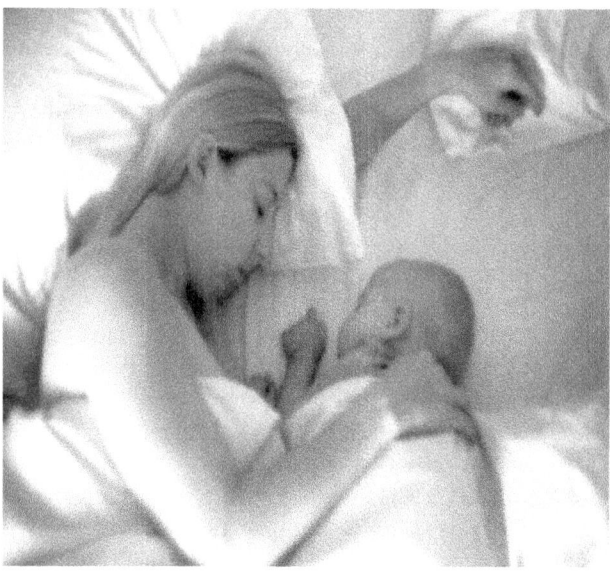

A baby sleeping with mother

3. Getting Baby to Sleep in Crib

Patting them, swaddling them, singing lullaby to them, taking them for a walk, and many more things just to make sure the little babies get some proper sleep. However, it is not an easy task. Babies are very choosy and restless when it comes to sleeping. During the first few days, you prefer making your baby sleep next to you. This is good for the baby as well, since he/she will need you around. The problem arises when you are planning to shift your baby to a nursery in a crib. Babies are very particular about their surroundings. They get used to a particular surrounding and then hate it later, when there are any changes in the setting. Sleeping beside their mother makes them feel safe and secure, a feeling they can't experience in a big crib. This is what makes them uncomfortable and they make a fuss about sleeping in a crib alone. This process of making them shift to a crib will take a persistent and patient trial on your part.

Tips to Make Baby Sleep in a Crib

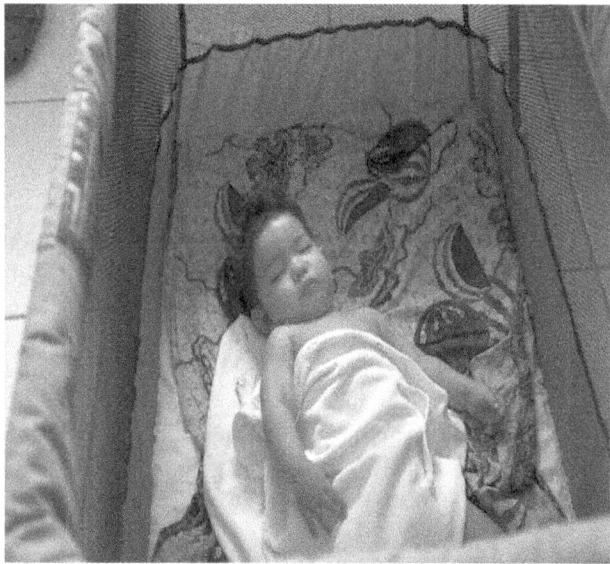

A baby crib

- ❏ Relax and don't get anxious. Take your own time, if you are not ready to shift your baby to a crib. Your baby might also be afraid of sleeping alone. It may take some time for this shift to happen.
- ❏ Babies don't usually prefer changes because they get used to a particular pattern and feel secured in the same pattern. So, any changes in the new room will make them uncomfortable. Try and keep the setting similar to the room in which the baby was previously sleeping. For example, if a ceiling fan was used in the previous room, run the fan.
- ❏ Use the same kind of bedding and swaddle the baby in the same blanket, in which he/she was sleeping before. This will make him/her get the same feel and he/she will not get affected by the change of place.
- ❏ Keep the bedtime routine same. Whatever you used to do before going to sleep with your baby, continue the same routine. If you used to play with the baby before going to bed, continue doing the same even now.
- ❏ All babies are different from one another. They might take their own time to get comfortable with the crib. Don't get angry with them if they are crying or refusing to sleep in a crib. You may seek some advice from mothers who were successful in shifting their babies to the crib.
- ❏ Make the crib a perfect place to sleep in. Make it cozy by putting rolled blankets in a circle; this will make the bed smaller. Newborn babies like having something close to their heads. Crib can be a scary place for them to sleep, make sure you don't put anything in the bed that can fall over their face.
- ❏ Babies are very sensitive to the change of temperature. It is advisable to make the temperature of the room, where the baby is going to sleep, warm and cozy enough for your baby to be comfortable. Before putting the baby in the crib, make sure the crib is not cold. You can use a warm bottle and place it on the crib for it to get warm, but make sure it does not become too warm. Make sure to remove the bottle before putting the baby in the crib. You can even use a sleeping bag, which is more comfortable for your baby. Your baby can enjoy the same kind of temperature throughout.
- ❏ Roll down one of your top or any other cloth in the crib where the baby is sleeping. Babies love to get their mother's smell. If the bed will smell of mom, they will feel much better and safer.
- ❏ You can also swaddle your newborn baby. Swaddling the baby will make him/her feel relaxed and cozy. In the beginning, you can swaddle the baby completely, but when the baby turns 6 weeks old, your baby's arms should be left free. Babies may use their hands for self-soothing or for communicating hunger by sucking their hands or thumbs.
- ❏ Make it a routine to put your baby in a crib to sleep. You need to be patient enough to continue trying. To make your baby shift to sleep in a crib will take time; you need to be persistent in implementing all the methods to make this happen.

4. Sleeping Safely

There is nothing more peaceful than the sight of a sleeping baby. At the same time, there is no thought more terrifying than having to see your baby hurt himself/herself, while sleeping soundly. Unfortunate as it is, there are a few instances of crib deaths. Every parent's main concern is to keep their baby safe and sound, even when he/she is asleep. Though numerous studies have been done on crib accidents and deaths, no one has been able to pin point the exact reason for the same. This fatality seems to be caused when a number of factors work together and affect the baby in some particular way. Researchers have come up with a few simple rules to be followed, which considerably lower the risk of crib death, while the baby is asleep.

Crib Safety Rules

- Make your baby sleep on his/her back.
- Make the baby sleep in the 'feet-to-foot' position and away from the end of the crib. Place the baby in such a way that his/her feet are facing the foot of the crib, but are not touching the end of the crib.
- The right temperature for a baby's room is 18°C (65°F). Babies should never rest in very hot temperatures.
- Do not use an electric blanket or a hot water bottle in the baby's crib.
- They should not be allowed to sleep either in direct sunlight, or near a fire or heater.
- The baby's clothes, sheets and blankets must be usually made of cotton only.
- All that babies need while sleeping is nappy, vest and sleep suit. If it is a hot night, make sure you dress the baby lightly.
- The room in which the baby sleeps must be smoke-free. Do not smoke or allow anyone to smoke near the baby.
- During the first six months, make sure that the baby crib is in your bedroom.
- Avoid sleeping with your baby on the sofa.
- If you smoke, drink alcohol, take medicines or drugs that make you sleep deeply, then do not allow your baby to share your bed.
- Do not cover the baby's head unless it is very cold, as they lose excess heat from their heads and faces.
- When the baby has temperature, his covering should be light and not heavy as is often believed.
- The baby's bedding, mattress, covering should be kept clean, sun-dry and aired.

5 Getting Your Baby on a Sleeping Routine

Rock them, cradle them or wrap them up, whatever you do your baby is not ready to sleep! This situation can occur with any parent. Babies are usually restless and getting them to sleep at night is very difficult, as they are still in an excited mind frame. It is beneficial for this reason to have a fixed sleeping routine for your baby. It will help both the baby and you. It will make the baby aware of what is coming next, it will also give them a sense of time and will help them put their body in a particular pattern. A routine will also make your work easier, but for that you need to keep repeating the same routine everyday till the time your baby gets used to it and no more requires your help. The sooner the better, start moulding your baby's day into a routine from when they are 6-8 weeks old, so that they get used to it and follow it as they grow up. This routine may vary, depending on your family's lifestyle and yours and your baby's comfort.

Tips to Establish Baby Bedtime Routine

Here are some tips to establish the bedtime routine for your baby :

- **Give Them a Soak**
  One of the most popular methods to get your baby follow a bedtime routine is by giving him/her a warm bath. Having a bath just before going to bed is quite soothing and relaxing. Make your baby sit in warm

water and clean them up. This will ease them up and make it easy for them to get a good sleep. Bath is also a good way to spend some special time with your baby. If your baby doesn't like having a bath, don't force it upon him/her.

- **Feed Them**
  Another way of getting your baby into a full sleep routine is by sending him/her to bed with full stomach. Feed them just before sleeping. This will help them sleep properly and will let others in the house to sleep peacefully as well.

- **Let the Energy Drown**
  It is better to allow babies to exhaust any pent-up energy out before going to sleep. So feel free to dance with them, play with them and let them bounce in a bouncer. All these activities will help your baby get exhausted completely, which will put him/her to a sound sleep easily.

- **Send Them to Bed Clean**
  Getting ready for bed routine can also include washing your baby's face, wiping or brushing gums and teeth, changing his/her diaper, etc. Send him/her to bed clean, so that he/she feels fresh and ready to doze off. It is important to develop the habit of brushing before going to bed at a young age, so that they get used to it as they grow up.

- **Chat with Them**
  You can even chat with your kids before sending them to bed. It is the best time also for the parents and kids to bond along well. Just speak to them about the entire day. No need to wait till your child is big enough to speak; you can chat with infants as well.

- **Sing a Song**
  You can sing a song for your baby. It can be any song and not just a lullaby. A slow soothing melody can put things on track. It can relax your baby and put them in a calm state. It can also be a signal for them that it's time to sleep.

- **Play Some Music**
  A soft slow music can ease the transition of your baby from a tiring day to a good night sleep. A slow soothing music from a radio or a stereo can calm even the crankiest of babies. Music will relax your baby and carry them to sleep. If your baby is really screaming and too tired, use a hair dryer or a vacuum to create noise to distract the baby.

- **Play with Them**
  Playing a quiet game with your baby in the room is a good way to spend some quality time with him/her. You can play any game that your baby enjoys, but not the one that gets them too excited. Playing a game will extract the leftover energy in them and will give them a sound sleep.

- **Say Goodnight Ritual**
  Many babies like roaming about the entire house and wishing goodnight to all the members and their favourite toys and belongings. It can be added on to the normal routine as a daily ritual, if your baby is pleased at the end of it and goes to bed with a smile.

- **Read a Bedtime Story**
  Another common and all time ritual is to read your kids a bedtime story. This will not only put them to sleep but will also help them to recognise and relate with words. It is an educative way to put your baby to a sleeping routine.

- **Take Them Out**
  Take your baby for a long walk. Make sure the stroller is positioned such that the baby does not face you. A walk with your infant in fresh atmosphere will prove to be really effective.

- **Get To Know Where Your Baby Sleeps Well**
  Get to know where your baby loves to sleep. There is no right or wrong place as such. Some babies like to sleep in their own crib in their own room, some like to sleep in their crib in their parent's room; some

of them like to sleep on the parent's bed with them. This habit of your baby may also change with his/her age. Be adjustable to your baby's changing style, and make him/her sleep as he/she wishes.

- **Dancing**
  Hold your baby and slowly dance around a low lit room. This will exhaust your baby a bit and help them have a good relaxed nap.

- **Massage Your Baby**
  Massage is an excellent way to relax a tensed baby. Use a little lotion or oil and rub it all over. It will relax the muscles and soothe them after a day full of activities.

- **Avoid External Aid**
  Many parents get exhausted after a day's long work and they prefer resorting to external aid to get their babies sleeping, for example using a pacifier, taking your baby for a drive, or rocking or nursing your baby to sleep. Though your baby might initially fall asleep quickly with these external aids, but this is just making your job more difficult. The problem that you will face is that your baby is not learning how to sleep alone. Instead, take some time off to get your baby to sleep without any help.

- **Be Flexible in Approach**
  Stay flexible with your sleeping program. A single approach may not work with all the kids. Don't stick on to a failing experiment. Use some other night time parenting style. Babies have different temperaments and families have different lifestyles. Adapt a night time strategy that will suit your baby's disposition and family's lifestyle. If the style is working, continue it, if not, drop it and be open to change in style.

- **Let the Baby Learn to Sleep Alone**
  Whenever your baby is going to sleep, be it day or night, take it as an opportunity to help your baby learn how to sleep without any help. It is a process which will take time to show result. It is not an overnight miracle, so there is a need for regular, patient approach.

- **Don't Get Upset**
  It may so happen that you try all the tactics to put your baby into a sleeping routine and they may not get used to it. Do not get boggled or impatient if something like this happens, as it is quite common and the kids take their own sweet time to fit into a routine.

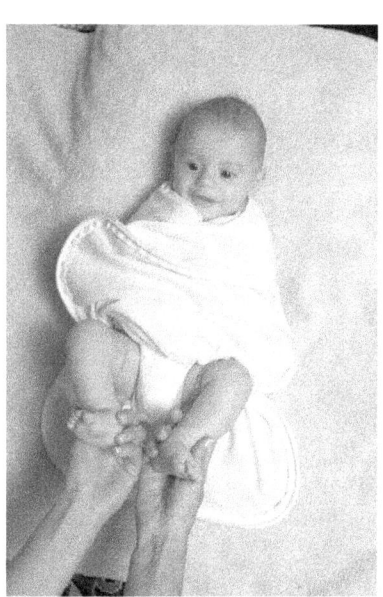 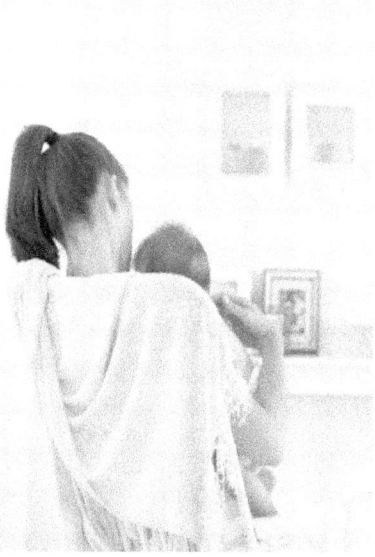 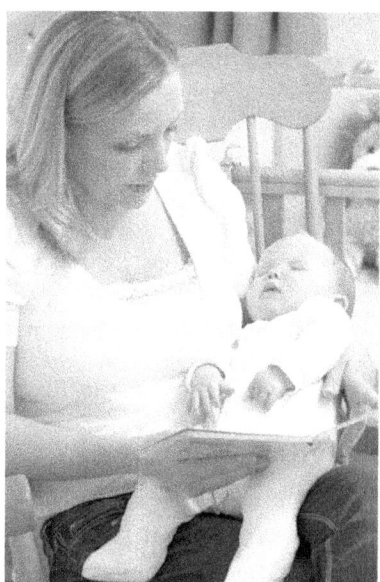

Tips to get Baby on a Sleeping Routine

6. Baby Sleep Problems

Nothing can be more pleasing than to see a newborn sleeping peacefully. A newborn needs 14 to 20 hours of sleep a day. It is essential for a baby to complete his/her cycle of sleep; otherwise, lack of sleep may affect his/her health adversely. Some kids get up from sleep, feed and go back to sleep. However, there are some that do not get a peaceful nap. Whatever the parents do to make them sleep, they will wake up in a few minutes and start crying. This is one of the common problems faced by parents of a newborn. The baby's sleep pattern can vary and parents may take some time to understand it. Their sleep patterns are subject to change at different places and time. The only time any parent can rest or do some other work is the time when babies sleep. But there are many problems that babies can face when it comes to sleeping.

Noise

Babies are very sensitive and even the slightest of disturbance or noise can wake them up from their sleep. Babies get restless and stressed if their sleep cycle is hampered. It is better to shut down all the disturbing noise when a baby is sleeping. Make your baby's room soundproof; so that nothing can spoil his/her sleep. A simple way to do that is to shut all the doors and windows.

Time

Your baby may sleep at any time. However, it is always helpful to have a fixed time schedule for the baby. Keeping the time of baby's sleep fixed will help the babies to get in a routine and once they are in a routine, it will become easier for you to plan out other works for the day. Nevertheless, there may be days when your baby refuses to sleep till he/she is too tired.

Bedding

Babies are not prone to changes and they love to stick to their routine. Any change in the discipline around them may make them unhappy. Similarly, the bedding on which a baby sleeps should also be the same. Try to have similar kind of bedding for the baby. This will make them comfortable and sleep peacefully.

Touch

It is nice to comfort the babies. So lie down with them and stroke them to make them go to sleep. However, do not make it a habit. If you make it a routine, the baby will expect the same routine by the same person every day, and if that will not happen it may lead to restlessness affecting his/her sleep. Babies tend to get dependent on one person (usually the mother) and feel protected and always want the same person around while sleeping.

Lights

Some babies may get used to sleeping in dark, while for some any condition is just fine for sleeping. Try to minimise the use of lights when a baby is sleeping.

Teething

If your baby is teething, it will be very painful for him/her and the pain will not let them sleep. Take advice from your doctor and use all natural remedies to ease the pain.

7. Getting Twins to Sleep

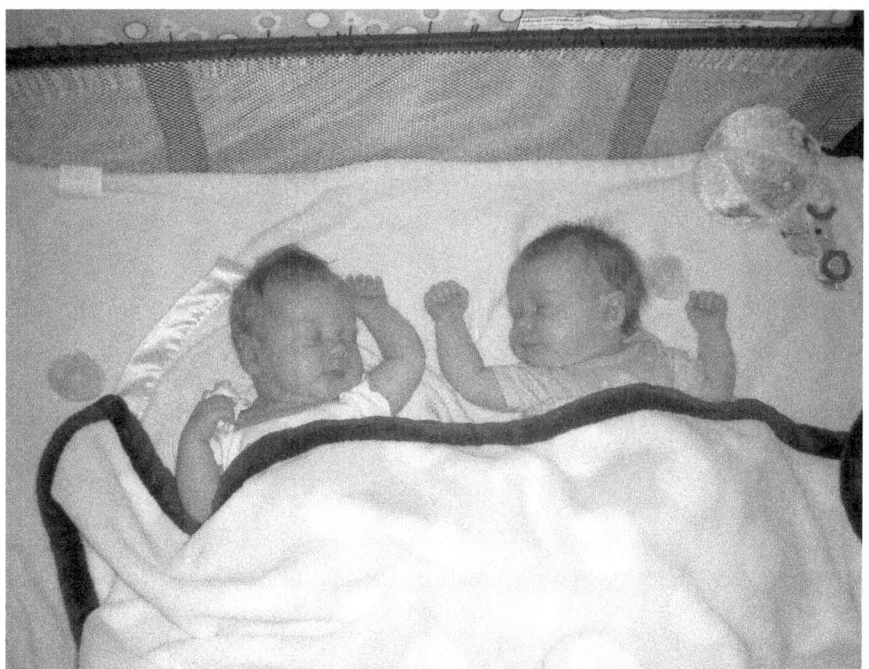

Baby twins sleeping

Twins are double delight, but this fun can also translate into problems and responsibilities as well. Having twin babies is quite lucky and can be a great fun only if you know how to handle them together. It becomes troublesome at times for parents to take care of twins, especially when both are as demanding and as fussy. There are a number of problems which the parents of twins might face. One such problem can be to make both the crying babies to sleep peacefully. It can get a bit difficult with twins, to make them get the required amount of sleep. They may be too restless and playful together and may just refuse to sleep. Here are some tips on getting your twins to sleep without any difficulty.

Put Them to Bed Gradually

Your babies should learn to sleep on their own the moment they get on bed. One of the ways to do it is to gradually and slowly help them get to sleep. Making them tired will not help much, as they may tend to get restless.

Take Them to Bed Together

You need to decide what is simpler? Your twins going to bed at the same time, or at different times! It is better and simpler for you if you develop a same time schedule for your twins. Keeping your toddlers on same sleep schedule is the key for developing a healthy sleeping pattern for them, and also giving you some time off.

Establish a Bedtime Routine

Toddlers love to have a fixed routine. Develop a simple and useful bedtime routine to help them get sleep easily. A warm bath, a bedtime story, cuddling, back rubbing and little talk can prepare your babies well for a good sleep. Sticking to the routine will also act as a signal for the toddlers that it is time for them to call it a day.

Be with Them

Along with soft music, if they have you next to them, nothing will be as soothing to them as that moment. Your presence will help them feel secure and will put them at ease. Try and sing some lullaby or a rhyme or read a book to them. All this will make them sleep faster.

Discourage Playing

When babies are together, they have many things to do. Discourage any night time play between the twins. You can keep them quiet as night. Let the room be dimly lit, do not encourage much playing. You can also provide self soothers like a soft toy, or a blanket to sleep with. These objects will divert their attention from each other and help them go off to sleep.

Attend to the Calmer One First

You may feel obliged to attend to the naughty one first and then go to the calmer one. but the truth is that you should always attend to the calmer one first, make him/her sleep and then go back to the brat. If you will always attend to the naughtier one at first, the calmer one will lose all attention which he/she should get, because all your time will go in calming down the noisy one.

8. Positional Asphyxia in Infants

Newborns need a lot of sleep. While this helps the child in his/her overall health and growth process, it also gives a little rest to the new mother. However, you need to consider if your child is safe while sleeping. This may sound a bit strange and out of place, because a baby can't be safer than when he/she is sleeping soundly. You might be thinking how your baby can not be safe while sleeping. What you miss here is that the position in which you make your baby sleep, which is of utmost importance to his/her safety. If your baby is not lying down in a correct position, it may add on to SIDS (Sudden Infant Death Syndrome). Infants are fragile and sensitive, so any kind of compromise with their sleeping position or sleeping place may cause them to suffer in future. It is important for the parents to get to know the right position for their babies to sleep, in order to save them from any risks whatsoever. Babies can pose a great risk to their life, if they happen to sleep in a way that might suffocate them. This leads to positional asphyxia, also known as *postural asphyxia*. It is a state of lack of oxygen to breathe, due to the sleeping position. Positional asphyxia happens mostly in infancy, when an infant is found dead with his/her mouth and nose blocked or their chest unable to fully expand. It can just happen suddenly, so parents need to be extremely careful while making their babies to go to sleep.

Keeping them Safe

- Provide a firm and proper bedding or mattress for your child to sleep. The bed or the crib where your baby is going to sleep should be properly and firmly laid down without anything loose lying on it.
- Make your baby lie down on his/her back and not on their stomach while sleeping. Research has proved that making your baby sleep on his/her back may lower the risk of SIDS.
- Remove unnecessary pillows, quilts, stuffed toys and other soft or furry items from the area where the baby is going to sleep. These items may lead to choking or suffocation for the baby.
- If your baby is a preemie, consult your pediatrician to know about any other sleeping position. If your baby went through any health hazards like respiratory distress, consulting a doctor will be a better option, to decide the right sleeping position for him/her.
- Purchase a newborn sleeping pillow to keep your baby from rolling down the bed, or to keep him/her from changing their position and moving from his/her back to stomach, which may cause breathing problems and choking.

- ❏ Use a sleeping suit rather than a blanket. It will remove all risks of suffocation and will also keep your baby warm. Blankets may make your baby grasp for breath. While the baby is sleeping, his/her face should not be covered by any quilt or blanket. The baby should also not be sleeping against any soft materials, such as toys. He/she should have enough space to breathe properly.
- ❏ Do not place your baby on a waterbed or sofa or any other soft mattress, soft surface or pillows for sleeping. This may lead to suffocation.
- ❏ Cribs though safe can also be dangerous, if you have not chosen the right one for your baby. The cribs should be of exact size with no loose ends. The mattress should be properly laid down. The bedding should be a perfect fit.
- ❏ The crib should also not contain any soft toys, sheepskins, quilts or any such material that can choke the babies during sleeping. There is also a risk of your baby getting some allergy or infection. The crib should be empty with the bedding properly laid down.
- ❏ Babies may love to share the bed with you. It can be dangerous at times and so, it is better to develop a routine for them to get sleep in their crib.
- ❏ Sleeping sideways or sleeping with the face down is a wrong sleeping position and can kill your baby. The ideal sleeping position would be sleeping on the back. Any other sleeping position just increases the risk of suffocation and choking.

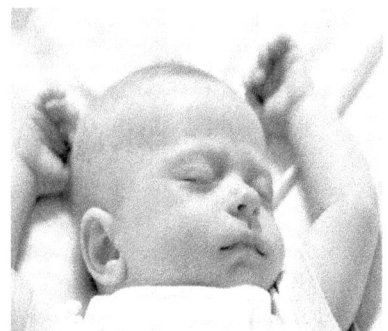 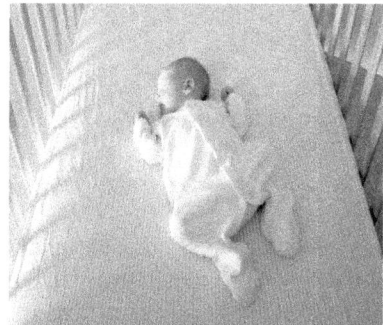 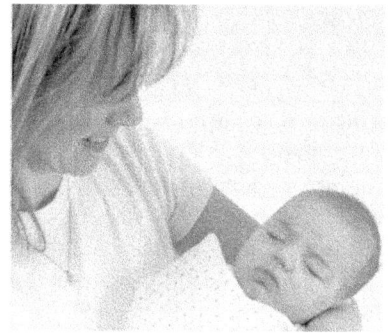

Right position of sleeping

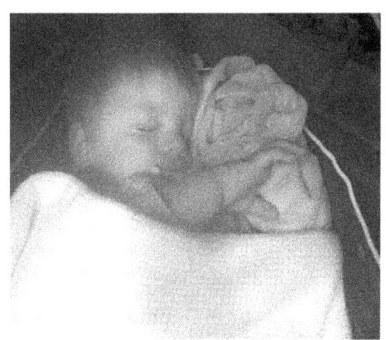 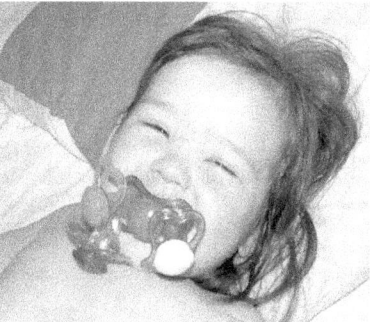 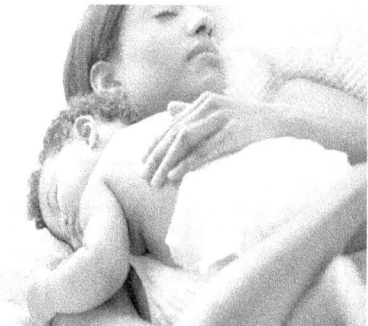

Wrong position of sleeping

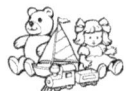

FAQs

Q-1. Why does my baby keeps waking up at night?

Ans. Generally newborns sleep for 14-18 hours but they keep waking up every 2-3 hours. They would take their feed and the sleep again after some time. This may cause a lot of worry and anxiety for the mother who herself feels deprived of sleep due to this sleeping-waking-sleeping routine. But this routine changes by the time your baby is 2-3 months old. Once the baby keeps awake for longer periods during the day, he/she will begin to sleep for longer periods at night.

Q-2. What is swaddling?

Ans. Swaddling is the process of bundling up the baby in comfortable clothes. Newborn babies get startled frequently during their sleep. By swaddling, mothers can minimise the baby's unwanted movements allowing the baby to sleep for longer period.

Q-3. What is the best way to put my baby to bed?

Ans. Although each baby develops his/her individual sleep pattern, but you may try the following pattern to help the baby to go to sleep. When the baby seems drowsy, darken the room and comfort, rock and cuddle the baby till he/she is drowsy. Then place the baby down in the bed and let him/her doze off.

Q-4. I put a curfew and do not allow any noise in the house when my baby goes off to sleep, which other members find very uncomfortable. What should I do?

Ans. If your baby is sleepy then he/she will doze off despite the sounds around. There is no need to impose a total curfew on all types of sounds in the house and disturb all the members of the house. Let the baby get used to the routine household sounds. However, loud, sudden noises should be avoided as they tend to wake up the babies from sleep.

Q-5. I am confused as to where to put my baby to sleep – in the crib or with me in bed?

Ans. Being close to mother is most comfortable for a baby. They definitely prefer to sleep in bed with their mothers. But there is a chance of accidental suffocation if the mother accidentally rolls over on to the baby. So only sleep the baby with you in your bed if you have a big bed. Otherwise put the baby to sleep in the crib in the same room near your bed.

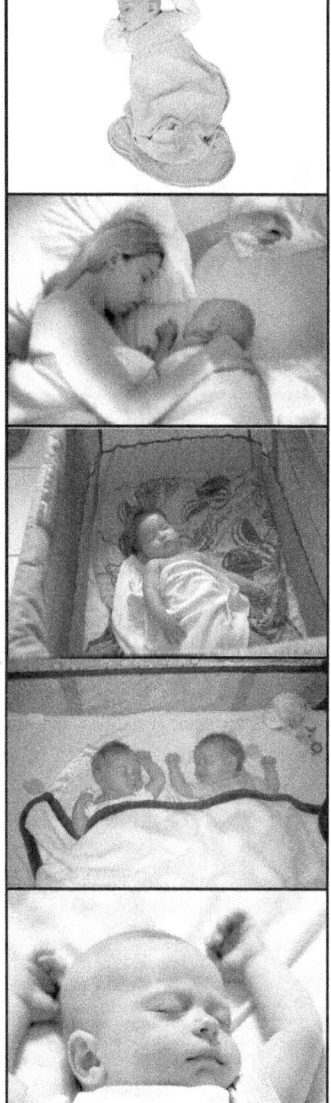

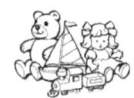

Baby Sleep Patterns

V
Baby Clothes

Talk about new born babies and the first word that strikes every mind is 'cute'. Right from the infant to the things that are purchased for him/her, everything around is cute and adorable. Add to this the loveliness of the vibrant colours. Usually *pink and blue* dominate the theme when it comes to purchasing things for the newborn. While pink is usually preferred, if it's a baby girl, blue serves baby boy the best. Amidst all the purchases, buying clothes is the most challenging. With commercialisation, the market has been virtually swamped with a wide range of options, as such making it confusing for the new parent to buy clothes for their little one.

At the time of buying clothes for the baby, parents are best advised not to be swayed away by the plethora of options available in the market. Though there are numerous designs and fabrics available for baby clothes, the best would be to pick the fabric which would ensure utmost comfort to the baby. Prickly accessories or small buttons should be best avoided. While these are some general consideration that parents should be cautious about, there are other things as well which should be adhered to while picking baby clothes.

1. Baby Clothing

Buying clothes for a growing baby is a bit challenging for many new parents. Today, the choice of baby clothing available in the market is unlimited. There are so many types of designs and so many fabrics available in baby clothes that choosing between them seems to be an impossible task at times. However, while buying clothes for babies, you need to keep certain basic conditions in mind. They should be comfortable, pose no hazard to the baby (such as buttons that might be swallowed) and be suitable for his/her age as well. Babies grow out of their clothes quickly, so you should not buy too many clothes at a time. In order to help you to buy clothes for newborns, we have provided a number of tips in the following lines, just for you!

Tips on Baby Clothes

- When buying children's clothes, the first thing to remember is that they must be easy and comfortable to wear and washable.
- It is always advisable to buy trousers or skirts with elasticised waistbands and shoulder straps, for a baby.
- Prefer buying clothes that can be stretched and have a wide neck for their easy accessibility.
- Avoid buying clothes that are adorned by lace, as babies can get their fingers caught in the lace.
- Always go for natural fibres as far as baby clothes are concerned, especially in summers.
- Clothes that open in the front and have poppers are easier to put on.
- Try to avoid buying clothes that have buttons.
- Never ever opt for clothes that have rough stitching. They can be uncomfortable for the baby.
- Since babies tend to be picked up by so many people, so many times, it is best to go for clothes that do not need ironing.

Basic Wardrobe for a Newborn

- ❏ 6-8 stretch suits (always buy according to weight, not age)
- ❏ 2 sets of night clothes (comfortable and easy to put on and take off)
- ❏ 4 sleeveless vests, with poppers under the crotch
- ❏ 3 pairs of socks
- ❏ 3 cardigans (for winters)
- ❏ A warm hat, mittens and snow suit (for winters)
- ❏ A sunhat and a light jacket (for summers)

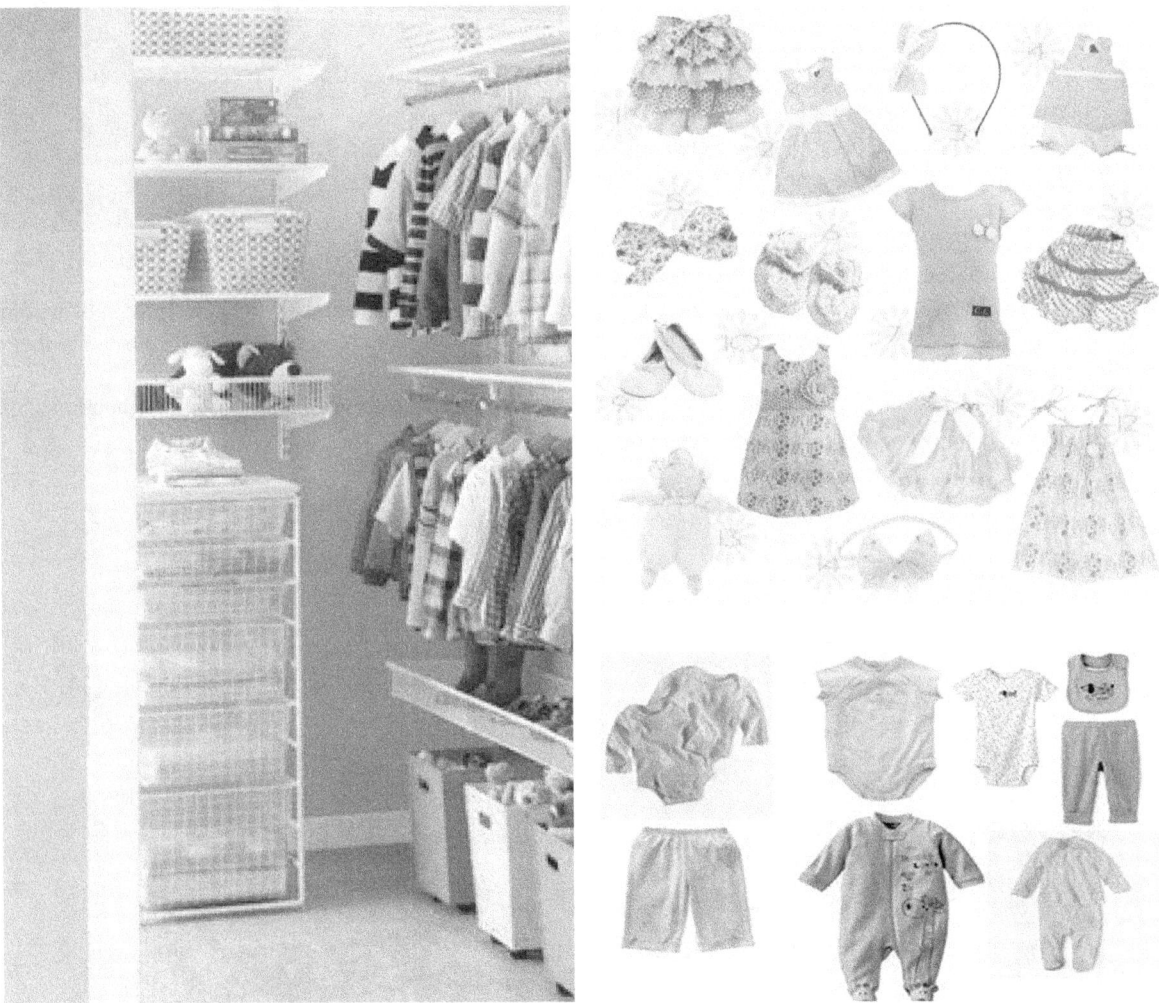

Different types of baby clothes

2. Buying Baby Clothes on a Budget

Babies outgrow their clothes so quickly that your head spins and your pockets wail. The anticipation of the arrival of a new one is the most exciting moment for all parents. Shopping for the new bundle of joy is equally exciting and fun. Parents enjoy shopping for baby clothes and buy expensive and varieties of clothes without realising that the babies grow rapidly in the first few months of life, outgrowing the size of all the clothes. As such, it makes sense to buy baby clothes on a budget so that it doesn't make a dent in your pocket every now and then.

Tips to Buy Baby Clothes on a Budget

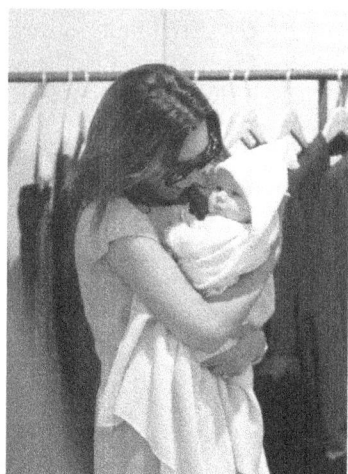

- You can shop for your babies from a store which does not have exorbitant prices. As babies outgrow their clothing very fast, it will prove to be a reasonable purchase.
- It is better and beneficial to buy clothes for your babies depending on their growth stage. What babies do the first few weeks is sleep and dirty their nappies. Four to six pieces of apparel for every three months of growth stage is a good idea.
- It is also beneficial to buy clothes in bulk. There are few brands that sell baby clothes in a pack of three or six. It will be easier and feasible to buy baby clothes from these brands.
- Hold a swap meeting with other mummies. Invite your friends, co-workers or neighbours who have babies of different ages and sizes. You can exchange worn-out or not in use clothes of each other's babies.
- Buy clothes well in advance. You can judge what size will fit your baby six to eight months later. So next time you hit a post-season or stock-clearance sale, you can buy clothes for future use as well. Babies need not be subjected to brands and fashion statements.
- You can even save a great deal of money by reusing old clothes. You can use your creativity in using old clothes to make new ones for your babies. For example, if your baby has outgrown the trouser, cut them to make shorts.
- You can even use internet to find out ways to go in for a budgeted purchase. There are many auction sites that offer lots of adorable baby clothes at good price.

Buying baby clothes

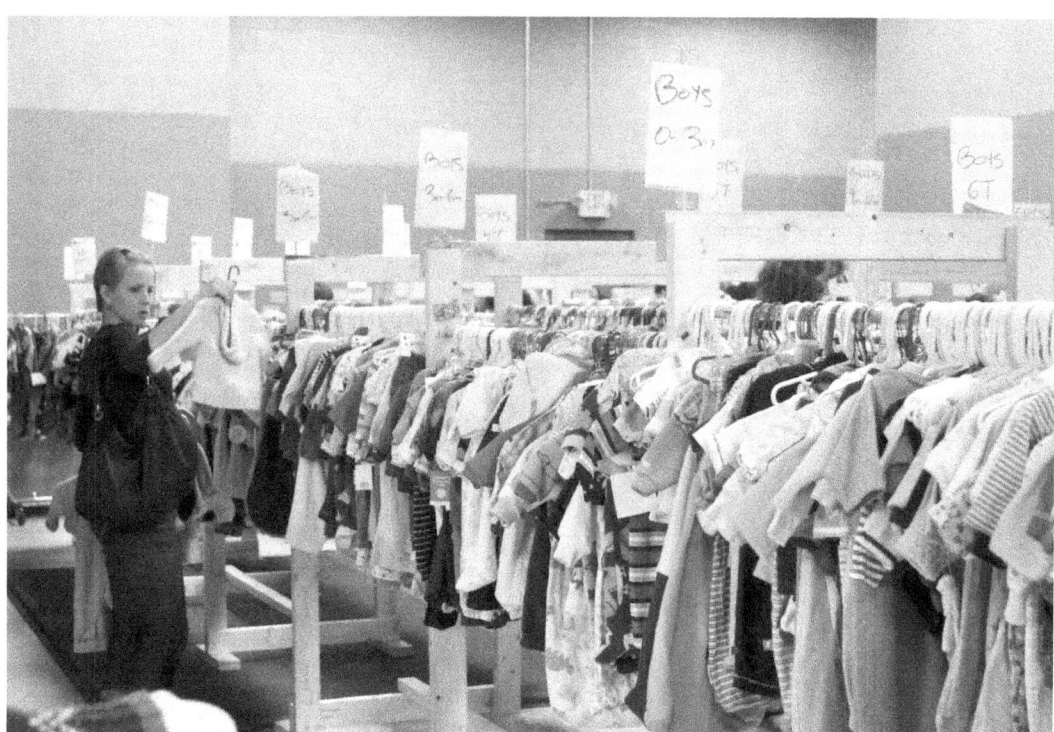

A baby cloth store

3. Buying Clothes for the Baby Boy

I like it blue, but he likes it yellow, but brown doesn't suit him! All these confusions arise when parents are planning to get the most adorable dresses for their charming little ones. Every parent desires to make their baby boy look like a little Red Riding Hood. Babies are cute beings, but there is lot of difference when it comes to choosing clothes for a boy or a girl. Apart from this, the place to buy, quality and quantity that you are buying matters a lot. Here are some ways and tips, which lead you to shop an astounding collection of clothes matching to your predetermined budget and mindset.

Decide What to Buy

Fancy baby stores can make you feel really tempted to buy those awesome looking stuff for your baby boy/girl. Think carefully and make a to-do list of those items which you wish to buy first, such as *pajamas*, *toppers*, *swimsuits*, *jumpers*, etc. elaborated in striking animal designs on them.

Go Simple and Easy

Creative outfits display a huge variety of those highly decorated costumes for babies having big buttons, fancy zippers, hangings and all. It is suggested not to go for such outfits as your baby boy or girl may feel uncomfortable in them and may develop a habit of tearing those delightful materials. Baby boys are much naughtier anyways!

Price Comparison

After you have chosen upon the kind of outfits and designs, it's better to go for a price comparison between the various store options, so that you don't simply burn your pockets at the time of buying clothes and later land up in compromising and picking low quality diapers!

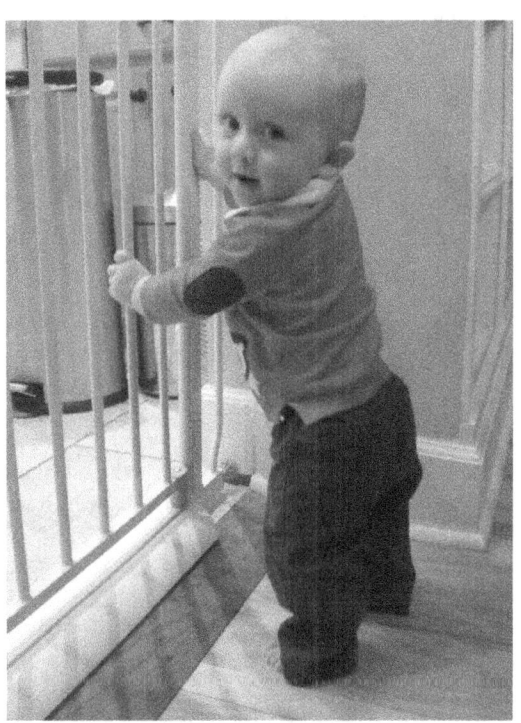

A smartly dressed baby boy

Seasons Matter

Before finally picking up outfits at the most feasible outlet, consider the seasonal criteria too. If its summers, go for cotton stuff as it is the most comfortable on your baby boy's delicate skin. If its winter or even autumn, choose some cuddling and warm stuff made from soft wool or hand-knitted sweaters.

Accessories and Special Clothes

Mothers decorate their baby girls like dolls, so why not sprinkle a little bit on cute baby boys! You can always get some cute soft animal shaped caps for them, gloves will be good as well and fur shoes would really make your baby boy look like a real prince. And yes of course, if any occasions are coming up then do get some special outfits for him and make him cast spell on others.

4. Buying Clothes for the Baby Girl

Imaginative ideas are galore as soon as the thought of buying clothes for your baby girl strikes your mind. Girls are always associated with soft colours, cutest designs and creative outfits including other accessories like hats and tiny cloth boots. As a parent, you would like to dress up your little girl like a tiny little angel. You start with categorising her cloth needs right from morning to night. You also need to decide that you have to buy clothes for the ongoing season or for the whole year, what kind of cloth you should buy so that she feels soft and cozy. One can refer to special baby shops to get the best buys.

Choose What to Buy

Choosing what to buy for your little princess is very important and you should plan her wardrobe accordingly. Starting from clothes to be worn in house to night suits, fancy clothes to tiny frocks, you have so much to decide on. Also, decide upon the number of clothes to be bought, so that you don't buy anything extra.

Decide Upon Colour Combinations

Baby girls always relate to soft colours, such as light pink, yellow, light green or white. You may take night dresses in darker shades. Choose glitter and glazy combinations for fancy clothes in light colours.

Creative Patterns

Babies are always amused from creative patterns. You can always choose strawberry patterns, flowers, animals, stars, moon and smileys on the clothes, which will interest the babies a lot and will keep them happy and smiling.

Soft Fabric Material

Babies are delicate beings and can develop sensitiveness or skin allergies to any fabric due to the presence of hard particles. Choose fabrics that are really soft to wear so your little girl/boy should feel comfortable wearing them.

Accessories

Now your baby girl or boy is all set and ready to take the form of a cute little angel/prince, so accessorise her from top to bottom with cute hats, cloth boots with different designs, colours and gloves.

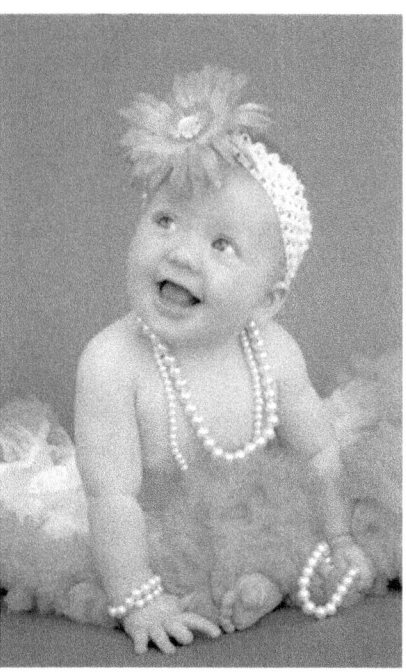
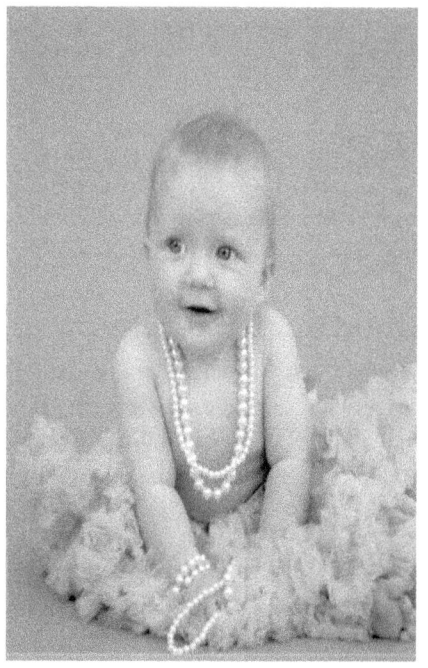

5. Taking Care of Baby Clothes

A new life brings along a lot of joy and happiness in the family. Everyone in the house is totally involved in taking care of the baby. It spreads a positive energy in the house. From the baby's cradle to the toys, everything is bought after a lot of argument and discussion. This is so because everyone wants to give the best to the baby. Likewise, taking care of a baby's clothes is also important. Clothes remain close to the baby's skin, therefore, it is important to keep them clean and tidy. It is essential to keep the baby's clothes germ-free so that the baby does not get affected by any infection or allergy. Clean, germ-free, soft and loose clothes will help your baby feel comfortable and stay cheerful.

Tips to Take Care of Baby's Clothes

- It is mandatory to wash any new clothes before your baby wears them. Your baby can be seriously harmed by new, unwashed clothes. It is essential to wash the clothes to get rid of all the dust, starch and germs that might have got accumulated in the manufacturing process.
- There is no need for any special detergent to be used for washing baby's clothes. The normal family detergents can only be used for washing your baby's clothes as well.
- Dealing with stains before washing them will help remove them properly and keep the clothes looking new. Formula, diaper accidents, and brightly coloured baby food can make stains that are tough to remove from baby's clothes, but if you take the time to work on these stains before washing, it will improve the success rate.
- Using a fabric softener will help to keep the baby's clothes soft and the baby will stay comfortable and happy.
- Do not mix baby's clothes with other clothes, while washing them. Always keep and wash baby's clothes separately, as adult's clothes may contain germs and dust that may be transferred to the baby's clothes. Also put 1 or 2 drops of savlon/dettol/or any disinfectent while washing your baby's clothes.
- Dry the baby's clothes in sun. This will ensure that all the germs and bacteria in the clothes will be killed and it will also give a fresh feel to the clothes.
- Soaking your baby's clothes in warm water before washing is also advisable. This will remove all the dust and kill all the germs.
- Keeping the baby's clothes after washing in a separate, clean place will ensure that the clothes remain germ-free till next use.

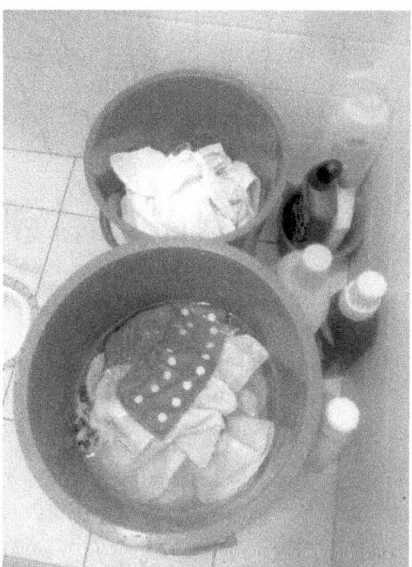

Washing baby's clothes

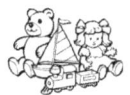

FAQs

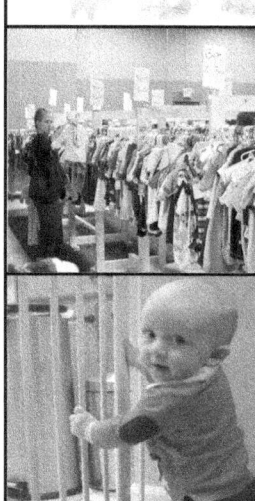

Q-1. During winter my baby's toes turn blue from time to time, whereas his fingers are normal. Why does that happen?

Ans. If your baby's toes turn blue but not the fingers or other parts of the body then the culprit may be the tight socks. Please check the size of the socks and make sure that they are fitting the baby properly.

Q-2. How warm should I keep my baby?

Ans. If the room temperature is around 27 degrees centigrade or more then do not clothe your baby in woollens. For summer season, use cotton clothes and for winter season, use cotton-woollen clothes.

Q-3. I dress my baby well in winters so much so that the baby sweats sometimes. Despite that my baby catches cold which does not go away throughout the season. What should I do?

Ans. In your effort to protect the baby from the cold, you are overdressing the baby. Common cold is caused by a virus in the environment. Keep the house clean, dust-free, wash your hands regularly and keep your baby warm and comfortable with enough clothes, but not overdress. Boost the baby's immunity so that he/she has a strong immune system to fight diseases.

Q-4. Should I wash my baby's clothes in washing machine or by hand?

Ans. You may use any or both the options so long as you rinse the clothes well and no trace of detergent is left. A final soak in antiseptic solution like dettol is very important for baby's clothes to disinfect them. In washing machine, this may seem very time consuming and tedious, so, you may wash the clothes in machine and then soak them in dettol in the tub before the final rinse.

Q-5. Some relatives have gifted soft, silky and lacy frocks for my baby. Can I put on those new clothes on her?

Ans. Babies feel most comfortable in cotton clothes as they are soothing to the skin. Lacy clothes for small babies should be avoided as their tiny fingers may get stuck in them. Always wash and disinfect all new clothes before the baby can wear them. This way the clothes are clean from all sorts of germs, dust and chemicals.

Q-6. What type of clothing material is the best for my baby's skin?

Ans. The clothing material for the baby should be light soft and porous to allow the sweat to dry. It should be non-irritating, non-inflammable and easy to wash. Cotton clothes are the best for the baby's sensitive skin. Do not buy synthetic clothes as they may cause allergy on the baby's skin.

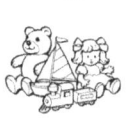

VI
Baby Furniture and Accessories

Once the baby is born, it is natural to get carried away while buying things for the newborn. There is no doubt that you will enjoy buying things for your baby, but you will have to be careful not to buy things the baby doesn't need. Also, it will greatly help you to assemble some of the most essential things even before the baby is born. It is important to remember that babies grow quickly and buying a lot of things that can only be used in the first few months will be a needless waste of money. It would be best if you could borrow some of the baby essentials from family or friends. Costly items like prams, rockers, high seats, etc can be bought second hand as they are used only in the first few months.

Your family and friends will gift a lot of the things that are required by the baby for the first few months. It is a good idea to talk to friends who have had babies before you and find out what they thought was necessary for the baby during the first few months. It is a good option to enlist the requirements of your baby and make your purchase accordingly.

1. Baby Bedding

Babies are small bundles of joy. Arrival of a baby fills the whole house with effervescence and colours. Baby bedding is an important part of the nursery and ensures absolute comfort and ease for the baby. Today, the market is stuffed with a lot of choices when it comes to baby bedding. If you are a new parent and are getting confused about what you should buy and what you should avoid, then read on to find what should be the best bedding set for your little one.

Tips for Baby Bedding Sets

- ❑ The first thing to keep in mind is that baby bedding is all about making your baby comfortable. So, at the time of purchasing, explore the plethora of shapes, colours and sizes available in the market keeping this in mind.
- ❑ At the time of selecting the bedding, consider the theme of your nursery. A nursery based on the theme, 'Cinderella' would have bedding that are in subtle shades of pink, green and yellow, while a nursery with the theme, 'Underwater Sea' needs bedding done in various shades of blue and green.
- ❑ The design would be another important consideration to make. Choose one that is lovely and pleasing to look at for both you and your tiny tot; after all, it is he/she who would be using the bedding.
- ❑ For the perfect baby bedding, you can select any one of the popular options, such as cartoon characters, candy colours, planes, automobiles, baby animals, calming tones, trains, fairy tales and wild forests.
- ❑ As for the size of the bedding, you should take care that it is neither too big nor too small. The bedding should be of the perfect size so that the baby can snuggle inside comfortably.

- Coming to the bedsheet and bedcovers, as it is popularly known as, should be colourful and stylish. The main reason for high demand of colourful bedcovers is that babies are always attracted to bright and vibrant colours. As for the style, the best preferred are printed bedsheets as they are easy to maintain and have no risks or hazards associated with them.
- Apart from the bedsheet, make sure that you get a bottom sheet for your baby's bedding. A bottom sheet is an absolute necessity as it helps keep the baby warm and also makes him/her fit snugly and cozily into the crib.
- Do not forget to get a cute-looking snugly blanket for your sweetheart. It would keep the little one warm and comfortable. However, while purchasing blanket for your baby, make sure that it is light in weight.
- Last but not the least, watch out for the amount of money you are spending on the baby bedding. The best bet would be to go for beautiful and comfortable baby bedding that are moderately priced. Such beddings would not only ensure pure comfort, but also would be light on pocket.
- There are innumerable fabric samples in the market. Don't be lured by the glamorous look, but also test the beneficial points.
- Baby-sleep Positioners may not be available to you within the bedding set and you may have to buy them separately. The side pillows and the head pillow with the foam support the head of the baby and also shape the sleeping posture of the baby. The advantage of these sleep positioners is that they go well with the bedding set. They can also be used with the bassinet* bedding set meant for infants.
- In the baby crib, bedding set you can also find crib bumpers, so that if your infant plays football on the crib, he doesn't get hurt. It can be of any tender colour like pink, blue or a mixture of both. A baby crib bumper, usually, comes in soft and supple colours, such as pink/blue, pink with blue stars or blue with pink stars. Foam-filled bumpers are more resistant to the kicks of your babies and the material also bounces back, thus giving a fresh look forever.
- Bassinets are actually meant for infants less than 6 months old.

A nice bedding can give just the right ambience to your baby for a peaceful and undisturbed sleep.

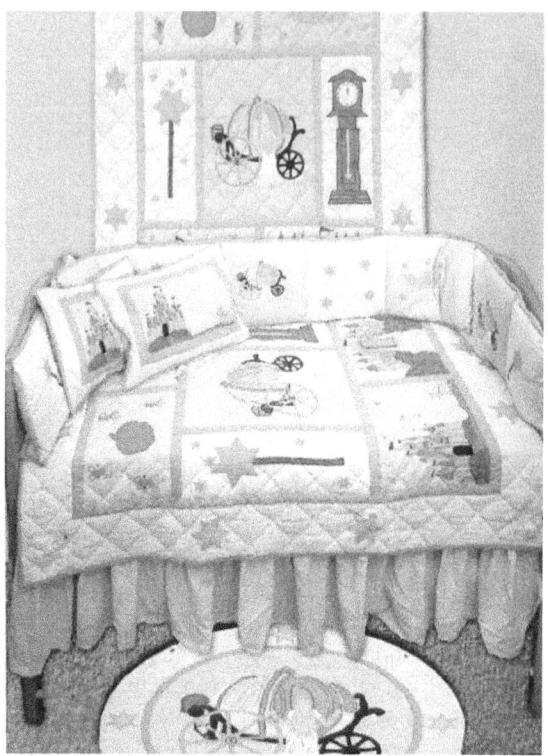

Decorating baby's bed

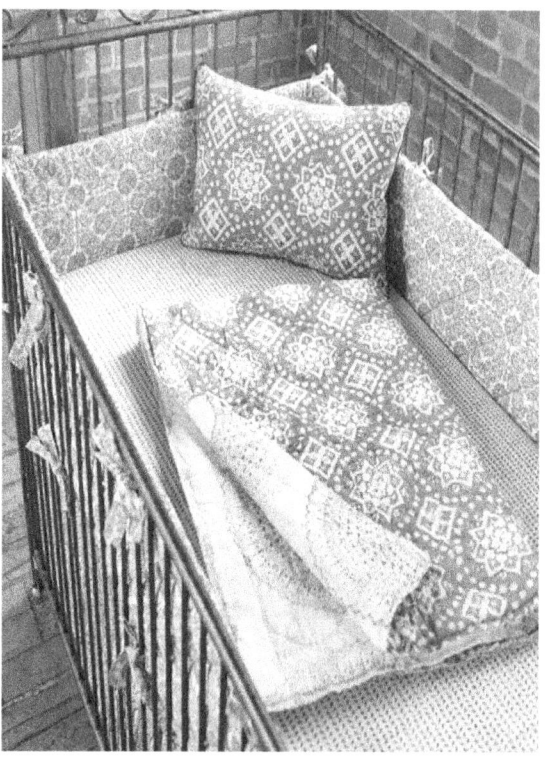

A baby crib bedding

2. Baby Carriers

Even with a newborn baby, there will be a number of errands that you will have to do. Also, you will have to take the baby with you wherever you go. The easiest and most cost-effective way of getting around with your baby is to place him in a baby sling or carrier. Both parents and babies like slings as the baby stays close to the parent's body and thus, both feel safe. Slings are easy to use while shopping, on walks and while using the public transport system. Slings can be used in places where it is difficult to use a pram or stroller. If used properly, the weight of the baby will be equally distributed and there will be no strain on your back.

Types of Baby Carriers

As various types of carriers are available in the market, it is best to try all of them and find the one you are most comfortable with. Find out from family and friends how useful they found the sling or carrier. If you can, try out a sling using an older child then you will get an idea as to how comfortable it feels.

- **Wrap-Around Sling**
  This consists of a large piece of cloth with a buckle you can adjust to make a cradle in which you put your newborn. It can be worn across the body like a sash to form a hammock in which the baby can lie. This can also be fastened to balance a toddler on your hip. Many women find this useful when they are breast-feeding. However as the baby grows older and weighs more, it becomes difficult to use.

- **Drop-In Baby Carrier**
  This consists of a pouch, which has arm and leg holes, and rests on the chest of the person wearing it. The baby is made to sit in this pouch with his arms and legs passing through the holes, so that he is secure as he sits. Newborns are made to face inwards and older children are made to face outward. Many parents prefer the drop-in carrier, as it is comfortable and less cumbersome than a pram. But once the baby is over six months, it is difficult to carry him like this.

- **Backpack Carrier**
  Once your baby can sit by himself without any support, you can use this carrier. This is worn on the back and usually has a metal frame; the baby gets a good view of what is happening around him. If you buy a raincover, you can use it in all kinds of weather. Some of the backpack carries have a pull along feature with wheels and a handle and can be used as a 'little-buggy' for short distances. Some come with stands, so you can grab a cup of coffee while putting the backpack down for a short time.

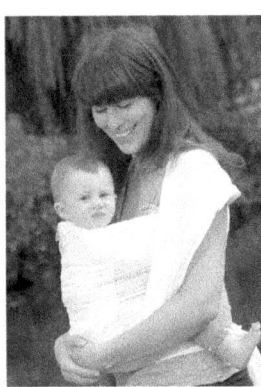
Wrap-Around Sling

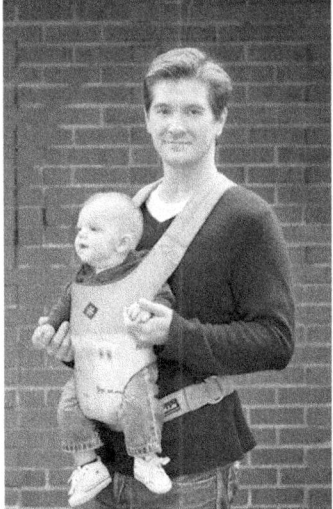
Drop-in Baby Carrier

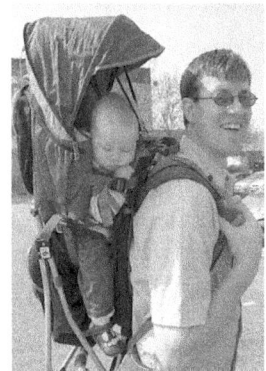
Backpack Carrier

Baby Furniture and Accessories

3. Baby Strollers and Prams

Carrying your baby yourself can be a bit hectic for you, though it is a universal practice. If both of you want to enjoy each other's company without disturbing the comfort of the other, you should opt for baby strollers. The market is flooded with a variety of baby strollers. As usual before paying for anything, you need to find the utility of the different strollers' type and select the right one for you, which can give comfort to your little angel and fulfill your purpose too.

Types of Baby Strollers

Here are different types of baby strollers from which you may choose the one which suits you the best.

- **Umbrella Strollers**
  Umbrella strollers are the ideal ones for travelling as they can be folded easily. Even if you are going for a long drive in car, these umbrella baby strollers are very useful as they can be used both inside and outside the car. They are the best for the infants.

- **Jogging Baby Stroller**
  The jogging baby stroller is meant for the parents who go for jogging or walking with the baby. Though these infant jogging strollers are light in weight, they are not meant for use in the shopping. You can find wheels of different sizes in the jogging strollers.

- **Standard Strollers**
  Standard strollers have a sturdy frame and are among the most durable type of strollers. Most standard strollers have fully reclining seats, which make them suitable to be used from the time of your child's infancy to the time he/she is a toddler. Standard strollers are easy to push and steer, especially when they are used on smooth surfaces.

- **Lightweight Strollers**
  A lightweight stroller is a good option as it, usually weighs less than 12 pounds. Most of the lightweight strollers do not have a reclining seat and are thus best suited for children, who are one year of age or a little older. They are also less expensive than most of the other types of strollers.

- **Combo Strollers**
  Combo strollers, being versatile, can be used right from the child's infancy to the time he/she is a toddler. A combo stroller features a toddler stroller base and a coordinating infant bassinet. Most of the combo strollers also come with extra seat padding and cup holders as well as many convenience features.

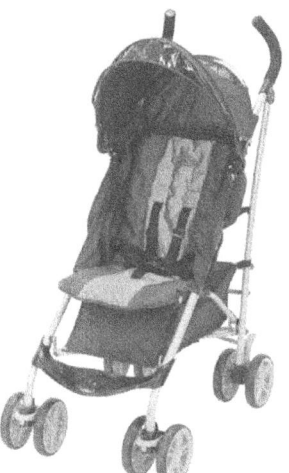

Umbrella Strollers

Baby Stroller Accessories

- Infant stroller has cover that protects your baby form rain. There are some strollers that have hood that covers the entire stroller till the wheels.
- There are also small umbrella in the baby strollers that protect the little angel from the scorching heat.
- These strollers are covered with fine wire net that prevents the small harmful insects to come in touch with the baby, but allow the baby to inhale fresh air.
- You can keep the food and any drink of your baby on the stands that are provided in the infant strollers, so that you don't have to carry it separately. There is also a provision of carrying basket with the stroller. However, be careful to hang the baskets low and light weight on the stroller or it may get misbalanced.
- There are also some attractive toys on the stroller, which are attached to them by a Velcro. Undoubtedly, they are within the reach of the tiny supple hands. And if desired, you can even use them in the car seats or cribs.

- In some baby strollers, there are elegant designed removable headrests and padding, so that your little one can find some comfort while experiencing the long tiring journey.

Baby Prams

Prams are normally the carriages in which new born baby lies down while going for a stroll. Babies outgrow them as they learn to sit. However there are some pram-cum-strollers available in the market which may serve dual purpose.

- **Coach-Built Prams**
  A coach built pram comes with a wide hood, a generous frame and large wheels. It has good suspension and good shock absorption abilities, which means comfortable ride for your baby. These kinds of prams are quite spacious and give enough space for your baby to stretch, turn and lie flat. It is very easy to handle these prams and it also takes care of the comfort and safety of the baby with its sturdy chassis and padded mattress. The only disadvantage of these kinds of prams is that they are very expensive and are not easily available. They are even bulky and once your baby grows up, you will need a stroller instead.

- **Three-In-One Prams**
  Pram style strollers are very common for newborn babies. They come with features like enclosed carrycots that can be pulled out and have swivel wheels. These models come with seats that can help you position the baby either facing you or away from you. They can even have a separate pushchair unit that can be securely attached and detached from the pram unit. The benefit of having a carrycot is that one can use them to carry the baby during naps or feeding time.

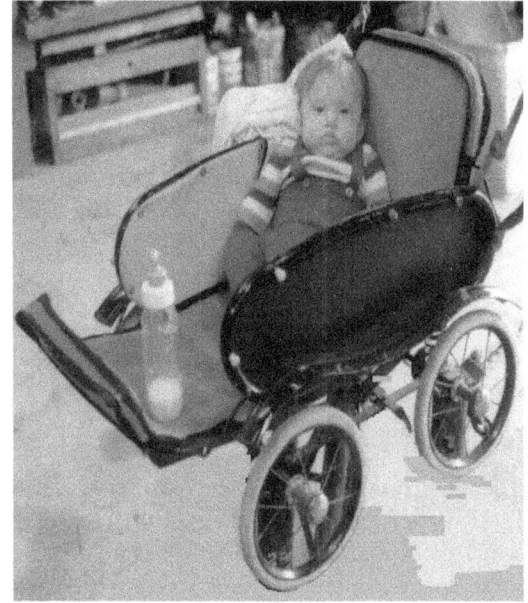

Coach-Built Prams

- **Two-In-One Prams**
  These are prams with a chassis and a seat with a hood. It can serve the purpose of both a pram, when in reclining position and a stroller when upright. The price tag is always a disadvantage for these kinds of prams.

Security Tips

- Make sure while buying a pram or a stroller that the belts are secure enough.
- The wheels and the support on the seat should be sturdy enough.
- Look out for carriages with breaks or other features to control and manage it.
- One more point to be kept in mind while buying a pram/stroller is that whether it can be maneuvered in all kinds of terrain.
- It should also be spacious and comfortable.

4. Baby Walkers

There is a constant demand of infant walkers in the market, though it is considered a risky item by many. If you have decided to buy a walker, do a brief research before selecting the right walker for your infant. You can get walkers that have an activity centre on the walker itself. Also, these infant walkers are available in different designs. Some are brightly coloured with all the funny cartoon pictures or designed with some lacy and satin material. There are also folding baby walkers available in the market that can be easily folded and carried over to any desired place. However, the security of your infant is the primary concern and you need to consider it before making a final choice.

Infant Walkers

Apart from some minor differences, almost all the infant walkers are basically circular in shape and designed in a way so as to enclose the baby. Some walkers come with central seats for baby to sit and totter around the floor, while some walkers are more traditional in their makeup and design requiring babies to stand and hold on to a handle for toddling about. Some traditional wooden walkers also feature a tray containing wooden blocks with numbers, alphabets, letters and mathematical signs. Electronic walkers are also available, which have activity centres so that babies can learn, discover and play even as they use them.

Toddler Walkers

The toddler walkers are meant for slightly older babies. In these walkers, the babies can grab the back of the walker, which gives them the option to hold on to the walker's back or move around a room. Toddler walkers may be designed in the shape of a car, truck or other popular vehicles to fascinate the young kids. The two-in-one walkers are also a good option for growing babies as they can be used for dual purpose: as a secure activity centre and for walking.

Infant Walker

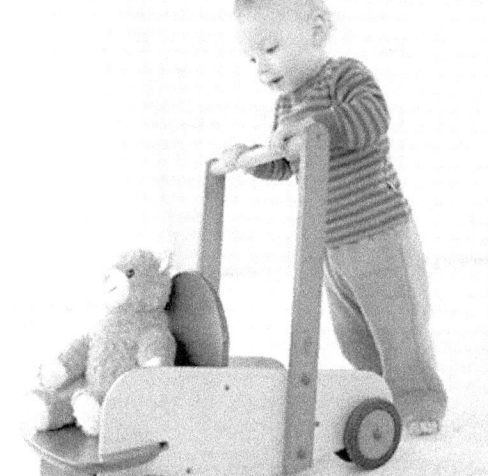
Toddler Walker

Tips to Use a Walker

- ❑ You should cover the electrical switches and plugs.
- ❑ The latches of drawers and cabinets should be covered.
- ❑ It is better that you either remove the furniture with sharp edges or smoothen the sharp edges.
- ❑ Remove all the breakable items from tables and shelves where your infant can reach safely.
- ❑ Don't carry hot water or food in vessel near the baby when seated in the walker. The baby might knock it against you with the thrust of the walker causing a dangerous accident.
- ❑ Don't allow your child near the stove heater or other heating appliances.
- ❑ Keep the house locked with a childproof lock, so that the baby can't go outside the main door of the house to the backyard or garage without the help of any elder person.

5. Baby Toys

If you think that your baby's toys are the luxurious items required just to decorate the room of your child, you will be pleasantly surprised at your ignorance. The first baby toys have a great potential to help in the overall development of the personality of the child. Baby toys are generally colourful, so that they appear attractive to the eyes of the babies. Infant toys are generally attached to the cribs or hung on the upper side of the child cot, so that the sound and movement amuses the little one.

Rattles and Teethers

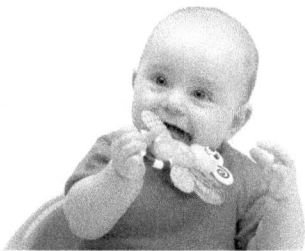

Rattles and teethers are great toys for children, especially when they are learning to chew. However, it is better to keep them in refrigerator when unused. The coolness of the refrigerated rattle will be a relief to the gums of the baby. Toys that make noise or move when squeezed also help in development of the child. Babies get to know that their act of squeezing the toy makes it move or creates some sound from the toy.

Nesting Cups

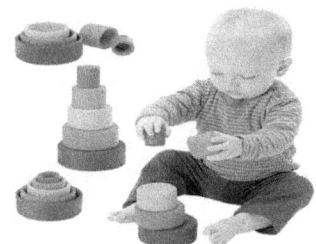

Nesting cups come in different colours and sizes, so that they can be stacked or nested. These toys can be used to develop the colour and size recognition abilities and hand-eye coordination of the baby. The best nesting cups are made of plastics that come in several solid colours and may consist of more than five cups.

Stacking Rings

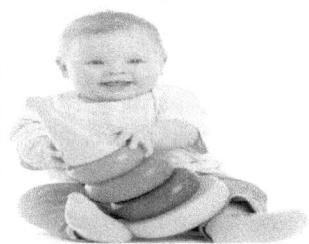

Stacking rings are as educational as nesting cups and come in different colours and sizes placed in a cone. These rings also help the child in colour and size recognition, hand-eye coordination and for pretend play as well. The most inexpensive stacking rings are made of plastics. You can buy the more fancy rings, which also contain other fun activities for the child.

Soft Building Blocks

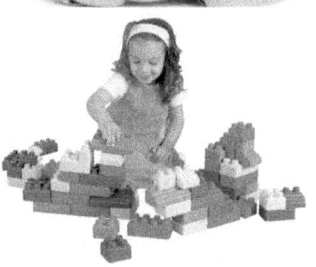

Soft baby building blocks help your child to develop motor skills. The baby will use his/her little fingers to grasp, lift and manipulate the building blocks. As such, they are considered to be one of the best toys for the little ones. For a very young age group, soft building blocks are preferable. You can also choose blocks with other activities embedded in them to increase their play value for the child.

Colourful Picture Books

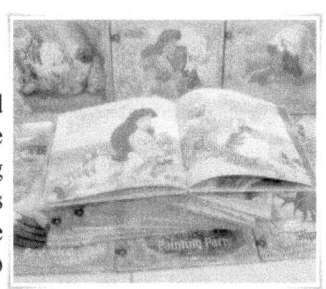

Another interesting way of developing the intellect and personality of the child is by reading simple short stories to him. However, this is only possible once the child is old enough to understand, at least, something from the story. Reading habit never goes without paying off and it can easily overcome all the obstacles that age creates. When he/she is little grown-up then you can give him the more durable rhyme books or other colourful pictured books. These books are made up of thick cardboard or hard cloth, and are specially designed for infants.

6. Baby Monitors

The universal problem that a mother of a newborn has to face is little or, sometimes, no sleep or rest. Also, it is simply not possible to stick around your baby during all the twenty-four hours of the day. At the same time, you can't stop worrying about the troubles that your little one can face when he/she is not under your careful observation. It is in this situation that the baby monitors prove to be the most helpful tool to make you aware of your tiny angel's needs.

Audio-Video Baby Monitors

These monitors are actually used to see or hear your infant when you are physically not present near him/her. These monitor have two sections; one is placed near the baby and the other remains with the mother. It can work both with battery and directly through electricity. One part of the baby monitor is to be placed in between 10 feet of the baby's crib, so that it can make you alert of the baby's moving or crying, etc. Though the widely used baby monitors are the audio monitors, but there are infant video monitors where you can view your baby on-screen with all his different gestures. You can also get to know the room temperature of the infant's room with a monitor.

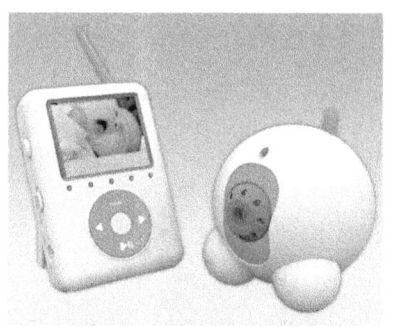

Audio-video baby monitors

Baby-Breathing Monitor

Another variety among the baby monitor is the baby-breathing monitor. Premature babies require these breathing monitors and the hospital authorities generally provide it, if they find such requirement. It might be, sometimes, possible that the walls or the cordless phones or even other baby monitor can be an obstacle and send you wrong alerts. So, it is better to have a frequent checkup whether your baby monitor is working properly or not. Also don't keep a baby monitor near the water, else there can be serious accident.

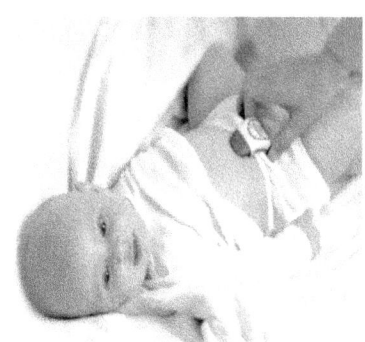

Tips to Choose the Best Baby Monitor

Baby-breathing monitor

- ❑ It is better to opt for a small size infant monitor, so that you can carry it in and around the house.
- ❑ There are some monitors that give you the alert regarding when your battery needs to be changed. It is better to use those baby monitors that contain this feature or you will not know about the battery replacement and it might be possible that you will stop receiving alerts even when your child needs you the most.
- ❑ See to it that your infant monitor has a light alert beside the sound alert. It might happen that you are busy watching TV or cleaning the house with a vacuum cleaner and the sound may not reach your ears. But as the monitor lights up, you become aware and rush to your infant's crib.
- ❑ You can also use monitors that have two receivers. You can easily leave one receiver in the room and take another with you outside, if required.
- ❑ There are some brands that have a high bandwidth compared to others. These powerful monitors are ideal for the remote areas where the technology development or usage is less, as these monitors give clearer signals compared to others. However in hi-tech places that are replete with technical devices, such as cell phones and computers, you require a baby monitor of low bandwidth.

7. Baby Safe Feeder

It is a real pleasure to see your baby grow. The first time he/she sits, stands, speaks and eats; are the special moments and they are cherished by you. Any tiny progress of the infant seems to be extraordinary to your eyes. As a parent, apart from enjoying the wonders of your baby's childhood, it is your duty to provide him/her a safe and secure growing phase. Apart from taking bigger financial measures, it is your duty to take care of the baby's smallest necessities. To ensure that he/she eats right, sleeps peacefully and play safe is your duty. One more tool that will help you ensure your child's safety is Baby Safe Feeder.

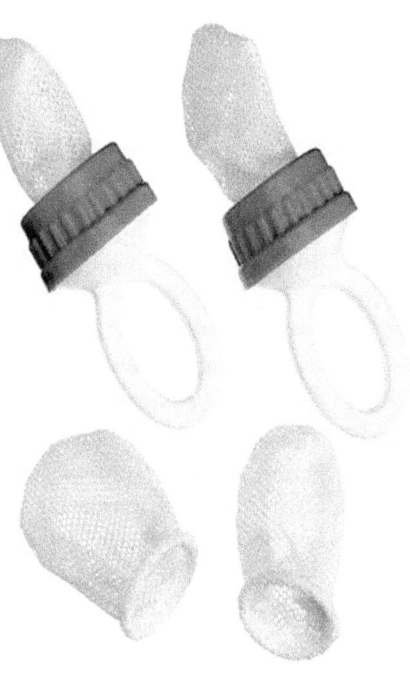

What is a Baby Safe Feeder!

A baby safe feeder is a disposable mesh bag attached with a plastic ring that helps in feeding the baby safely. The food items are stuffed in a mesh bag and given to the baby who sucks them according to his/her own wish. The plastic ring attached at the end of the mesh bags assure that your baby does not gulp up the entire food piece at a go. It is also an easy way to keep a baby engaged. Using the baby safe feeder is also a nice way to feed baby with fruit piece, vegetable piece, meat or any sweetener.

Baby Safe Feeder as a Teether

It is a very painful phase for a baby when his/her teeth begin to come out of the gums. To overcome the uneasiness and pain caused during this period, the baby develops a tendency of chewing and eating all solid things that come in his/her way. However, at times, it becomes very dangerous because the kids gulp up big pieces of food or any uneatable item that can make them choke. To avoid this, one can always offer the baby a safe feeder that will keep him/her away from all these dangerous items. A baby safe feeder is also a terrific soothing teether, if filled with ice or frozen fruit.

Tips for Using Baby Safe Feeder

- ❑ Always make sure that the safe feeder you are using is of good quality. The mesh bag attached with the feeder should be gentle in touch.
- ❑ Try to keep the safe feeder away from the reach of dirt, dust and pets.
- ❑ Clean your baby's safe feeder with lukewarm water after every use.
- ❑ Stuff the mesh bag of the safe feeder with food of your kid's choice, so that he/she does not throw it anywhere and get engrossed with something else.
- ❑ Keep, at least, half a dozen of safe feeders with you, so that you do not have to rush to wash one when it becomes dirty.

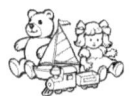

FAQs

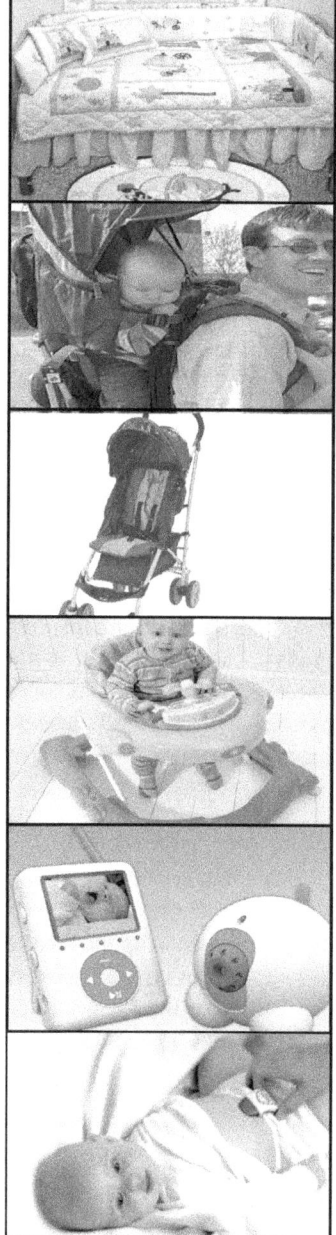

Q-1. I have a wrap-around sling to carry my baby in, but I am fearful of using it as my baby may feel suffocated in it. What should I do?

Ans. A wrap-around sling is a very comfortable baby carrier both for the mother and the baby. Once your baby grows up, it may be a little difficult to use but for newborn babies, it is quite comfortable. In the wrap-around, the baby will feel your warmth and remain snug and happy.

Q-2. The sheets on my baby's bassinet bedding get loose easily on the rubber sheet under them and every now and then I have to tuck them all over again. What should I do?

Ans. The sleeping sheets on the bassinet should fit perfectly. If they are loose then the baby may get entangled in the sheets which may be harmful for the baby. So get a few well-fitting sheets for the bassinet.

Q-3. How do I protect my baby from mosquitoes?

Ans. The safest way of protecting babies from mosquitoes is using mosquito net. There are specially designed mosquito nets for babies available in the market. Do not use mosquito repellant on the body of the baby as they can cause allergy. Using mosquito coils, mats and liquid vaporizers are also not advisable as they can also cause breathing problems.

Q-4. I am afraid of buying any rubber and plastic toys for my baby due to the fear that they may contain some toxic component. What toys should I buy for my baby?

Ans. There is always a fear in the mothers about the quality of material used in baby toys owing to toxicity of many materials. However, you cannot altogether avoid buying toys for the baby. So go in for toys from those company which have a safe label on them. Always buy toys of a renowned brand and do not go in for local ones as they may not have the material and other specifications printed on their label. Rattles and teethers from a well-known brand may be safely given to the baby.

Q-5. I would like to give my baby a baby safe feeder. Please tell me what all I can put in it?

Ans. A baby safe feeder is a disposable mesh bag attached with a plastic ring. It helps in feeding the baby safely. The food items are stuffed in a mesh bag and given to the baby to suck them. you can place any sold food item like a piece of fruit, vegetable, sweetener etc which the baby can chew and suck through the mesh bag. Any of these things can be placed in that bag depending upon your baby's liking. However, try to keep the safe feeder away from the reach of dirt, dust and pets so that the baby does not catch any infection by chewing on the dirty feeder.

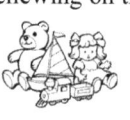

VII
Premature Baby Care

Every parent-to-be naturally hopes for a baby to be born healthy and full-term. But even with modern medicines and hi-tech facilties, seven percent of babies are born prematurely. A premature baby is born before the 37th week of gestation and is sometimes nicknamed as a 'preemie'. Babies can be born prematurely for different reasons like pregnancies with twins, triplets or more babies, stressful events like long distance air travel, emotional stress of the death of someone very close, etc. However, normal day-to-day stresses of living have no evidence on inducing premature labour. Mothers who deliver premature babies are often scared and nervous as their newborns have a higher risk of developing complications. The earlier the baby is born, the higher the baby is likely to develop complications.

Since premature babies are not fully equipped to deal with the outside world, they require special care. Their little bodies have areas that are yet to mature and fully develop such as lungs, digestive system, immune system and skin. A baby born healthy requires special and extra care and attention. Here comes the role of the parents to keep their baby as healthy and comfortable as possible. A few tips are required on the parents' part to smooth out the process of caring for a preemie. This chapter of baby care will help you out with feeding your premature baby and the needs demanded by a preemie. Also look out for the growth chart of a premature baby and the various health problems faced by such a baby.

1. Feeding Your Premature Baby

Before your baby was born, you might have probably dreamt about how it would feel to hold him/her in your arms and feed him/her. You might have already decided and planned out what all to feed or how to feed him/her a nutritious diet. However, if your baby has been born prematurely, you may have to reconsider your plans. Feeding a premature baby can really be a stressful task for any parent. It becomes an issue of daily care and concern. In the womb, the baby might have got all the nutrients and fluids via the placenta and umbilical cord. But when a baby is born premature, this chain of receiving nutrients and fluids is broken. As such, the deficiency that results can be taken care by nursing the baby or by feeding him/her formula, or by following other methods as prescribed by the doctor to fulfill the baby's basic requirements.

Total Parenteral Nutrition

Total Parenteral Nutrition (TPN) is a method of feeding used for extremely premature babies or one who are very sick. In this method, nutrients, such as glucose, protein and fat solutions are introduced directly into the baby's bloodstream through a vein. Babies have an immature digestive system, so this method is brought to use. This method also helps the kids to preserve their energy. TPN provides all the necessary nutrients to your baby to help him/her grow and thrive.

Tube Feeding Method

Supply of adequate amount of nutrients to the baby is necessary for them to grow properly. Tube method makes sure that the baby gets enough nutrients. Babies have a higher metabolism, their brain is developing and they are growing fast. However, premature babies have limited supply of energy and nutrients. Thus it becomes important

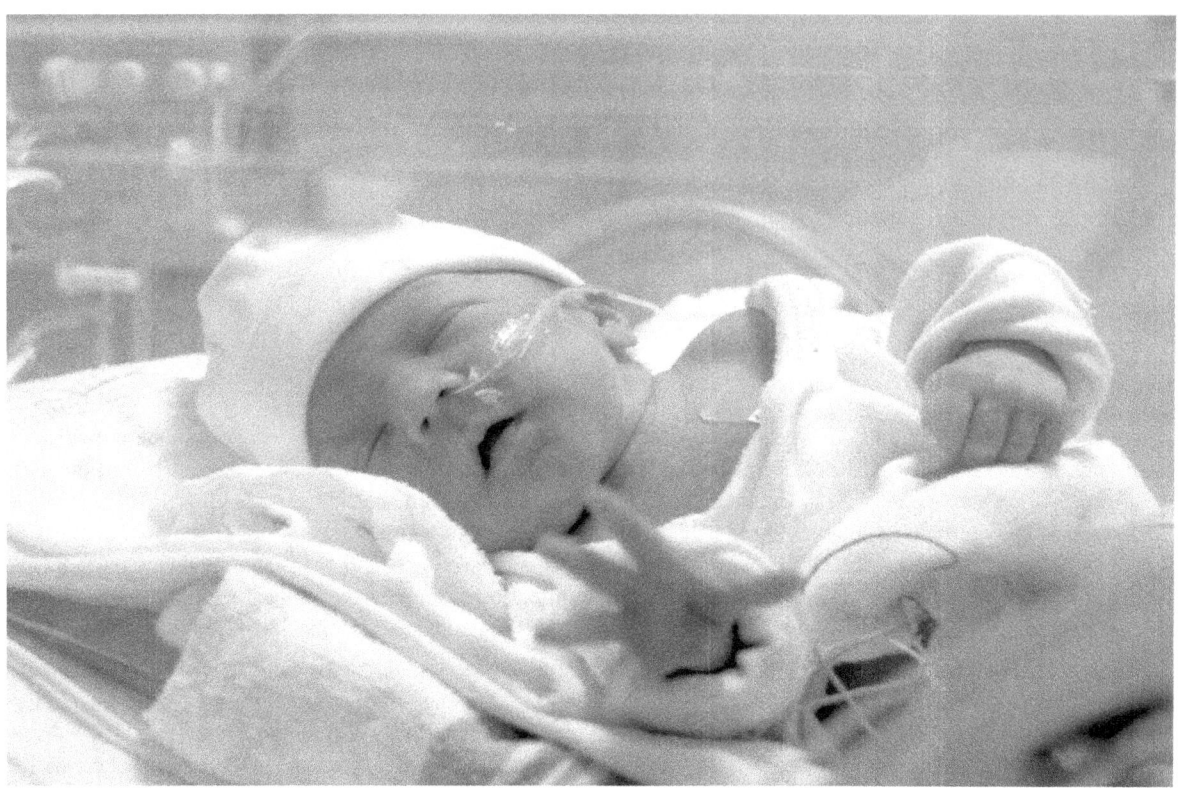
Premature baby being fed with tube

to tube feed them, so that they can take in small intake of nutrients without using too much of energy. The coordination of sucking, swallowing, and breathing needed for feeding is not developed in babies born before 34-36 weeks, so a tube is passed through their nose or mouth down to their stomach.

Nursing
Nursing is the best way to protect your kids from different illnesses. Your body produces specialised proteins called *antibodies* to fight off infection. Mothers transfer these antibodies to their babies through placenta during the last three months of pregnancy. This process is broken if a baby is born prematurely. Mothers also can transfer these antibodies through breast-feeding. This will help in providing immunity to the babies against any virus or infection.

Supplementary Feeding
In the early stages of your baby's development, proper supply of enough energy and fluids is important. Sometimes, it may get difficult for mothers to express enough milk because of some illness during pregnancy. Two of the alternatives that can be used in such a case can be to use additional breast milk donated to some hospitals by other mothers, or to use formula milk. This is a temporary method to be adopted. Full inspection of the donated milk will be conducted by the doctors before feeding it to babies.

Bottle Feeding
When in hospital, babies are fed on formula milk, made particularly for their nutritional needs. When your baby is out of hospital and ready for coordinating sucking, swallowing and breathing, he/she can be fed by a bottle. These

formulas or formulae contain more of nutrients that a premature baby requires, such as iron, fat, protein, several vitamins, calcium, phosphorous and magnesium.

2. Premature Baby Growth Chart

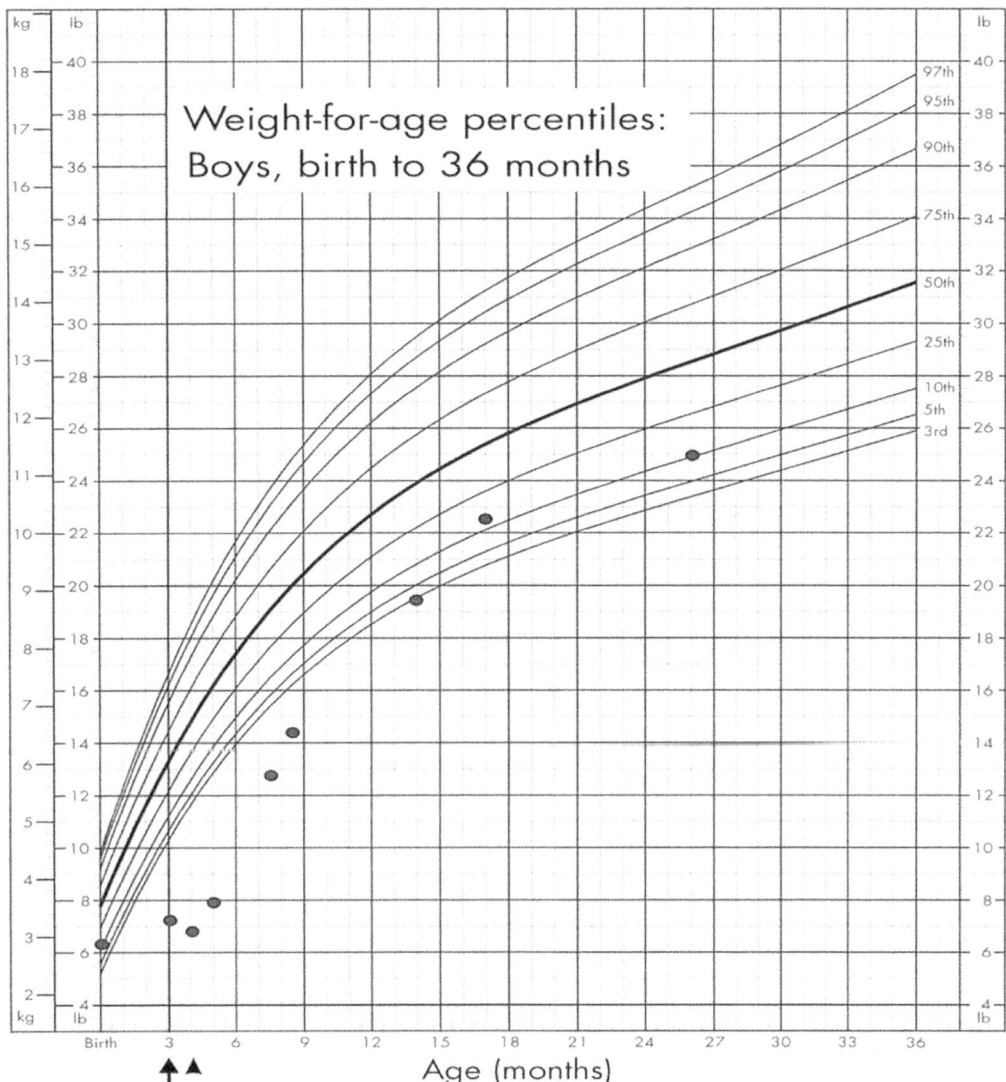

You can measure your premature baby's growth by a growth chart. A growth chart is a tool that the specialists use to evaluate and keep a track of your baby's physical growth. Parents at times get worried with the results of this chart, especially if the baby is premature. They should remember that their child will grow at his/her own pace, and that this test is conducted to get the data, so that you can work towards better growth of your kid if he/she is lagging behind. Growth chart is just a normal guide for you and your doctor to keep a track of your baby's growth, there is nothing to get worried with the result. What a growing baby requires is just the intake of all necessary nutrients and fluids. If the baby is getting these nutrients in some form or the other, there is nothing to worry, as the baby will grow at his/her own pace.

Doctor's Way of Measurement

❑ **Weight**
The doctor or the nurse will put your baby on a scale, either a traditional beam scale or an electronic model, to weigh them. Both the types will be set to zero before your baby is laid down. Your baby should not be wearing any clothing during this test. The measurement is usually taken in kilograms and recorded to the tenth of a kilo. The doctor or nurse will tell you your baby's weight in pounds to the closest ounce.

❑ **Head Circumference**
The doctor will measure your baby's head with a flexible measuring tape. He will place the tape at the area where the circumference is the largest, like just above your baby's eyebrows and ears, around the back of their heads. It is important to measure your baby's head circumference to get to know whether your baby's brain is growing properly with the right pace or not. The brain growth is reflected in the size of the skull. So, if your baby's brain is not growing normally, his/her head circumference may not be increasing as it should. There is even a problem if the circumference of the head is increasing very fast. This means your baby's brain is growing very fast, which may be an indicator of problems like hydrocephalus (the formation and buildup of fluid in the brain). Both the ends are quite dangerous and alarming, so the brain growth should just be apt. But do not get alarmed if your baby's head looks big. If you have any doubt, go for a checkup, as the head may look big even because either of the parent's head is big.

❑ **Height**
The doctor or the nurse will measure your baby from the top of their head to the bottom of their heel. Some practitioners use a special device with a headboard and a movable footboard for accurate results. There is again nothing to get worried with the measurement, as your baby will grow only as much he/she should. The length of the baby is also affected by his/her genes.

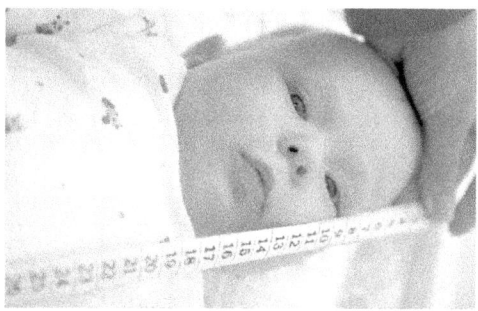

Growth Measurement at Home

❑ You can weigh your baby at home by using a weighing scale. Get your baby on the scale and note the number. Then, put your baby down and you get on to the scale without the baby. Subtract the number from your combined weight and get your baby's appropriate weight.

❑ Also measure your baby's length. Lay your baby down, take a measuring tape and stretch it down from head to toe. It is better if there is someone to help you. Your results will not be the same as the doctor's figures, but you will get a rough idea.

❑ Wrap a flexible measuring tape over your baby's head to measure his/her head circumference. The goal is to measure the head at the spot, where it has the largest circumference. After all the results are there with you, place them on a growth percentile calculator to find out whether your baby is growing properly or not.

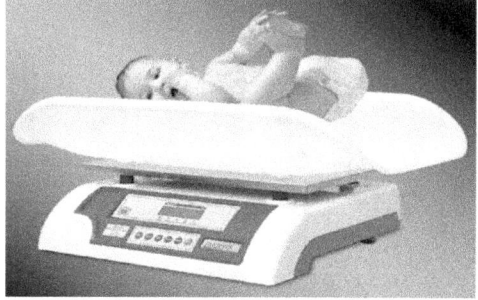

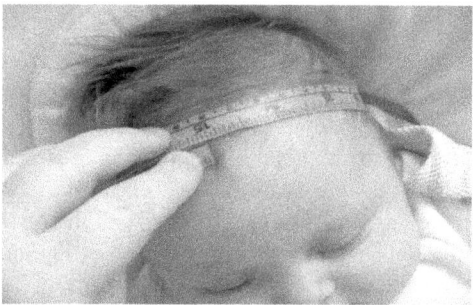

Baby Profile Measurements		
Weight	Height	Head
EAT Six Months		
8.1 kg	69.1 cm	41.5 cm
EAT Five Months		
8 kg	67.32 cm	41.4 cm
EAT Four Months		
6.3 kg	61.4 cm	39.2 cm
EAT Three Months		
5.56 kg	58.5 cm	36.9 cm
EAT Two Months		
4.4 kg	54 cm	36 cm
EAT One Months		
3.1 kg	48 cm	34 cm

3. Premature Baby Health Problems

Bringing up a baby is a great but difficult experience, because a parent needs to take many health and safety precautions. If the baby is premature, the difficulty, the precautions and the care to be taken, increases. Parents of a premature baby have only one question to ask, what the different problems are that their babies will encounter. There is a stage of development that all babies go through inside the womb. However, a premature baby will not be able to complete the development cycle, facing multiple problems after birth. This will call in for extra care and effort on parent's part. The parents should not only take good care of a premature baby and get him/her medical attention, but should also make an effort to learn about the different diseases that their babies may face. This will help them understand their baby's problem and get him/her the right treatment.

Health Problems in Preemies

These are some common health problems that the premature babies are more prone to have.

- **Respiratory Problems**
  Respiratory distress is the common problem faced by as many as 43% of premature babies born between 30 to 32 weeks, or before that time. For lungs to inflate properly, a chemical called *surfactant* is needed, which a full-term baby or a normal baby can produce, but a premature baby can't. They may need artificial surfactant, or might need breathing help till the time they and their lungs grow up.
- **Jaundice**
  It is caused by a product of *red blood cell* called *bilirubin*. Preemies are the most affected by a rapid rise in bilirubin, and are treated more often than full-term babies to prevent a risk of high number of bilirubin damaging the brain.

- **Apnea**
  Babies born before 34 weeks of full gestation period develop Apnea, or a period where breathing stops, because their brains and lungs are not developed fully. Apnea may be accompanied by Bradycardia, where the heart slows down. Stimulation or other respiratory help may start the normal breathing process again in babies.

- **Gastro Esophageal Reflex Disease**
  Gastro Esophageal Reflex Disease (GERD) affects half of the premature population. In this disease, the babies throw up whatever they eat due to the stomach contents coming up the esophagus. The infants suffering with GERD have many other symptoms too, such as they spit up, lose weight, or may have respiratory problems like cough or pneumonia.

- **Intraventricular Hemorrhage**
  Preemies born before 30 weeks have fragile blood vessels in their brains. An Intraventricular Hemorrhage may occur if these blood vessels break. This bleeding in the brain may be mild or severe. This bleeding may also have serious consequences, such as developmental delays. A mild bleed does not usually have long-term effects.

- **Retinopathy of Prematurity**
  Retinopathy of prematurity or ROP is the abnormal growth of blood vessels in the eyes of premature babies. This abnormal vessel growth may lead to retinal detachment and blindness. The disease affects half of the babies born before 26 weeks, but only 1 % of them born before 30 weeks.

- **Patent Ductus Arteriosis**
  Before birth, the babies depend on the placenta for oxygen and have a different circulatory system after the birth. They have *ductus arteriosis*, an opening between the major vessels. This ductus usually closes after birth for food to flow in normally. However in preemies, this opening might not close even after birth. This causes Patent Ductus Arteriosis or PDA which occurs in younger preemies and leads to abnormal circulation. Medication or surgery will be needed to close the ductus.

- **Necrotizing Enterocolitis (NEC)**
  Necrotizing Enterocolitis (NEC) occurs in as many as 13% of babies before 26 weeks, and 3% babies born between 30-32 weeks. NEC affects the intestine of the infants. Various symptoms of this problem are a distended belly, lethargy and feeding intolerance. The early it is tracked, the better and safer it is for the preemies. It can be treated by antibiotics. A severe case may also require surgery.

- **Sepsis**
  Sepsis is a serious problem in preemies and is caused by bacteria in blood. It may occur earlier by exposure to the bacteria in the womb or birth canal, or later from contaminated equipment or IV lines. The symptoms may include breathing problems, swollen belly and lethargy. If caught early, it can be treated very easily with antibiotics.

- **Broncho-Pulmonary Dysplasia**
  Broncho Pulmonary Dysplasia (BPD) is a chronic lung condition caused by airway inflammation. It affects those babies more who were on ventilator for a longer time. It may cause difficulty in breathing and low blood oxygen levels. Babies with BPD need extra oxygen, till the time the condition subsides.

4. Premature Baby Needs

What babies look for in their parents is a secure and caring hand. Babies really do require that extra bit of care and concern. When a baby is premature, he/she requires even more care and protection. Premature babies often are lacking in some or the other aspect, as compared to a normal baby. Special care for preemies is required to overcome any developmental loopholes. Premature babies face a number of physical and emotional challenges, such as impaired vision and hearing, jaundice and anaemia, etc. These are definitely situations to be handled medically, but parents also play a major role in promoting healthy development of their babies. Parents can help the premature babies to give emotional strength to develop both mentally and physically. However, there are times when the parents may not know what their babies need or expect from them, and how they need to take care of their premature babies.

Tips to Take Care of Premature Babies

- Learn more about your baby. Always, be aware about your baby's condition and medical assistance given to him/her. Uncertainty or lack of knowledge can be a risky situation. Ask as many questions as you can and seek answers for all your queries, because it is the question of your baby and their health.
- Be an observant parent. Know about each and every move and action of your baby. Do share your concerns and any change in your baby's condition with the medical team. Bring to their notice all recent developments in your baby, so that they can function accordingly.
- Breast milk is a must for a premature baby, as it contains proteins that will help in fighting infections. Your baby may not be able to take breast-feed initially but do not let the milk supply dry up. Once the baby is strong enough put him/her exclusively on breast milk.
- Provide lots of love and concern to premature babies. Speak to them in a loving tone. When they are ready, cuddle them, hold them close to you, turn their head so that they can hear your heartbeat, try and make skin to skin contact. All this gives them a sense of security.
- Dress up your baby comfortably. Premature babies are small in size and they lack in body fat, so they need special clothes. Their clothing should be such that it fits them properly and keeps them warm. The warmness will make them comfortable, relaxed and happy. Their clothes should also have easy openings for easy diaper change and hook up to any hospital equipment.
- You can bond very well with your baby at time of feeding him/her. Mothers develop skin to skin contact during nursing; this increases the bonding between the baby and the mother. Some babies may also require gavage method (tube feeding) to feed them. When solid food is introduced after 4 or 6 months, the meals should be small and frequent.
- A premature baby needs diaper change around 5 to 6 times a day. Don't get worried, as it indicates that your baby is getting required amount of nutrition. There are special diapers available for premature babies, which fit them well and can be removed without undressing them.
- Premature babies have a different sleeping pattern. They sleep for longer hours because of their developmental needs. To make sure that they get adequate amount of sleep, limit their exposure to stimulating environment and outsiders. They are also at greater risk of SIDS. Make sure they sleep in a proper position, i.e. on their backs and not on stomach. Also check that their bedding is firm and without any loose or suffocating items.

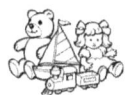

FAQs

Q-1. What are the common causes for premature birth of babies?

Ans. Any baby who is born before the 37th week of pregnancy is termed as a premature baby. In india, about ten percent of all births are premature. The main causes of premature births are malnutrition, infection, high blood pressure, toxaemia of pregnancy, diabetes and severe heart and lung diseases in the mother. Sometimes a baby is delivered prematurely if the doctor finds the baby suffering from lack of proper oxygen supply in the mother's womb.

Q-2. What are the problems a premature baby has to face?

Ans. The earlier the premature baby is born, the lower would be his/her birth weight and the greater would be the severity of the handicaps the baby may have to face. Such babies are likely to have difficulties in breathing, maintenance of body temperature and feeding.

Q-3. What is an incubator?

Ans. An incubator is a machine which has the environment similar to the mother's womb. The incubator's inside temperature and the humidity can be controlled as per the needs of the baby. The oxygen content of its air can be adjusted externally. The nutritional requirements of the baby who is kept in the incubator are met through intravenous feeding or feeding through a tube passed into his/her stomach.

Q-4. What is the care required by a premature baby on reaching home?

Ans. Premature babies have a reduced ability to maintain their body temperatures. The room in which they are kept should have a comparatively higher temperature. The baby should be covered with proper clothes at all times. Since the immune system of a premature baby is deficient, he/she needs extra-protective measures. Always handle such a baby with clean hands after washing them with soap and water. The number of visitors must be severely restricted. Anyone suffering from throat or respiratory infection, fever or any other communicable disease should not be allowed to come near the baby.

Q-5. What kind of nutrition is required by a premature baby?

Ans. Breast milk is the best for a premature baby. If the baby is unable to suck at the breast, then the milk may be expressed and given to the baby with a bottle having an extra soft nipple. Since premature babies are deficient in body stores of vitamins and iron, they should be given vitamins and calcium and administered iron supplements from the age of six weeks onward to prevent the development of anaemia.

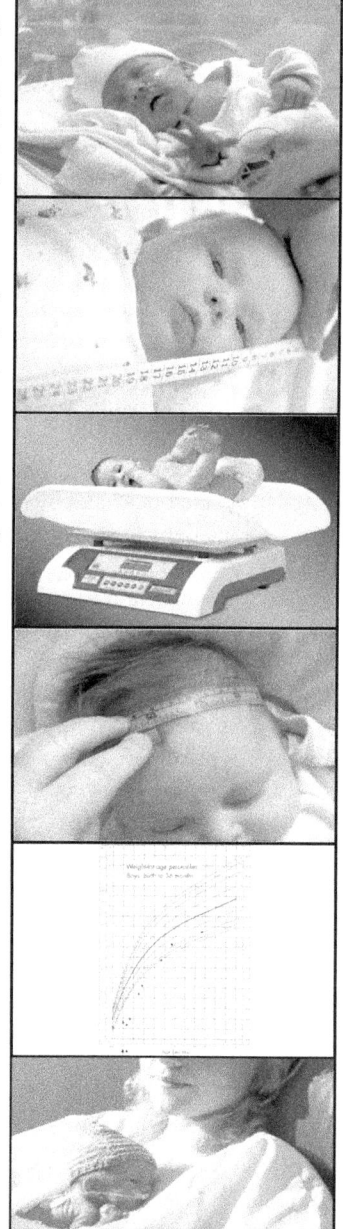

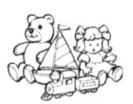

VIII
Tips for New Mom

One of the greatest milestones in a woman's life is becoming a mother. No other single event brings about as many changes and as much responsibility for her, as this one. Having a baby gives a woman a sense of fulfilment and enormous joy. At the same time, it has been seen that the first-time mothers get overwhelmed by the changes that take place in their life as well as their body, after the baby is born. The life of a woman changes completely with the arrival of the baby and the amount of work she has to cope with, leaves her completely exhausted. While nothing can equal the joy that motherhood brings, new mothers often find themselves in a demanding situation.

New mothers have the challenging task of caring for their babies, even as they have to care for themselves and ensure that they recuperate from the strains of delivery as soon as possible. After all, only a healthy mother will be able to ensure a healthy growth and development of her baby. However, a huge responsibility, such as that of a child, can certainly baffle the new mother and make her feel anxious and frustrated. In order to help all the new moms out there, we have provided a number of tips in our related chapters. These tips will prove extremely useful for all the women in the world, after the birth of their child.

1. Going Back to Work after Baby

Some new mothers will not be able to stay at home with their babies for long. They may have to return to their jobs after three or four months. However, you should try to stay at home for as long as you can. If you can work part-time or from home, nothing like it! The newborn needs your attention and care and no one else can give your baby the motherly care that only you can give. At the same time, you will have to get back to work sooner or later. You can't avoid work for long no matter how much you want to be with your little baby. Eventually, both the mother and the baby will have to learn to live without each other for 8 to 10 hours of the day. Here are some things you can do to prepare yourself and your baby, so that going back to work after baby is easier for both of you.

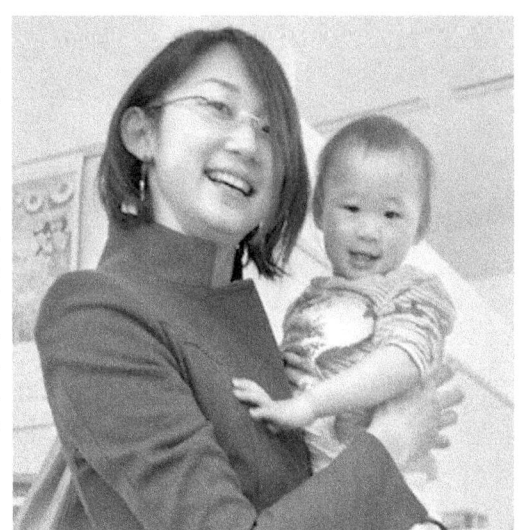

A working mom with baby

Working after Having a Baby

- ❑ Before you join work, start leaving the baby for some time with someone who would be with the baby in your absence. This will make them get used to each other and the baby will not miss you terribly, when you are not around.

- ❑ You could even give yourself a trial run of travelling back to work. This will give you confidence that you can travel again. Since you have been at home for quite some time, it is better to get a hang of office work once again.
- ❑ These physical separations will help both the mother and the baby, once the mother returns to work.
- ❑ During your maternity, keep in touch with your colleagues by phone or by e-mail. This will help you to maintain the same comfort level in rejoining after a long period of time.
- ❑ Be aware of what is going on in the office. Keeping yourself informed will only help you to be in touch, so that you look forward to joining office after the break.
- ❑ You can make some short visits to the office before your official joining date. This will help you get to know what is happening at office and will be seen as a proactive step to getting back to work.

2. Health Tips for New Moms

New mothers need to take special care of their health, along with attending to the needs of the new born. Since they have also gone through a lot during their pregnancy and delivery, physically as well as emotionally, it is important to give ample attention to the health front, so that recovery is quick and you are back to your normal healthy shape in just a matter of some days. Keeping hale and hearty is essential as a new baby can exhaust you very soon, making you feel tired and jaded. Here are some very useful health tips for new moms.

Keeping Fit

Nowadays, everyone wants to get back into shape soon after the baby is born. Mothers would like to regain their original slim figures within a few months. Though it maybe difficult to find time and exercise with a newborn, mothers who make the effort feel much better, as your energy level increases as well. If you cannot go to an organized exercise class, find time to do a few exercises at home or simply dancing at home can do the trick. Other ways to exercise are:

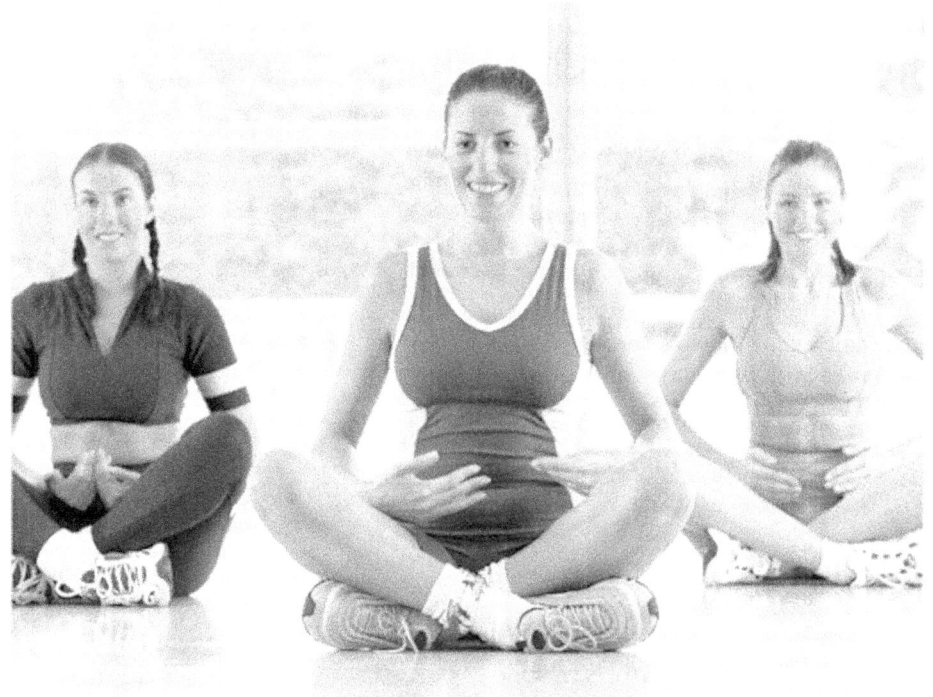

Getting back into shape after child birth

- ❏ Taking a walk is a good option; you could take your baby along. If the local park has a smooth pathway, you can use a pram or a baby sling.
- ❏ Some pools have crèche facilities, so you can leave your baby there and swim without worrying. Swimming once or twice a week is good enough.
- ❏ Join other postnatal exercise classes at the local gym.
- ❏ Attend postnatal exercise classes conducted by the child health clinic.

Healthy Diet

As you will be breast-feeding the baby, you will have to eat well. It is possible to lose weight by following a healthy diet. Even while snacking, make sure that the snacks you eat are healthy. Try some of these:

- ❏ Vegetable soup with whole wheat or whole meal roll.
- ❏ Hummus eaten with breadsticks or sliced raw vegetables.
- ❏ Toast and baked beans.
- ❏ Toast and scrambled eggs.
- ❏ Tuna sandwiches.

Eat plenty of vegetables, fresh fruits and drink enough water. Increase your calcium intake by drinking a lot of milk and increasing consumption of dairy products.

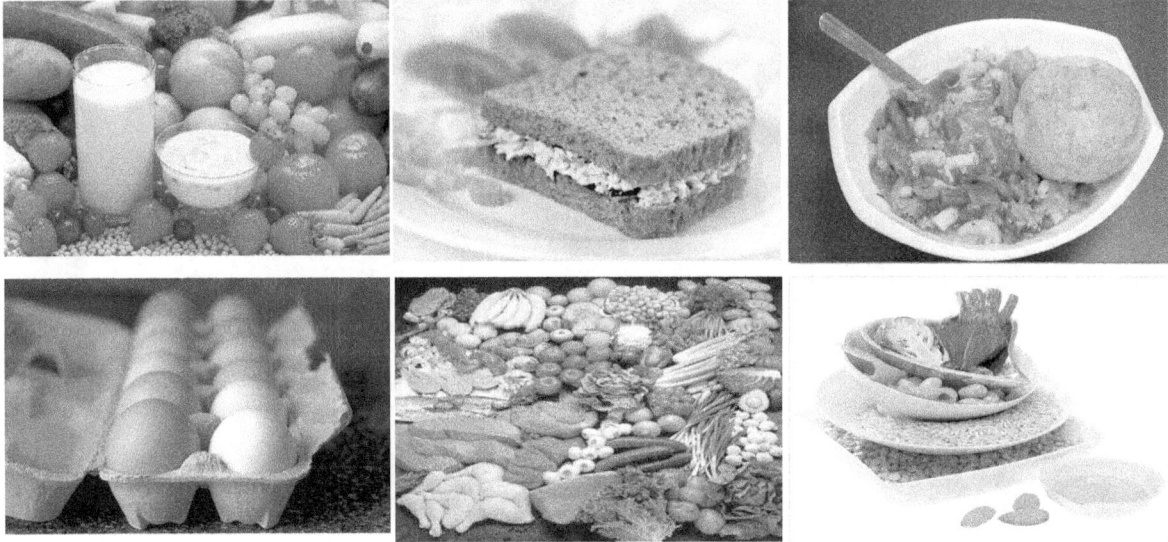

Socialising

Most new mothers feel more reassured and gain confidence when they interact with other women in the same situation as they are. Try to form a group of new mothers, discuss problems and share solutions with each other. Others ways to socialise with new mothers are:

- ❏ Meet regularly at each other's house.
- ❏ Establish a babysitting circle.
- ❏ Take care of each other's children.
- ❏ Go out together.
- ❏ Having a well-established social circle and play group for your children.
- ❏ Visiting mother and baby clinics together.
- ❏ Joining together local sports centre for postnatal exercises or baby swimming classes.

3. Marital Relations after Childbirth

With the arrival of the baby, the relationship between husband and wife will undergo a change. There may be some initial strain and tensions in the relationship, though there is nothing that the two partners cannot solve by taking out time for each other and talking things out. After childbirth, each partner has his or her own expectations and apprehensions. Some of the things that men worry about after childbirth are earning enough for the family, the kind of father they will make and the fear of feeling left out as his wife will be devoting all her time to the baby. At the same time, a woman too has her own apprehensions and fears regarding whether her husband will support her for whether the baby will affect her relationship with spouse.

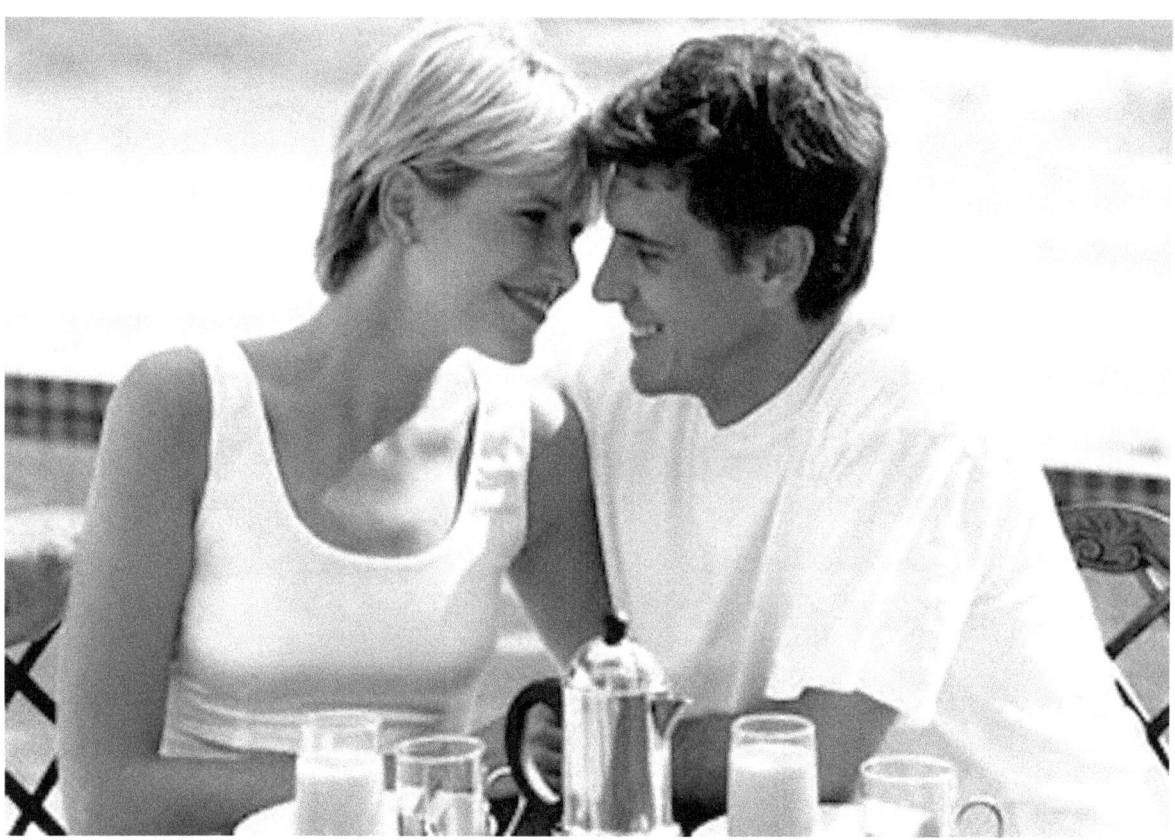

Relations with Spouse after Baby

After parenthood, it becomes very difficult for both partners to find time to spend together as a couple. A newborn baby takes up all the time of both the mother and the father. Though it may seem that the baby is affecting your relationship, it is not so. Neither does a baby damage a good relationship, nor does he/she improve a bad one. It is ultimately up to the partners to find time for each other, no matter how difficult it is or how tired they are. Here are a few things you can do to keep your relationship alive.

- Talk to each other about how you feel and also regarding your problems.
- If you disagree on something, then just agree to disagree. Do not try to always have the last word. This will make things worse; do not let your ego get in the way of the relationship.
- For some time, each day, continue to think of your partner as your lover and not the father or mother of your child.

- ❏ Spend time with the baby together, play and cuddle the baby together. This will give you quality time as a family.
- ❏ Once a week, ask a friend or a family member to take care of the baby for a few hours, so that both of you can spend some time together alone.

Sexual Relationship Post Childbirth

Sexual relationship maybe affected to a great extent once the baby is born. Since this important aspect of your relationship is affected, it may take a toll on your bond. As a new mother, the demands of your baby, exhaustion, unhappiness with bodily changes after childbirth and the effect of breast-feeding on sex drive can make you feel withdrawn from sex after childbirth. Your partner may feel that you have only time for the baby and not for him. While you may feel that everyone is only making demands on you and you don't have any time for yourself. Taking out time to improve your sexual relationship will help you and your partner.

Let's Remember

- ➢ **There is no right time to restart your sex life. You can begin wherever you left.**
- ➢ **Just lying together, cuddling together and spending time together can improve your relationship and make you comfortable with your body.**
- ➢ **If sex in painful even after the vagina heals, you should consult your doctor.**
- ➢ **The vagina is an elastic and supple tissue, which heals quickly.**
- ➢ **A woman's body was created to bear children and the human body has great recuperation powers.**
- ➢ **If you still feel that you and your partner are having problems with your sexual relationship, take advice from an expert counsellor.**

4. Travelling with a Baby

Though you may be travelling less frequently, once you have a baby till he/she is a little old, it does not mean that you stop taking holidays because of the little ones. But, you will have to make elaborate plans well in advance. It is quite natural that you will want to go for a weekend outing nearby with your family and the little one. Travelling with your baby can be really enjoying if he/she luxuriates the surrounding with you. And your baby can only enjoy the outing if he/she finds the atmosphere compatible. Being away from home is a big change in routine for both, you and your baby, so you will have to plan ahead, even anticipate problems and be prepared to deal with them, so that the entire family enjoys a good holiday. Taking advice from parents, who have taken their children on holidays, is a good idea. Here are a few tips about things that worked for other parents while travelling with a baby. To make the journey comfortable and enjoyable for him/her, you need to carry some safety accessories necessary for your infant.

Travel Accessories for Babies

- ❏ You will have to pick up some baby wipes for a quick wipe-up for infant while travelling in the flight.
- ❏ While selecting the baby travel safe seat prefer the bulkhead seats, if your baby is an infant. These seats are meant for babies kept in bassinet.
- ❏ It is a better idea to carry milk and other food for your babies, as your baby may feel hungry anytime during the journey.

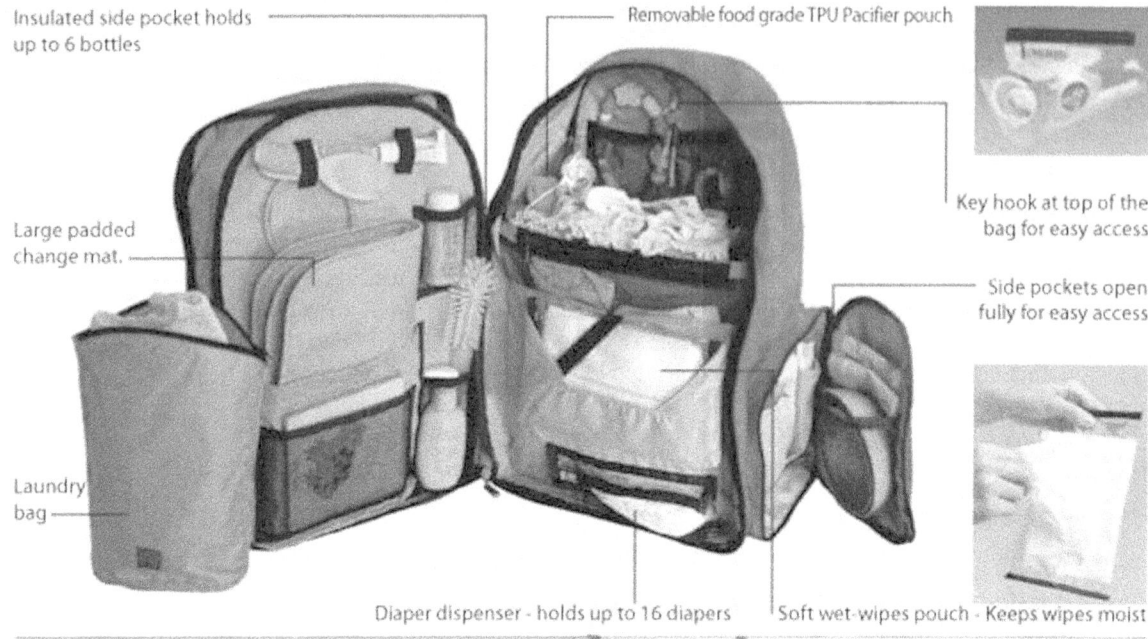

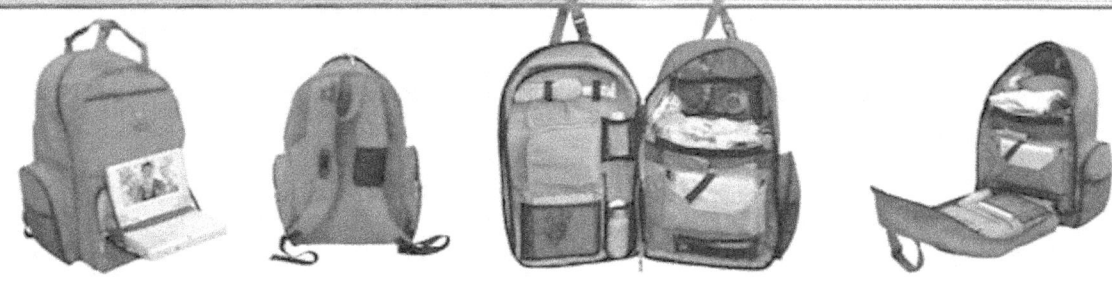

Baby's travel bag

- If your infant is breast-feeding or bottle-feeding, feed him/her during take-off and while landing. It will prevent the noise to reach his/her ears and he/she will feel comfortable while having milk.
- Carry fragranced bags so that you can dispose the diapers in the toilet bin after putting the diapers in the bags.
- Carry a set of clothes for your infants handy as you might need to change in the flight. He/she may spoil the dress while being fed or otherwise. Therefore, be prepared for such a situation.

Tips on Travelling with a Baby

- You may use the toilet before boarding the plane, as the bathroom in the aerodrome is quite spacious and clean compared to the flight toilet.
- Before going to catch a flight, check the health of your child with a doctor. If he/she is unwell, it is better to postpone the trip, till the baby recovers fully.
- Don't depend on the flight attendant for heating the milk bottle. They may not understand the adequate temperature required for the milk bottle of a baby.
- You can carry some books specially meant for infants, as they can be a good pastime for them while travelling.
- While booking a holiday, find out what facilities the tour operator provides. Children, who are two years or below, usually travel for free. Also check whether your baby will require a passport.

- Find out what kind of childcare facilities the operator provides, such as baby cots, prams, highchairs, etc., so that you do not have to carry these things with you.
- Once you decide on the holiday location, consult your doctor about the vaccination your baby requires before you decide the holiday dates. If there are vaccines to be taken, it is best to take them a little before the holiday date. Some vaccines cannot be taken together and may need a few weeks in between. So, you will need time to vaccinate your baby.
- The most difficult part of your holiday will be the journey, and with a small baby, it will not be easy. You should book an air cot well in advance. Get seats that are together, so that you have ample space on the flight. Book meals for your children in advance, it would help if they could be served before you are served.
- If you are hiring a car, ask the company to provide you with a baby seat, so that you don't have to carry one.
- Take toys for the journey, old and new ones, so that the baby will be occupied and will not get tired of the journey.

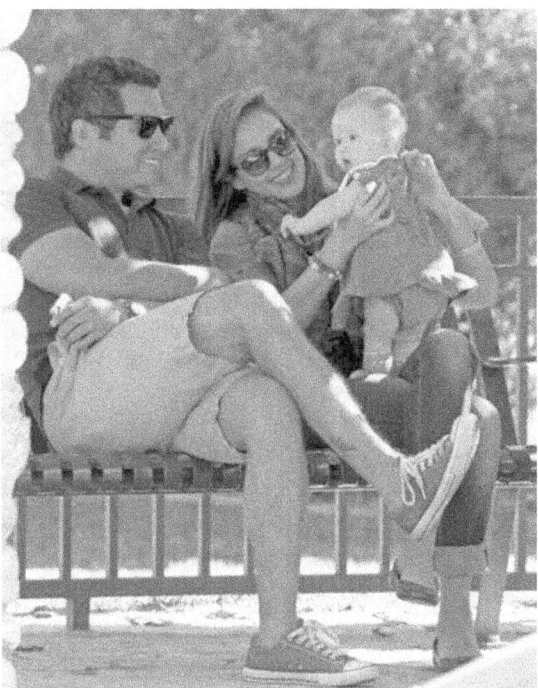

A couple with small baby on a trip

- There could be delays on the way, so you should carry enough snacks for the baby, especially drinks, milk powder, hot water etc. It is better if the snacks don't consist of sticky food, as they are messy.
- It is easier to travel if you are breast-feeding, you don't have to worry about sterilized bottles or clean water to make bottle-feeds.
- Take your baby sling or back carrier, it will occupy less space and it will be easy to carry the baby around.
- If you are holidaying in a place where the weather is hot, make sure that you carry sun block for your baby as his/her skin is delicate and more likely to get sunburns.
- While booking your holiday, you can book a hotel that provides childcare facilities such as nannies, crèches, etc. You should check them before using them and only avail them when you are sure your baby will be well taken care of.
- You may use the toilet before boarding the plane, as the bathroom in the aerodrome is quite spacious and clean compared to the flight toilet.
- Don't depend on the flight attendant for heating the milk bottle. They may not understand the adequate temperature required for the milk bottle of a baby.

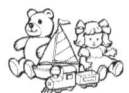

FAQs

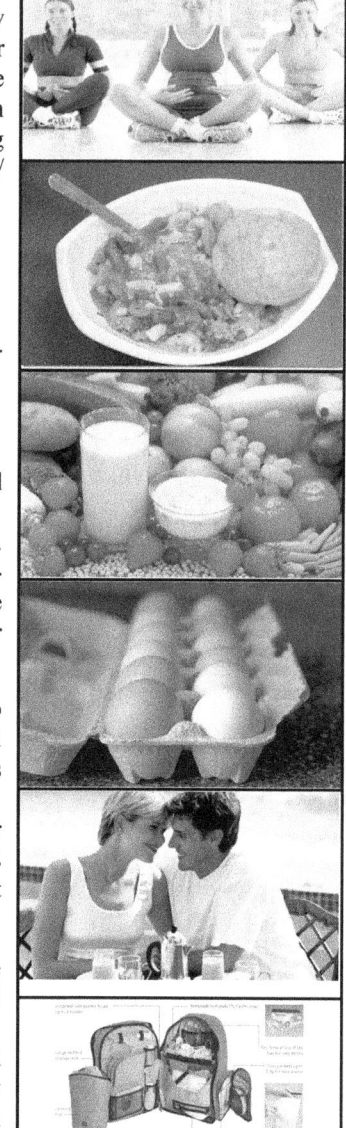

Q-1. I am a working woman. My daughter is now four months old. I have to join work soon. When can I put her in a care centre?

Ans. If yours is a joint family, then it would be better if you could hire a nanny for the baby who could care for the baby under the vigilant eye of other members of your family. But if you have to put your daughter in a care centre, then it is advisable that you wait till the time she weans away from exclusive breast-feeding. Although it is preferable that you delay sending the baby to the baby care centre at least till the baby is toilet trained and he/she is able to tell you about her day at the centre to some extent.

Q-2. How do I choose a good care centre for my baby?

Ans. While choosing a care centre, keep these things in mind:
- ➤ The centre should be close to your home or workplace.
- ➤ The cetnre should have a favourable child and child caretaker ratio e.g. 2:1 for very small babies is better.
- ➤ The place should be clean, spacious and well-ventilated.
- ➤ The kitchen and toilets should be hygienically maintained.

Q-3. My baby is eight months old. When I get back home from work, I feel too tired to breast-feed the baby. What should I do?

Ans. Your baby is old enough to not to depend exclusively on breast-feeding. Give her other foods along with breast-feeding. Completely stopping breast-feeding would not be advisable as mother's milk is highly nutritious for the baby. Rearrange your work at home in such a way that you get some time for breast-feeding the baby.

Q-4. I have a demanding job, a small baby at home and household chores to attend to. After completing all these tasks, I get so tired that hardly find any time for my husband. This has irked my husband and lately he has begun snapping at me and the baby. What should I do?

Ans. You cannot do everything alone. You are also a human being. Make it clear to your husband that he must share some of your responsibilities if he expects some time lone with you. If he agrees to share your responsibilities, then it would be better for your relationship.

Q-5 After my delivery, I have put on lot of weight. In a month, I will be joining office but recently I found out that I do not fit in any of my old clothes. What should I do?

Ans. You have two options – either get back into shape by exercise and controlled dieting or buy new clothes which may fit you. The first option is definitely better though it may not be as easy as it sounds. However, some effort on your part may show you good results. Join a Yoga or Aerobic class. Go for regular walks. Do postnatal exercises which keep you fit. Eat healthy diet and avoid snacking on high-carb foods.

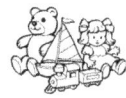

IX
Raising a Green Baby

Environmental issues have become a major concern in today's world. We have to make conscious efforts to take the pressure off the environment. Well, if you thought that your newborn baby cannot contribute his/her bit towards restoring ecological balance, you are definitely in for a surprise. Your little one can be made eco-friendly right from his/her birth. This is the only way we can safeguard the planet resources and ensure that our children's future is safe as well.

Environmental consciousness can begin right from the time of birth of your baby. By being eco-friendly, don't assume that you are not doing the best for your kid. You just need to follow the basics and buy products that are both suitable for your baby and the environment.

You also need to change your habits in order to be environmental friendly. It is not only good for the baby but for your ownself. While feeding the baby if you consume organic foods which are free of chemicals like pesticides and insecticides, then it is good for both you and your baby.

1. Raising Eco-Friendly Baby

Raising an eco-friendly baby is not a tough task. All that you need to do is change a few habits and get the baby accustomed to the things that are environment friendly.

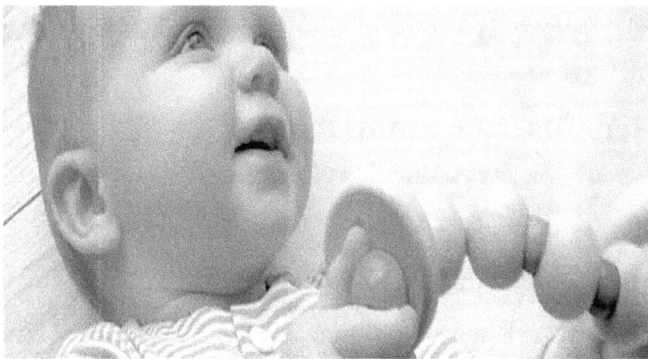

Baby playing with wooden toys

- ❑ The first step would be to make a list of the things that your baby would require. Certain things like cots, beds and cupboard can either be borrowed from friends and family or you can buy them second-hand.
- ❑ Next in line, comes the type of items you buy. Rather than buying things that can be exclusively used by a boy or girl, buy things that both can use. This will lead to saving resources as well.
- ❑ Breast-feeding qualifies as the most environment friendly food for your baby. Mother's milks is deemed as the most sterile and healthy food for a toddler. Feed breast milk to your baby instead of formula food, as long it is practicable.
- ❑ Do not opt for disposable breast pads. Instead, use washable breast pads, as they are eco-friendly.
- ❑ When it comes to infant's nappies, get reusable cloth nappies made of cotton. These are simple to use and long lasting and can be used for more than one child.
- ❑ You can get your baby wooden toys rather than the plastic ones. This is an effective way for being eco-friendly parent.

- In terms of clothes, the best bet would be to buy secondhand baby clothes. Since babies grow very quickly, the clothes are hardly worn.
- Some of the other items which you can get second hand include cot linen, soft furnishings, bouncy chairs and inflatable baby nests.
- While getting wooden objects, such as high chairs and baby toys, keep away from tropical hardwoods. Instead, look for ones made from trees grown in sustainable forests.
- In terms of baby care toiletries, use the ones that are eco-friendly. These items use natural ingredients that are soft and kind to baby and toddler's skin.
- Once you baby has grown and can consume solids, make him/her your own baby food rather than getting packaged ones.

2. Organic Diapers

In the tug of war between the cloth diapers and the disposable ones, it is the more recently introduced organic or biodegradable disposable diapers that seem to have won conclusively. With cloth diapers being messy to handle, and the disposable diapers considered to be ecological threats, the organic diapers seems to be a perfect solution to all of these problems.

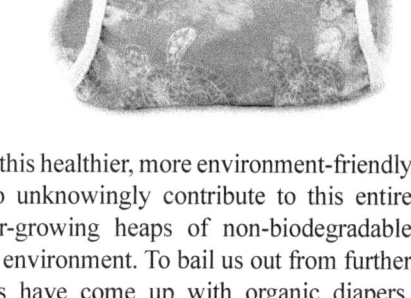

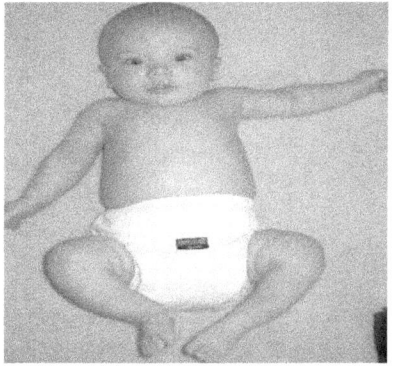

A baby with an organic diaper

Organic diapers are believed to be made of biodegradable materials that decompose easily and can be easily flushed or composted.

Concerned parents now can opt for this healthier, more environment-friendly option for their little babies, who unknowingly contribute to this entire biodegradation process. The ever-growing heaps of non-biodegradable diaper waste are a big threat to our environment. To bail us out from further damage, concerned manufacturers have come up with organic diapers, also called the *smart cloth*. Organic diapers have all the benefits of their disposable counterparts, with the added advantage of being eco-friendly. They can be flushed or changed into compost for your garden.

Benefits of Organic Diapers

- The greatest advantage of organic disposable diapers is that you can trash it in your garbage can without worry.
- An organic diaper comes with the goodness of both cloth and disposable diapers. They are easy on your baby's skin.
- Organic diapers are much more absorbent than their cloth equivalents, and hence help in keeping your babies dry and comfortable for longer hours.
- The best thing about organic diapers is that they are 100% natural and non-allergic. They are the best choice for your baby's tender skin, as they are softer and run no risk of rashes and skin irritations.
- What more, you don't have to wash these disposable diapers. Just flush them or use them as compost.

Tips to Choose Organic Diapers

- If cost is a concern for you, you can go for the organic pre-fold diapers. Apart from being affordable, these diapers are easily adjustable and can be used from birth till toilet training and beyond. However, there is a flipside to these diapers. Tying pre-fold organic diapers can be a time-consuming affair, and they are a bit difficult to handle. They are also more susceptible to leakages than the more fitted ones.
- If you are looking for options on organic diapers, totally-organic fitted cloth diapers are the ones to go for. Available in a variety of sizes these diapers are adjustable and can be used till your baby gets toilet

trained. However, you would need pins or diaper fasteners to secure them. These nappies are less prone to leakages because of elastic fittings, and run a lower risk of rashes.
- If time is a concern for you, then you can opt for all-in-one organic diapers that are easy to fix and are available in a host of different colours and sizes. These have strong built-in moisture barriers and are washable. All-in-one organic diapers come with Velcro or snaps and can be easily adjusted to your baby's size. The downside is that they are more expensive than the regular pre-fold diapers and can cause skin rashes at times.
- Pocket all-in-one diapers are a better option than the normal all-in-one diapers. They are available in a variety of colours and sizes and are moisture-resistant.
- Organic diapers are usually made of cotton, hemp, bamboo and soya fibre. To know what is best for your baby, pick a sample of each fabric. Hot wash the fabrics with mild detergent and dry on medium heat in order to understand how soft these fabrics are and how absorbent they can be.

3. Organic Baby Clothing

Amazingly soft, naturally made fibre without the use of chemicals are healthier for your baby. This is not a figment of imagination or a fairy tale to be told to your baby. In reality, you can gift your adorable loved ones these organic clothes that are extremely durable and have micro-bacterial properties, which shield them against germs. These small activities also give rise to more attachment and bonding. Your baby can be a good example for others to go eco-friendly. Conventional baby clothes come dyed in chemicals and contain pesticides, which do not go away in one wash. If you think that organic baby clothes do not offer many varieties in clothes, you are in for a surprise! From diapers to jackets to swimsuits to jumpers, just about anything is available in organic clothing shops.

Organic Clothes for Babies

- Cyanazine, dicofol, naled, propargite, and trifluralin are some dangerous chemicals, which can cause cancer and are most commonly involved in fabricating cotton clothes. Avoid these.
- Allergic reactions can be triggered out of using clothes on which many manufacturers use dyes and chemicals to impart good colour and look. Therefore, go in for pale colours, as this eliminates the chance of harmful side-effects of dyes.
- Organic clothing is high in style and you can clad your babies into creative and natural outfits and make them feel different from others. They are available in varied colours, shapes, designs and patterns.

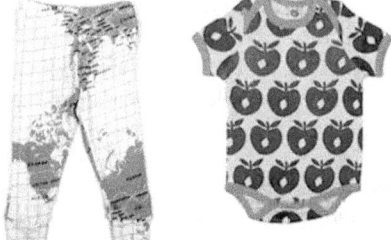

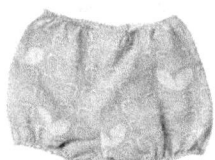

Organic clothes

- Organic clothes for babies can also form a memorable and unique moment in the life of parents, as they always think of getting the most special, safe and amazing gift for their babies and organic clothing provides them the opportunity to make clothing a special experience for their babies.
- Parents can bring in various baby gifts in the form of a complete range of baby products, such as clothes, bedding material, toys, etc and rest assured that organic clothing will be an eye-catching idea to flaunt around a bit.
- The main purpose of organic baby clothing is to create a natural care criteria, which includes everything, right from clothing, toys, bedding or food. As the world has grown highly inorganic and almost everything is polluted, it's better that the parents of newborns decide to go natural and save their babies from chemicals, pesticides and pollution. After all, nature is all about creating a balance in the world and these small acts can add to it.

FAQs

Q-1. I would like to buy best and most expensive things for my baby and at the same time I would like to be environment-friendly. But it seems the two do not mix. What should I do?

Ans. If a thing is expensive, it does not necessarily be good for your baby or environment-friendly. So choose those things which are healthy and useful for your baby and favour environment as well.

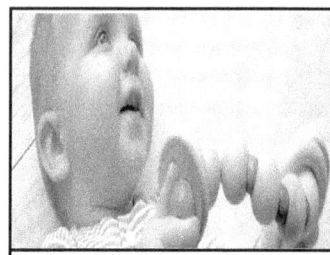

Q-2. I would like to buy organic clothes for my baby but they are not easily available in the market. Sometimes people dupe in the name of organic cloth. What should be done?

Ans. For buying good organic clothes for your baby, go to well-established stores or shopping malls which have a reputation of selling such products. There are no chances of cheating in such places. You may choose from different designs and variety there.

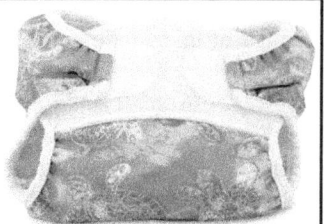

Q-3. The organic diapers available in the market are very expensive and short in supply. What alternative do I have?

Ans. If you cannot find the organic diapers in the market easily, then the next best option is the home-made cloth diapers which are inexpensive, easy to make and readily available. These diapers are soft on your baby's skin and environment-friendly too.

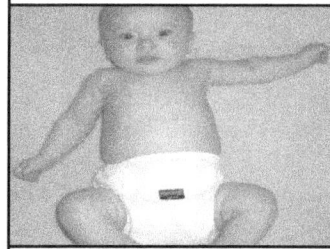

Q-4. Wooden toys are said to be environment-friendly toys. But will they not hurt my baby?

Ans. Do not buy heavy wooden toys which may hurt your baby. Buy the light ones with rounded edges. If the baby is very small, then just place them above the crib from where the baby can see them and play from a distance.

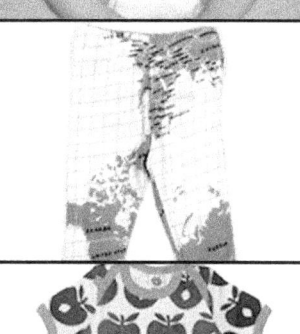

Q-5. How should I dispose of organic diapers?

Ans. Organic diapers are made from biodegradable material. It is safe to dispose them off with other biodegradable waste. Do not wrap them in plastic bags instead wrap them in pieces of newspaper and throw them along with biodegradable wastes.

Q-6. Whenever my baby wears dark, printed, colourful clothes, he develops a rash all over the body. Why does this happen?

Ans. Many dark-coloured dyes and chemicals used in coloured clothes can trigger an allergic reaction in children. So go for white or pale colours which will eliminate the chances of any allergic reaction on your baby's sensitive skin.

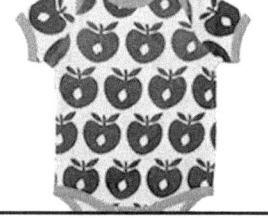

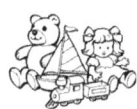

Part II
CHILD HEALTH PROBLEMS

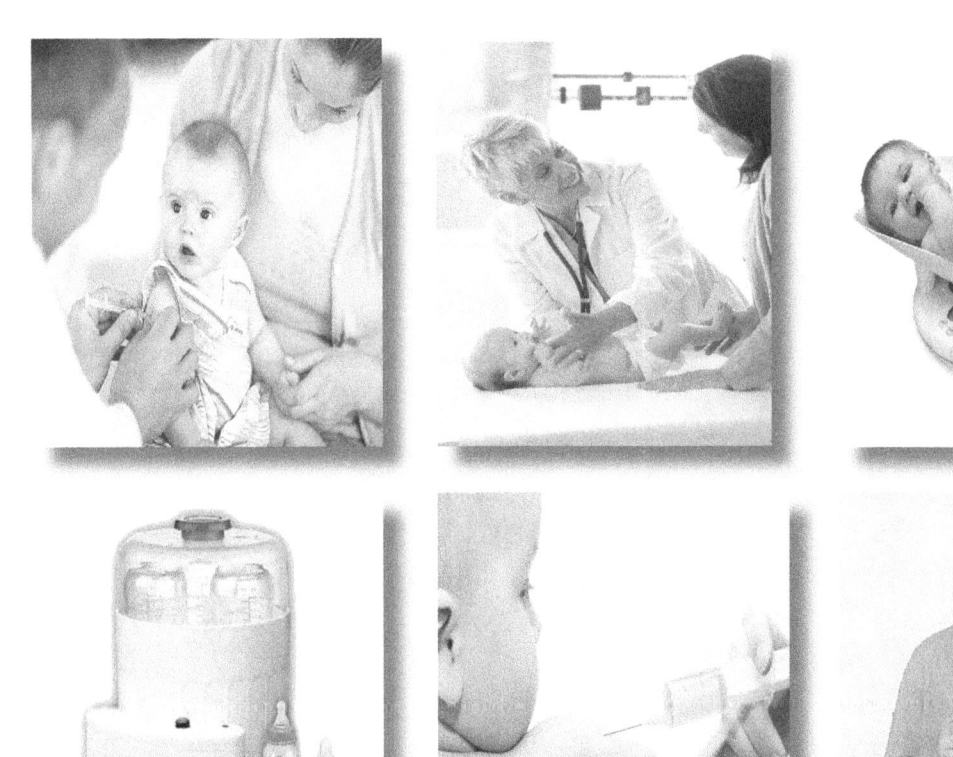
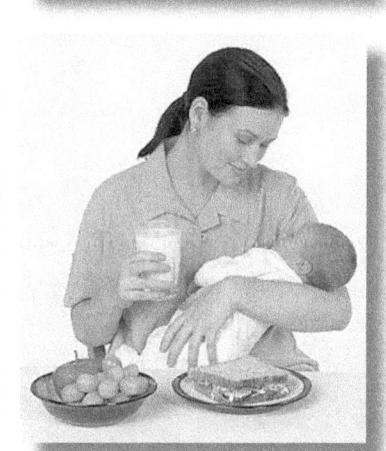
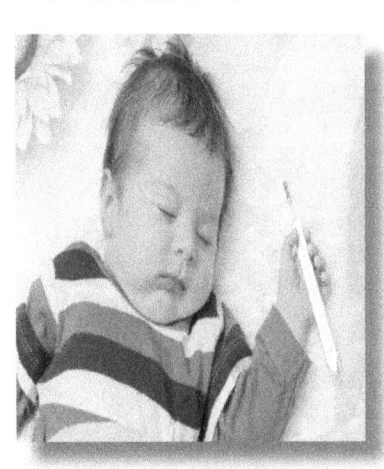
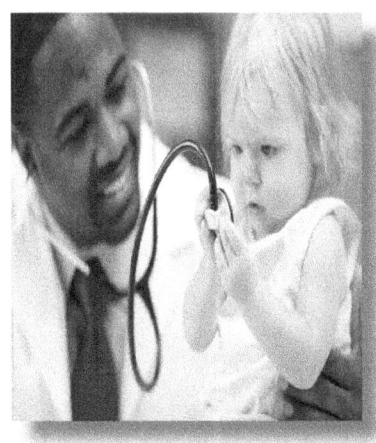
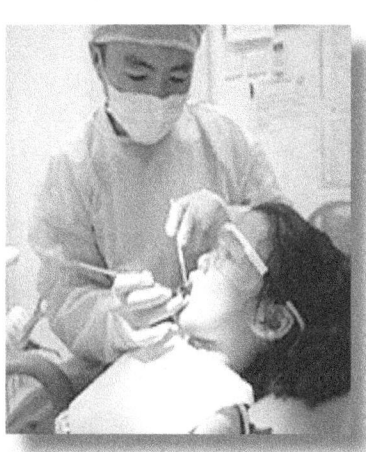

I
Baby Feeding

The right start can help your baby develop a lifetime of healthy eating habits. The first year of a baby is very crucial as it is all about development, nutrition, exploration, sharing and learning. Feeding your baby is all the more an adventure for a mother. While feeding, breast milk is the best food for your newborn for the first six months of his/her life as it includes the right amount and quality of nutrients to suit the baby's first food needs. Breast milk contains antibodies and other immune factors that help your baby prevent and fight off illness better. Though breast milk is the best food for your baby, it does not meet all the baby's nutritional requirements.

As far as feeding your baby with milk is concerned, cow milk-based infant formula milk is the next best choice. At six months, it is advisable to introduce your baby to other foods. In fact, your baby will indicate you when he is ready to take on other foods. These include your baby will start feeling hungry frequently, he/ she is able to sit up without support, shows interest in food when others are eating, and lets you know that he does not require more food by leaning back or turning his head away. This chapter of baby care deals with introducing your baby to formula milk, tips on bottle feeding, and sanitizing those bottles. It also covers how to choose nipples and bottles and problems related to feeding your baby.

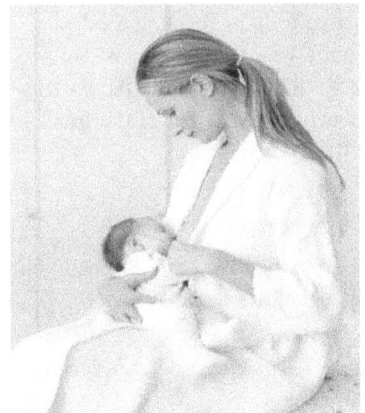 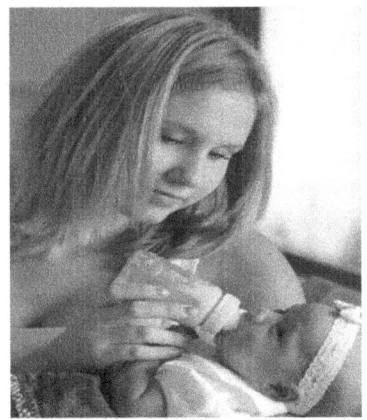 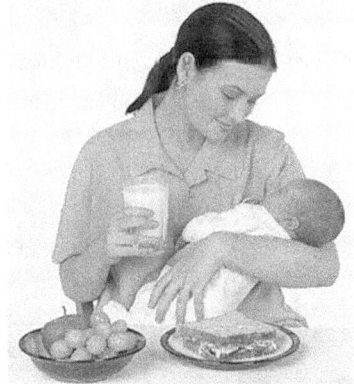

Different ways of baby feeding

1. Food Guide for Babies

Anxiety over feeding your newborn can drive you into frenzy! Most new parents are often worried about how often and how much they should feed their little ones. What more, contradictory advices from friends and folks like feed your baby when hungry or feed your newborns after every two hours can make you feel quite helpless? Coming up with the right feeding chart for your baby can be quite an accomplishment. Babies are highly erratic and vary from each other in more ways than one. So what works for one baby may not work for the other. This surmounts the confusion for the parents who are left unsure about the right feeding chart for their babies and which feeding plan to follow.

Here is a complete food guide for your little one. This chart is meant to be a rough guideline on what and how much to feed your baby from birth to 12 months.

From Birth – 4 Months

A newborn baby's stomach is roughly the size of a grape and requires very little food in the beginning. During this stage of infancy, a baby turns towards nipple for sustenance.

Tips to Feed

- The best recommended food during this stage is mother's milk or formula food. As your baby's digestive tract is still developing, solid food is a strict no-no. Also, avoid feeding your baby on cow's milk before 12 months.
- During this stage, your baby needs to be nursed more frequently if put on breast-feeding. Since breast milk digests easier than formula milk, your baby is likely to get hungry faster. A one month old baby needs to be breastfed for seven to nine times a day. As they grow old, the newborn need to be nursed less frequently. While some babies may wail for food after every one hour, others may go for a 2 to 3 hours gap between each feeding.

From 4 – 6 Months

This is the stage when your baby shows signs of development. Apart from significant changes in relation to growth and other vital changes, your baby will show a considerable rise in his appetite too.

Tips to Feed

- During this stage, you can introduce your baby to semi-liquid, iron fortified food, such as rice cereal or other grains cereal like oats or barley, apart from feeding him/her on breast milk or formula food.
- You can start with giving your baby 1 tsp of dry rice cereal mixed with 4 to 5 tsp of breast milk or formula food. Keep the consistency light in the beginning and gradually thicken it, as the baby grows used to it. You can also increase the feeding duration to two once your baby grows fond of the food. In case your baby refuses to take in the cereal at first attempt, try again after a few days.

From 6 – 8 Months

This is the ideal stage to introduce your baby to solid food. You can continue to breast feed or formula feed your baby. However at this stage, you can add other food supplements like fruits and vegetables to his/her diet.

Tips to Feed

- You can introduce your baby to pureed or strained fruits and vegetables like banana, peaches, pears, carrot, potato, avocado, squash, etc.
- You can increase the quantity of cereals to 3 to 9 tbsps in 2-3 feedings, during this stage. For fruits and vegetables, you can start with one tsp fruit and slowly increase it to ¼ to ½ cup in 2-3 feedings. Also, while introducing new foods to your baby, make sure to start with a single variety and wait for three days to ensure that your baby is not allergic to that particular variety of food.

From 8 – 10 Months

At this age, a baby shows appetite for solid food and other finger foods. You can continue to breast feed your baby along with feeding him/her on other essential food items.

Tips to Feed

- You can start with small amounts of soft pasteurised cheese, yogurt, cottage cheese, cereals like rice, barley, wheat, oats, mixed cereals, mashed fruits and vegetables, finger foods like small pieces of ripe banana, well-cooked spiral pasta, crackers, small amounts of protein like egg, pureed meats, poultry, and boneless fish, mashed beans with soft skins, such as lentils, split peas, black beans and non-citrus juices like apples or pears.
- Start out by feeding your baby with ¼ to 1/3 cup daily. For cereals, you can opt for ¼ to ½ cup iron-fortified cereal daily. The fruits and vegetables should be kept to an amount of ¼ to ½ cup every day. You can give 3 to 4 tbsps of juice to your baby.

From 10 - 12 Months

This is the time by which your baby's teeth appear and he/she can swallow food more easily.

Tips to Feed

- During this time you can introduce bite-sized, soft-cooked vegetables, such as peas and carrots to his/her diet. You can also introduce him/her to tastier combo meals like *macaroni* and *cheese*.
- You can increase the quantity by ¼ to ½ cup combo foods, ¼ to ½ cup iron-fortified cereal, ¼ to ½ cup fruits and ¼ to ½ cup protein foods.

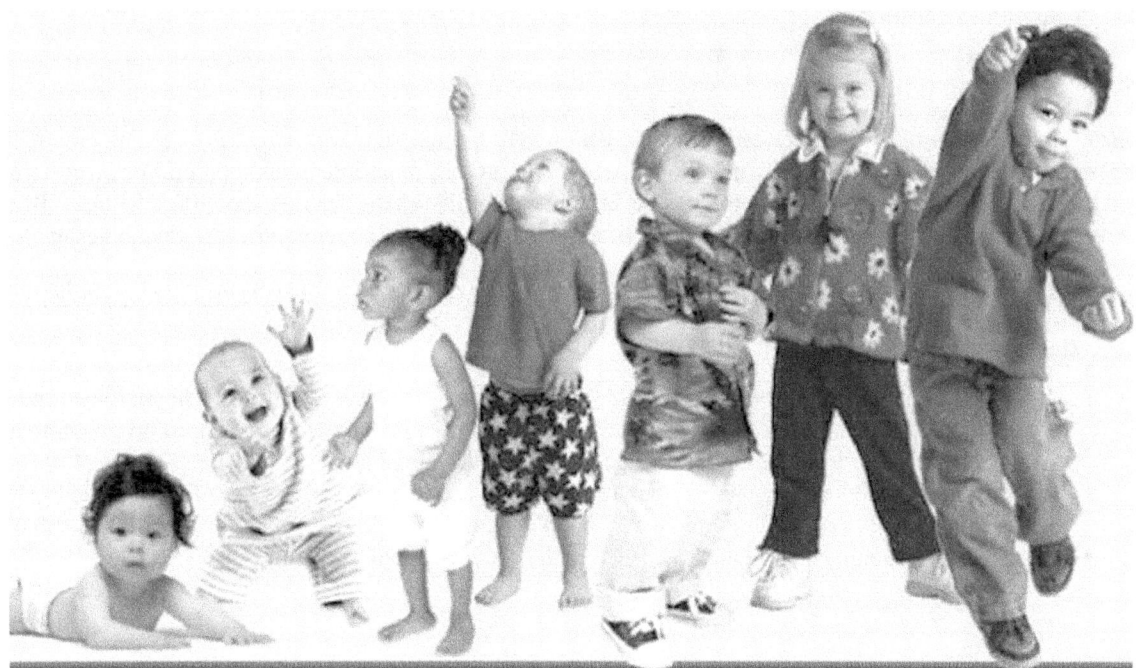

Baby in different stages of growth

2. Feeding Problems

If you are seriously bothered with your little one throwing up or gagging every time you feed him/her, reading this article will surely help. Feeding problems is very common among babies, although it might trigger panic button in mums at times. Choking while eating or refusing to eat are some of the characteristic plights of baby feeding woes. Feeding is the ultimate bonding experience for a mother and her baby. So, every time your baby refuses to be nursed or eat, or puke and poop after meals, it is likely for you to curl your brows with worry. Feeding problems in babies can lead to gastro-esophageal reflux, gastroenteritis or dehydration. Proper nutrition and suitable feeding techniques can allay your problems to a certain extent. Understanding what leads to feeding problems can help to ease out your stress and take an action. Here are some common feeding problems and ways to deal with them.

Spitting Up

Most mothers are often troubled with their babies spitting up every time they are fed or nursed. This is one common problem with babies since they cannot sit straight during and after feeds. As the sphincter that separates the esophagus and stomach is still immature, it becomes difficult for the babies to keep their food in place and thus it runs up the mouth or nose each time after they are fed. It generally worsens if a baby eats too fast or sucks in wind. However, this problem is likely to fade away by the seventh month.

Tips to Manage

- You can cut down spitting up of food by feeding your baby before he/she is extremely hungry, making him sit upright after every feed, burping him for three to four times, and checking the flow of your feeding bottle.
- Spitting up can sometimes lead to gastro esophageal reflux that might need medical help. In such a case consult a pediatrician.

Throwing Up

Your baby may often throw up after eating, which isn't a very normal sign. Vomiting after feeding can be the outcome of acute viral gastroenteritis, infections, ear or even urinary tract infections. Forceful throwing up of food can also be the result of blockage of the stomach outlet. Vomiting after feeding should not be treated very lightly, since it can be indicative of serious health disorders in your baby like meningitis, intestinal blockage, and even appendicitis.

Tips to Manage

- A baby suffering from gastroenteritis might throw up very frequently after feeds. The best way to deal with it is to keep him/her on fluids, so that he/she doesn't get dehydrated. It is helpful to give him/her smaller amounts more frequently than larger amounts given at once.
- If your child has abdominal pain, is unable to swallow and keep fluids, has high fever, is lethargic or acting extremely ill, vomits for more than 12 hours, vomits blood or green material (bile), or is unable to urinate, he/she should be immediately rushed to the doctor without any delay.

Overfeeding

Overfeeding is another common feeding problem among babies. Most parents tend to feed their babies every time they cry, or give them a bottle to distract them even if they aren't hungry. Overfeeding can lead to spitting up and diarrhoea and can also lead to obesity in the longer run.

Tips to Manage

- Do not try to feed your child every time he/she cries. At times, you can try to distract his/her mind with toys and other things.

Underfeeding

Some babies fuss a lot while feeding. Result? Underfed babies. Some babies tend to fidget while eating or have difficulty in swallowing or sucking. Improper feeding techniques or poorly prepared formula milk that has lumps can cause the baby to spit up. Also, abusive and irresponsible parents may sometimes deliberately withhold food from their little ones leading to hungry, underdeveloped babies.

Tips to Manage
- It is important to know which formula milk to pick and how to prepare it as per your baby's convenience.
- If your baby is undernourished and underweight, medical intervention might be required to resolve this problem.

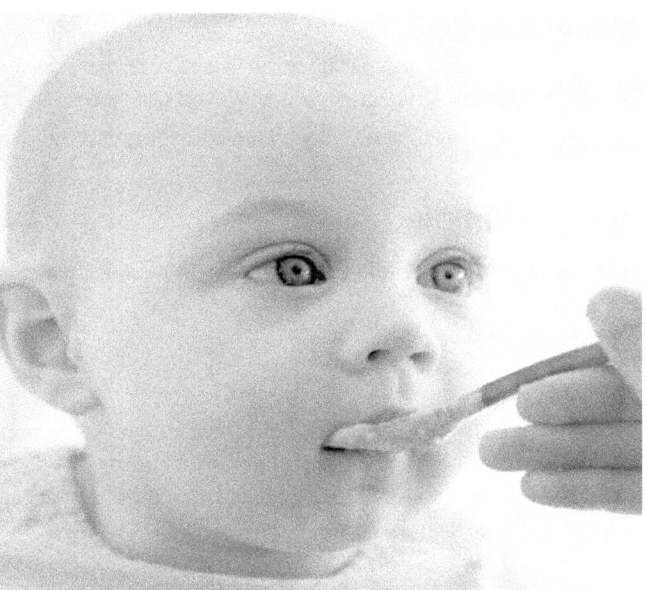
Underfeeding in babies

Dehydration

Dehydration is one of the most serious complications that might occur as a result of poor intake of fluids or breast milk in babies. A dehydrated child can show symptoms of dry mouth, less active and playful, sleepy and lethargic, cry without tears, less urination. Severe dehydration can cause the concentration of salt in the blood to drop or rise significantly, and at times, lead to seizure and cerebral hemorrhage.

Tips to Manage
- Dehydration can be successfully dealt with by feeding your baby on fluids and electrolytes, such as sodium and chloride.
- If the condition is severe, intravenous fluids may be needed. In such a case, it is better to consult the doctor.

Always Hungry

Your little one may always appear hungry, no matter how frequently fed. If your baby appears to be hungry despite of frequent feedings, he may have difficulty latching on properly. It could be also be the result of insufficient milk production or even a sore mouth.

Tips to Manage
- Learn how to breast feed properly. You can talk to your doctor if your child has problems latching on. Frequent feedings, pumping and even drinking enough fluids may help in increasing the milk supply.
- Look for small white patches or sores in and around your baby's mouth. Consult a doctor in case your child has a sore mouth.

Sleeping Soon after Meals

It is normal for your baby to fall asleep soon after feeds. Also if your baby fails to latch on properly while feeding, he/she might fall asleep.

Tips to Manage

You can check out with your doctor to make sure there are no other severe complications involved. However, if your baby is unable to latch on properly, you can release the suction and reposition your child again.

Give frequent feeds to your baby so the baby does not remain hungry.

Passing Motion

If your baby passes motion every time he/she is fed then this could be the result of lactose intolerance or some other allergy.

Tips to Manage

- ❏ It's better to seek advice from a doctor in case your baby is suffering from allergies. Babies suffering from lactose intolerance can benefit by switching over to soy formula milk.
- ❏ If the doctor is not able to detect any of the above causes then wait for a few days and see if the situation changes with time.

3. Transition to Bottle-Feeding

Making your baby shift from breast-feeding to bottle might be a tedious task. Almost all the parents face the problem ensuring a smooth transition pertaining to this. Babies who are breastfed find it very difficult to digest a sudden change in the schedule. They may refuse the bottle when introduced to them for the first time. It is very difficult to make babies get used to something, and when they get used to something, it becomes very difficult to make them shift to another schedule. It may take a long time for you to make your baby get used to the bottle. You should understand the fact that your baby was used to your warmness and coziness, and it will be a bit difficult for them to get introduced to a totally different pattern or technique of feeding. You need to have some patience and accept the fact that this process will take some time.

Be Patient

Do not hurry, be patient and keep the process of shifting your baby from breast-feeding to bottle-feeding a bit slow. It is better to wait a bit before you introduce the bottle to your kid. There is a difference in nursing and having milk from a bottle. Therefore, the baby might reject the bottle when you introduce it for the first time. It is advisable to apply the bottle rule at the third or the eighth week.

Maintain Consistency

Babies don't like changes and even if there are any changes they don't get used to the change very soon. So, it is better to keep everything same even during bottle feeding. You can boil the bottle nipple to body temperature; this will give a same feel to the baby. Give breast milk in bottle for the first time, if that's what the baby is used to. If you are feeding some formula, warm it up to the body temperature.

Calm and Cozy Affair

It is a common practice to bottle feed in a peaceful and quiet place and time. Another thing that can make bottle feeding easier is to have a body contact that will be a mimic for breast-feeding. Sometimes, it is advisable to take tour baby to a quite place and just be with them. This cozy and calm way of feeding should be applied at times to make the process easy. It also will increase the bonding between the baby and the mother.

Change of Guard

A baby who is used to nursing might find it a bit odd to find a bottle instead. It is better to let someone else start with bottle feeding for the first time. Go for a walk and let the father handle the baby for some time while feeding. Any other person can also take up the job for the first time.

Switch Arms

While breast-feeding you need to change sides while feeding and even during different feedings. Do the same when feeding with bottle. This will give the baby the same feel, and is also good for your back and the baby's neck and vision.

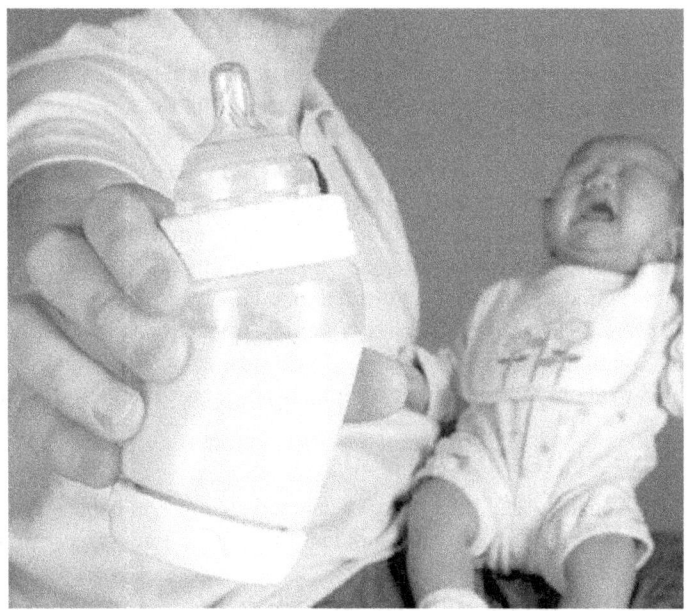

Bottle-feeding

Don't Measure

When nursing, you don't know how much does your baby has consumed. However, while feeding the baby with a bottle you can measure the quantity. Don't try to measure as to how much your baby had? Let the baby decide as to how much milk he/she wants. If the baby is drinking more or less according to you, it is just normal.

Use the Right Nipple

The nipple that you use to feed your baby should be the right one with the correct hole in it. The nipple hole should not be too small or too big. If it is too small, it will make it difficult for the baby to suck the milk, leaving them with no option but to give up. On the other hand, if the hole is too big it might choke your baby as the flow will be too fast. Turn the bottle upside down before feeding. If milk flows instead of drips, the nipple hole is too large. If the baby tries too hard and gets tired during sucking, it means the hole is too small.

Make Them Burp

Babies may swallow a lot of air while drinking from a bottle. Make it a habit to burp your baby half way to make them get rid of the air swallowed and also to avoid stomach pain. To minimize air swallowing, tilt the bottle, allow the milk to fill the nipple and the air to rise to the bottom of the bottle.

Making Night Feeding Easier

To make night feeding easier, keep boiled water with right temperature in a thermos used only for the baby's water. Keep the water bottle and the formula you need in the bedroom, so that you can mix the formula real fast when the baby wakes up.

4. Choosing Formula Milk

Deciding on whether to breast-feed or formula feed your baby is one of the first major choices that you have to make as parents. Although nothing can equal the advantages of breast-feeding, it may not be possible for all women to nurse their little ones consistently. Comfort, lifestyle, and at times, medical concerns require us to make that big decision for our babies to switch from breast-feeding to formula feed. In case you have to go for formula food, it is important to consider that the baby's nutritional demands are adequately met. Breast milk has all the vital nutrients required for your baby. For all mothers who cannot breast feed or choose not to, infant formula is the next best nutritional alternative. But for this, it is important to educate yourself on the kind of formula food that is good for your baby. Formula food are usually based on the nutritional standard of human milk and are rich in proteins, fats, carbohydrates, vitamins, minerals, and water. They contain vital ingredients which match up to the rough proportions of human milk. Here are some formula foods for you to choose from. Scroll down to know how to choose formula milk for infants and watch him/her grow into a happy healthy child.

Premature Infant Food

This is made to suit the exclusive demands of preterm babies. Premature infant formula food is heavy on calories and other nutrients essential for the proper nourishment of premature and low-weight babies.

Cow Milk-Based Formula Food

This is the kind of formula food that an average baby should be on, if not breast fed. However, it is medically advised not to introduce your little ones to cow's milk before 12 months as your baby's digestive system is not suitably developed to handle the complex balance of nutrients contained in it.

Soya-Based Formula Food

For babies suffering from lactose intolerance or milk protein allergies, soya based formula milk is the best option. Replete with essential nutrients, this formula food is made of soya beans. However, this milk should be given to your babies only after medical consultation.

Gentle Formula Food

This kind of formula food is generally lower in lactose content than the general milk based formula food and is best recommended for babies with gas problems, or those babies who generally fuss over milk.

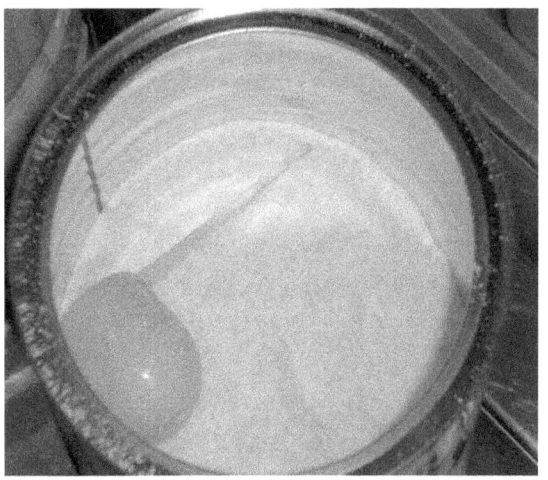
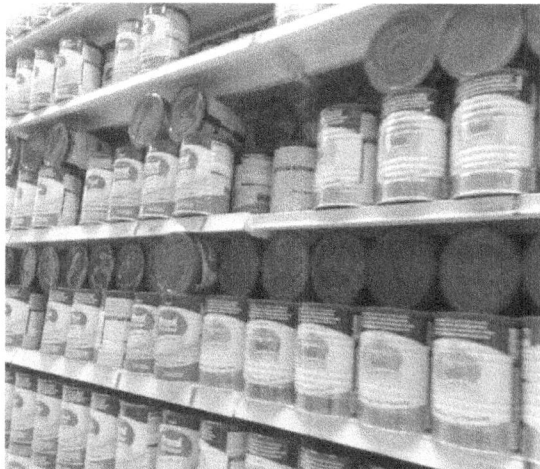

Boxes of formula milk

Lactose-Free Formula Food

Lactose free formula foods are the perfect pick for babies with zero tolerance for lactose based food. Some babies are born with lactose intolerance. In this case, lactose free formula food is the right choice.

Toddler Formula Food

This kind of formula food is best given to toddlers aged between 9-24 months. As this milk is specially designed for a specific age group, it is sated with all the necessary nutrition and prebiotics required for your growing child. It is easy to digest as well.

Elemental Formula Food

For babies suffering from milk and soya allergies, elemental formula food is the best source of nutrition. You can choose this to ensure that your baby has the best in nutrition as well as taste, and also to ensure that its health is not adversely affected.

5. Guide to Choose Nipples and Bottles

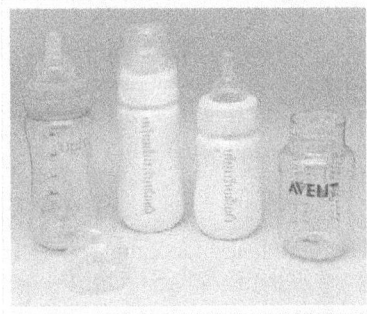 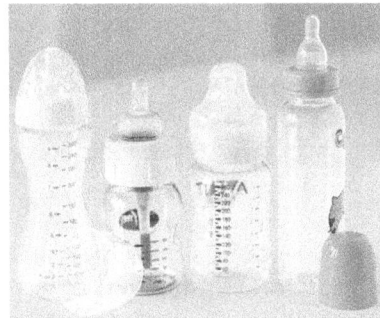 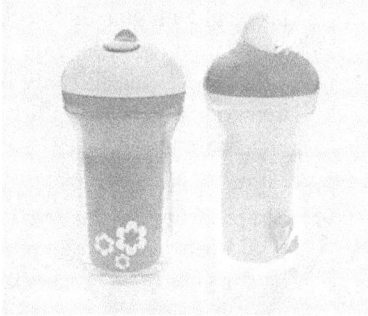

Do you wish to get a feeding bottle for your baby but have the least idea on what to buy? Feeding bottles can play a crucial role when it comes to feeding your child and parents are usually anxious to make the best pick. Choosing the right bottle can make the challenging work of feeding your little one a child's play. For some parents, figuring out their child's preference can be an easy bet, while for some, especially the new ones, it can be quite an uphill task. New mothers often struggle in choosing what is best for their baby. Contradiction of views in regard to feeding bottle can just add to their plight. With so many options to choose from, picking the right bottle for your baby is never an easy win. There are certain crucial things to be considered while buying your feeding bottle – the size, shape, material and types of the bottle and the nipple. Being aware of the little niceties about feeding bottle can actually bail you out from the gargantuan pressure of choosing your bottle. Here is a brief guide on how to choose the best nipples and bottles for infants.

The Bottle

- **Finding Best Bottle**
  The first big challenge is always to find out the right kind of bottle for your baby. You will find a great variety of bottles available in the market ranging from the basic ones to anti-colic bottles, sterilizer bottles, disposable bottles, and glass-feeding ones. Basic feeding bottles are easy on your pocket and easy to maintain. Sterilizer bottles and glass bottles, though little expensive, are a healthier option to go for. Anti-colic bottles are the best bet for babies who suffer with heavy and queasy stomach.

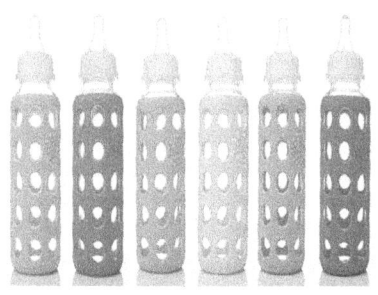 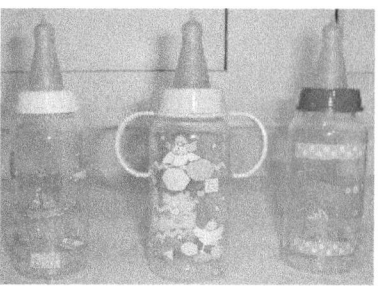 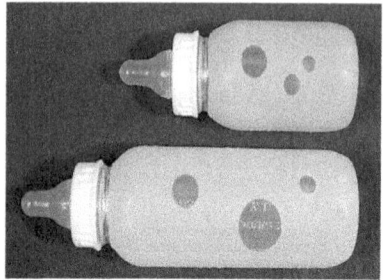

❑ **Size Matters**
The next important thing to take into account is the size of the bottle. The appetite of a baby usually varies with age. While a newborn may need a smaller bottle, the slightly older ones may want a bigger size. However, it's wise to go for a bigger bottle as your baby will need more food per meal, as he/she gradually grows up. Never try to fill the bottle all the way up from the beginning. Also, it is advisable to go for bottles that have colourful, easy-to-read measurements on them rather than the colourless ones as they are difficult to read once the bottle is filled.

❑ **Glass versus Plastic**
Are you still undecided on whether to opt for a glass bottle or a plastic one for your little one? The basic problem with glass bottles is that they are heavy, expensive and cumbersome in comparison to the light weight, unbreakable, chic looking and more economical plastic bottles. But think twice before picking your bottle! Recent study reveals that the plastic found in baby bottles can cause potentially harmful damages to your child. In case you still wish to go for plastic bottles, it is best recommended to go for any bottle that has "#7" recycling symbol or "PC" on the bottom. Also, discard any bottles that look scratched and cloudy.

❑ **Shape of the Bottle**
If your baby suffers from post-meal fussiness, the shape of the bottle is what you should concentrate on while buying your bottle. Some babies ingest more air while feeding that can cause tummy discomforts. In such cases, it is advisable to opt for bottles with an air vent system. Bottles with unusual shapes, such as the angular shaped bottles prevent air from entering into baby's stomach, thereby reducing all discomforts.

❑ **Drop-in Bottle Liners**
If you are much terrorised with the thought of washing and sterilizing the bottle each time your baby feeds, check out for the drop-in bottle liners. These bendable plastic bags easily fit inside the feeding bottles and are disposable. This reduces your chore to just cleaning the nipple and rinsing the other parts. Also, these drop-in bottle liners allow lesser air into the bottle making them safe for babies who suffer due to wind. A drop-in bottle does not contain harmful chemicals and is safe for your babies.

The Nipple

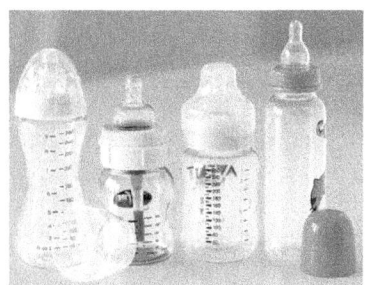 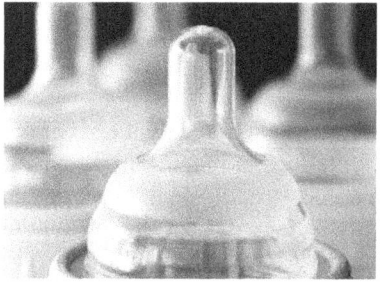 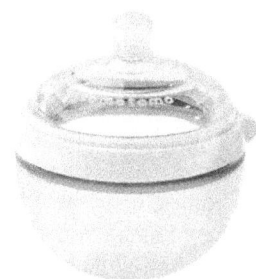

- **Shape of the Nipple**
  While deciding on your bottle, stress should be laid on finding the right shaped nipple for your baby. The choice varies from- traditional, orthodontic, or flat-topped nipples. You need to understand your child's comfort level. Orthodontic nipples are shaped to support your child's palate and gums. If the baby had been weaned earlier, he/she would prefer a fuller sized nipple against the flat artificial ones. In that case, it is advisable to opt for flat topped nipples that resemble the shape of a mother's breast.

- **Choosing the Right Flow**
  You should always check the speed of the fluid coming out of the nipple before picking your bottle. Most brands sell nipples designed for slow or fast flow. Nearly all newborns need a slower nipple in the beginning. Make sure that you don't choke your little one with excess inflow of food. For growing babies, however, you need a faster nipple with a wide hole for convenient sucking.

- **Material for the Nipple**
  There are plenty of options available in the market when choosing for nipple- latex, silicone, rubber. Latex nipples are soft and wear out easily. While picking up the nipples, always go for the silicone ones over the dark-coloured latex nipples. They don't pick up smell or taste and aren't potential carriers of allergies too.

  Also silicone nipples are hard to chew, thereby making them a safe option for your precious little ones.

6. Sanitising Baby Bottles

Babies are quite vulnerable to viruses, bacteria and parasitic infections. These infections can lead to any mild attack of thrush to the more serious conditions of gastroenteritis. So to save your babies from these infections, it is important to keep them in a clean and healthy environment. One of the very important items that need utmost care is your baby's feeding bottle. Baby's bottle should be properly sanitised. Some people think that a bottle just bought from the store is clean, so what is the need of sanitising it. The newly bought bottles are actually not clean. The bottles and nipples are coated with many chemicals, while they were being manufactured. Thereafter, they are packaged by people, sent to stores and then stocked on the shelves by people, thus travelling through many hands. Another important reason for which you should sterilize the bottles is *bacteria*. Have you ever forgotten the bottle in the diaper bag? Have you ever left the bottle unwashed for a certain time period to wash it later? Bacteria can grow in these bottles very easily, due to the milk particles left in the bottle, the warmth inside the bottle, and the dampness inside. So, to keep away these bacteria and infection from affecting your kid, it is advisable to sterilize the bottles properly. Sterilizing the bottles will keep them germ-free and fresh, and will save your baby from any risk of getting infected.

Tips to Sanitise Baby's Bottles

- **Boiling**
  One of the simplest ways to sanitise the bottle and keep it germ free is by boiling it. All the bottle-feeding equipments should be boiled for, at least, 10 minutes. The utensil you use should be for this purpose specifically. All you need to do is to wash the baby's bottle first and then, place it in a pan of boiling water. One precaution that needs to be taken is that the rubber nipple of the bottle should be replaced on a timely basis, as it can get sticky due to constant heat exposure.

  You can even sterilize the bottles and nipples by placing them at the bottom of a deep pot and covering it with water. Place a lid on the pot and bring it to boiling point. The bottle should be allowed to simmer for about 20 minutes before removal and then, put it for drying on a clean towel. If it is a glass bottle, place a wash cloth underneath it, in the pot, to prevent breakage.

- **Sterilising in Microwave**
  These days, there are bottles available that are microwave resistant. These bottles can be sterilized in the microwave on their own. It just takes 90 seconds to sterilize a bottle. One precaution to be taken while

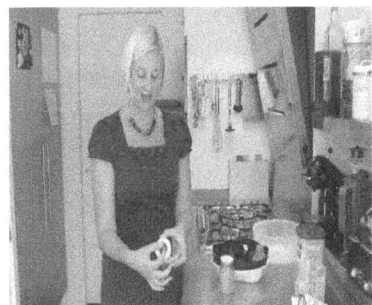 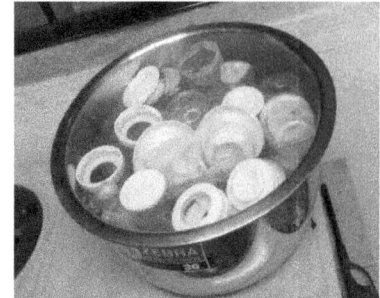 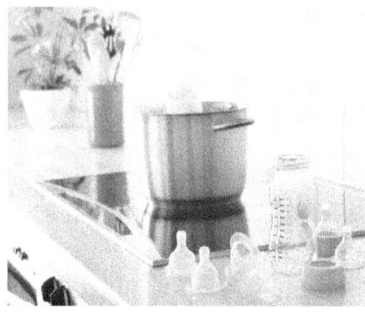
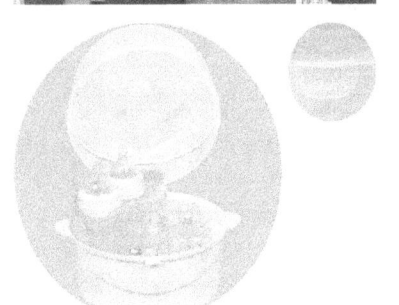 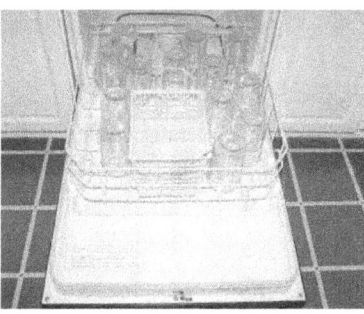 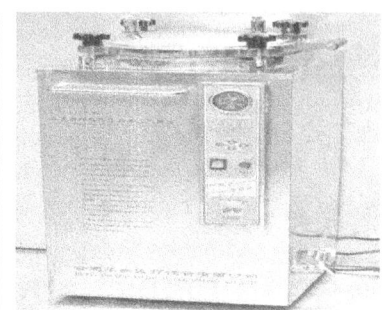

Different ways of sanitising bottles

putting the bottle inside the microwave is that it should not be sealed, as pressure might build inside during the heating process.

❏ **Bottle Sanitisers**

There are many bottle sanitisers available in the market that are designed by using the method of steam sterilization. In this method, the bottle and the rubber nipple should be kept in the upside down manner. Precaution should be taken while opening the lid of the steamer, as the insides might get pretty hot. This entire process takes 15 minutes for proper sanitisation of the bottles.

❏ **Cold Water Sterilizing**

Another method of sanitising baby's bottles is the cold water sterilising. This method uses non-toxic, chlorine free solutions or tablets for sanitising the bottles. These tablets are so safe that they can be applied on the skin or even swallowed without any harmful effects.

❏ **In Dishwasher**

Select the hottest cycle on your dishwasher and choose the drying option. The heat generated in the process acts like a sterilizer. If your dishwasher does not have an upper rack with its own water source just below, choose a different option for cleaning baby bottles.

❏ **Stove Top Sterilizer**

You can use a stove top sterilizer. It uses a rack to hold the bottles and other equipments and proceed with the sterilizing process. Do not leave the sterilized bottle for a long time in your working place as it may again get contaminated.

❏ **Electric Sterilizer**

An electric sterilizer is specifically designed to hold more than one bottle. It can also be carried out while travelling, this adds to its benefit.

7. Weaning to Solid Foods

Your baby cannot derive all the nutrition from milk all his/her life. After 4-6 months of exclusive milk-feed, the baby needs to be introduced to solid foods. It is a great experience for the new mother to cook tiny, special meals for her little one. But after spending hours in the kitchen slicing, dicing, sautéing and sweating, you prepare a nutritionally balanced, delicious delight only to realise that your baby is not enjoying it. While eating solid food is a new experience for your toddler, he/ she require time to get used to the various colours, textures and tastes of new food. As toddlers crave consistency and familiarity, most of them do not try on new foods unless you serve them numerous times. The best way to provide them with wide variety of healthful foods is to serve them in a positive, relaxed environment so that everyone can enjoy the meal. Give them food when they are likely to be hungry so that they can dig in immediately with whatever they are served.

Tips to Feed Picky Eaters

- Introduce a variety of healthy food to your baby at each meal. While offering a new food, simply add to your baby's highchair table making a fuss about it. Ensure that the food is age-appropriate.
- Start introducing new foods one at a time and in small amounts. Do not offer an entire meal of unfamiliar foods. Instead, offer the standards with something new.
- While serving your baby or toddler, always use toddler-size portions. For example, a serving size of bread for a 1-year old is only ¼ slice. Serve only 2 tablespoons of rice, potatoes or pasta as the serving size.
- Some kids have more sensitive palates than others and hence, they do not like texture, colour or taste of some foods. With such toddlers, try to make food that looks creative and tempting when served so that they are naturally attracted towards it.
- For toddlers that are picky eaters, food should contain the desired nutritional value your baby requires. You can add some wheat germ or tune to his/ her macaroni and some little chunks of fruit to their favourite cereal.

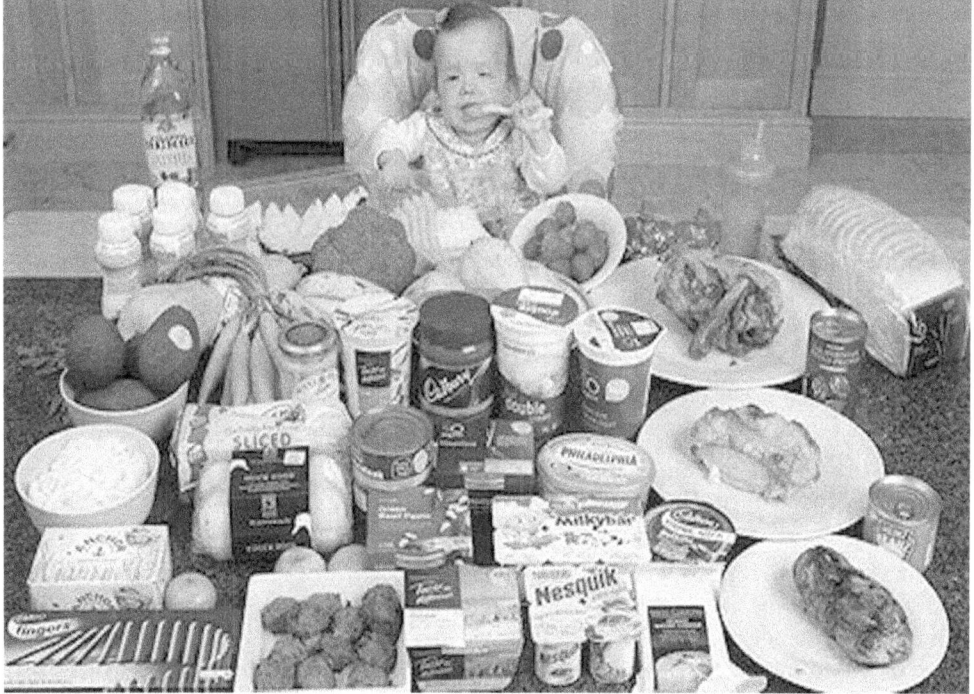

Baby surrounded by many foods

- Avoid serving sugary foods just for the sake of fulfilling his/ her diet. Remember that the food your serve should develop his sense of culinary adventure and not his sweet tooth.
- Keep the distractions at the dinning table at the minimum. If you have other kids running round the table or a cartoon is beckoning in the background; your baby is bound to lose interest in the food being served. Try making your baby's meals relaxed and quiet.

8. Healthy Diet for Toddlers

If you have seen the movie, Baby's Day Out, you would know it is not at all easy to handle kids. Ask the mothers how difficult it gets for them to feed their child, especially if their kid is a toddler. Babies grow at lightning speed, almost 3 inches every 3 months, but after a year or so they grow only 2 to 5 inches a year. While growth process slows down, nutrition remains the top priority. This is also the time when the kids are learning to eat and drink food other than bottle milk. This is the period of transition for the kids and, hence they require more attention with regard to their diet. If they get adequate intake of proteins, iron, vitamins and carbohydrates now, they will grow up to be a healthy boy or a girl. Even a little negligence at this stage will cost the kids their entire life. So it becomes necessary for the parents to plan out a proper food intake for their babies so that they can get the required amount of nutrition on a daily basis.

Nutritional Foods for Toddlers

- **Chocolate Milk**
  Milk is an important part of a kid's diet. Milk provides calcium and vitamin D to build strong bones. Children will gulp down plain milk without any complain, but it is better to add in some flavour to make it appealing and not boring. Why chocolate? Because there is a popular belief that chocolate does not hinder calcium absorption.
- **Baked Potatoes**
  Baked potatoes are rich in potassium and fibre. It is any day better than greasy and oily fries. It is lower in fat than any other form of potatoes.
- **Baby Carrots**
  For babies and toddlers, steam the carrots until soft and then cut them into small pieces and feed them.
- **American Cheese**
  One slice of this cheese has about 125 milligram of bone building calcium. Children between 1 to 3 years need 500 ml a day while 4 to 8 years old need 800 ml a day.
- **Fortified Cereals**
  Fortified cereals are another rich source of numerous vitamins and minerals, including iron and vitamin B, which build blood cells. There are two brands of cereals: ones with less sugar content and ones with normal sugar content. You can choose depending upon your baby's taste.
- **Broccoli**
  Broccolis are rich in vitamin A and C and with every bite, your child will get healthier and stronger. Many kids like it raw or lightly steamed. You can use the vegetables in other dishes as well.
- **Eggs**
  Eggs are packed with protein and vitamin D. They help in building muscles and provide calcium to the body. So an egg a day will complete your kid's diet requirement.
- **Mixed Vegetables**
  Mixed vegetables include a combination of different vegetables with different vitamins and proteins which the body requires on a daily basis. Peas for e.g., provide proteins and foliate and vitamin B. Green beans on the other hand provide potassium. You can either serve them all together in a bowl or toss them all in a soup.

- **Ketchup**
  Usually you might get worried with the fact that your kid eats everything with sauce. Let them continue eating ketchup as it contains a natural cancer fighting compound called *lycopene*.
- **Kiwi Fruit**
  This fruit has more vitamin C than orange. It is rich in fibers and antioxidants that help protect the body's cells from getting damaged.
- **Orange Juice**
  Out of all the natural juices, orange juice is the most nutritious. It contains lots of vitamin C, foliate and potassium. The calcium, fortified one is the best for kids who don't want to drink milk.
- **Sweet Potatoes**
  Slice it into strips, use little oil and bake into fries which will be serving all the vitamin A that a kid requires in a day.
- **Whole Wheat Bread**
  It is rich in fibre. Start with wheat bread first. When your kids transform into toddlers, get them used to whole wheat bread. Other such options may be brown rice, whole wheat muffins, etc.
- **Tortillas**
  These are low in fat. Roll them up with ham or turkey, slice into wheels, cut them into wedges, and then bake to make low-fat chips. You can also top with chopped vegetables and melted cheese.
- **Cantaloupe**
  It is one of the rare fruits containing both beta carotene and vitamin C. It is a great substitute for kids who are not vegetable eaters.
- **Peanut Butter**
  Peanut butter has become very popular among kids. It is rich in protein and a good source of fiber. Spread on bread or thin with water to make a tasty dip for your toddler.
- **Parmesan Cheese**
  Each serve of this grated cheese provide close to 10% of daily requirement of calcium. You can sprinkle it on top of pastas, pizzas, vegetables, salads and eggs.

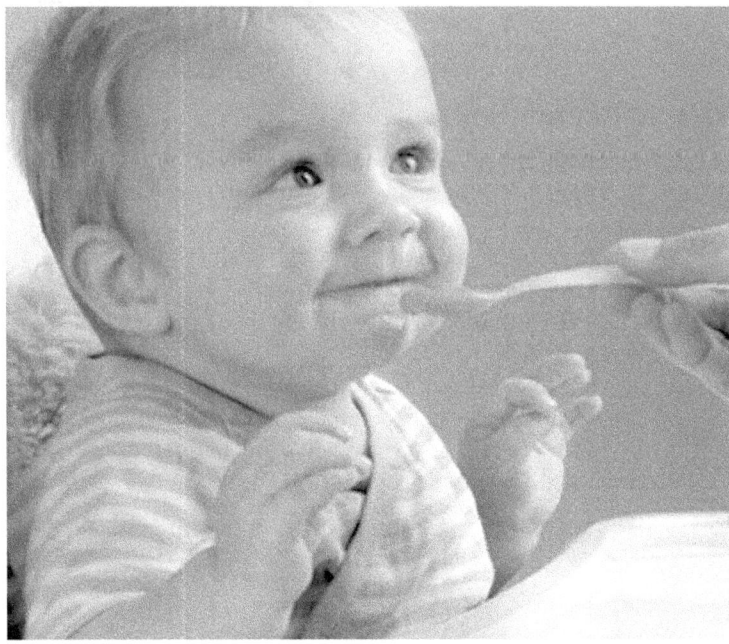

Food for toddlers

- **Yoghurt**
  Yoghurt is good for babies. Eight ounces of yoghurt provides around 250 to 450 milligrams of calcium. While purchasing, look for the ones that are low in fat. These beneficiary bacteria in yoghurt boost the health of your child's intestine.

- **Porridge**

  Porridge is very light and healthy food as it contains both milk and cereals. You may begin with porridge prepared with *suji* (semolina) and milk. Later you may prepare it with ground rice, ragi, millet, oats, etc.

9. Feeding Schedule

A baby, who is between 7-9 months old, should be given semisolid and solid foods with milk feed. A schedule given below may provide an idea as to how and what kind of foods may be given.

6.00 am	Breast-milk feed
8.00 am	Porridge/ Biscuit
10.00 am	Half boiled egg
11.30 am	Juice of any fresh fruit
12.30 pm	Khichdi/soft rice and dal/curd
2.00 pm	A piece of cucumber or any hard vegetable to munch on
3.30 pm	Milk feed
5.00 pm	Mashed banana
7.30 pm	Boiled and mashed vegetables/ rice/curd
9.30 pm	Breast-milk feed

Tips to Remember

- Be careful about the hygiene while preparing foods for the baby. The cooking and serving utensils should be thoroughly clean and you should wash your hands with soap and water before handling and preparing the food. Lack of hygiene may cause contamination of baby's food with germs causing diarrhea.
- The food for the baby should be cooked just before serving. In case of delay, the food may be stored for a few hours in a refrigerator.
- The half-eaten food or milk of baby should not be kept for later use as germs may grow in it and cause contamination.
- The intake of salt and sugar for baby should be minimum. Do not put extra fat, sugar or salt in baby's food as this may lead to blood pressure problems and obesity.
- Do not leave the baby alone while feeding because of the risk of choking. Do not give finger food in small size so that the baby may not swallow it the wrong way and choke.

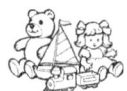

FAQs

Q-1. How do I start weaning my baby?
Ans. You may start by giving a teaspoonful of rice water and gradually increase its quantity. At the same time, you may also introduce other liquid foods like lentil water, thin soup, fruit juice in very small quantities. This may gradually be replaced with semisolid mashed foods. Slowly you may skip one entire milk feed with one of these foods.

Q-2. When can I give water to my baby?
Ans. Breastfed babies do not require water while they are on exclusive breast feeds because the breast milk contains sufficient water. Once the process of weaning starts, they may be given water to drink. If the baby passes urine 6-9 times a day and the stools are soft then you may consider the baby's water intake to be adequate.

Q-3. My baby does not like to eat cereal or other semisolid foods with spoon. Can I give her such foods with milk in bottle?
Ans. Do not mix cereals or other solid foods to the milk in the baby's bottle. Given them separately with a bowl and a spoon. Feed the baby playfully and at a time when the baby is hungry. After a milk feed if you try to feed the baby, she is more likely to reject the spoon as her hunger is satisfied.

Q-4. How much milk should I give to my baby after he starts taking semisolid foods?
Ans. Milk is an important dietry requirement for meeting the baby's nutritional needs. The milk intake can be reduced once the child starts taking solid and semisolid foods. Between 9 to 12 months the baby may be given about 750 ml to 1 litre of milk till he is five years old.

Q-5. My baby has just begun the weaning process. Can I give her fruit juices?
Ans. Fruit juices are good source of vitamin C. You may begin by giving orange or sweet lime (mosambi) juice. To start with, offer just two teaspoons of juice diluted with equal amounts of boiled and cooled water. Gradually increase the amount of juice still diluted with water. Once baby can manage to drink 50-60 ml of diluted juice then start giving undiluted juice in small amounts. Do not warm up the fresh fruit juice before giving it to baby as the heating may destroy the vitamin C present in the juice.

Q-6. My baby always leaves some milk in the bottle. Should I force-feed her?
Ans. Do not force-feed your baby by insisting that she should finish all the milk left in the bottle. She might vomit out extra milk which she does not need. So keep a note and give her less milk in the bottle next time so that she can finish it.

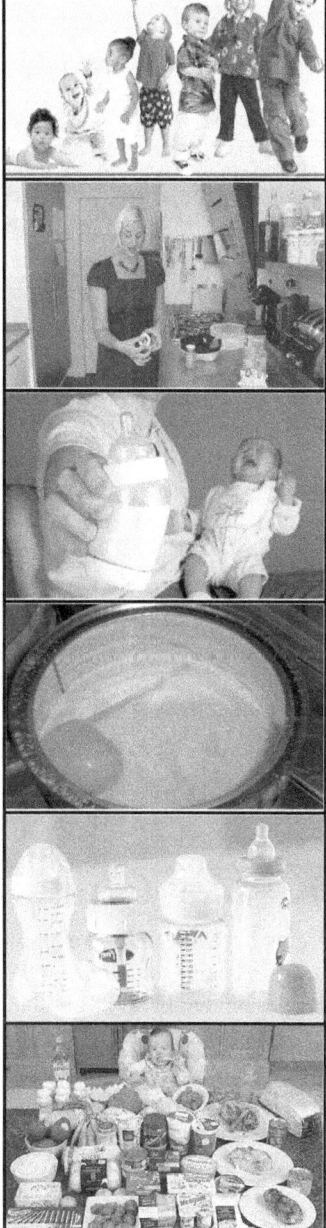

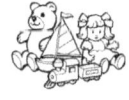

II
Baby Hygiene

The best way to keep your baby happy and healthy is to practise good hygiene. It comes out naturally to protect our baby from germs which urges us to great lengths to do so. And for doing so, we sterilize our baby's feeding bottle, use anti-bacterial soaps and cleaners, everything that can bar germs from our baby's world. But still, a number of babies suffer from different allergies. Reason? Without being in contact with germs, your baby's immune system will not function properly. Although breast milk provides protection through the antibodies passed on, but at times, the bacteria wins out and the baby gets infected to an illness. However, this does not stop us from providing basic hygiene to our baby.

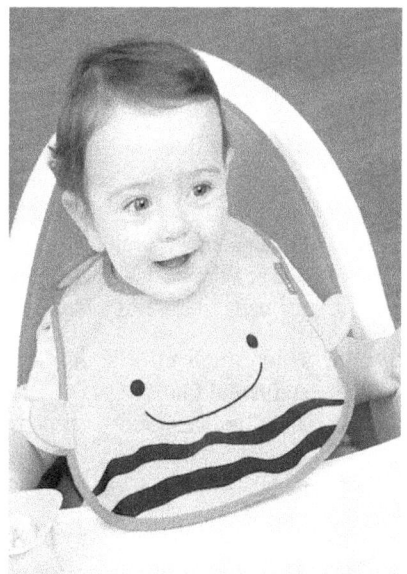

Apart from a nightly bath, there's more to keeping your baby clean and well groomed. Their fingernails need constant trimming, their hands should be washed regularly and hair definitely needs a frequent cut. And as your baby grows older, cleaning their gums and later brushing their teeth is an excellent start to teach your baby the hygiene rituals. To prevent from the hassle emerging at a later stage, it is best to start at an early age. For example, if you start cleaning your baby's ears right from the time they are newborn, by the time they are 18 months old, they will be habitual to it and won't mind getting it done. This chapter deals with the various parameters of cleanliness of a baby such as nails, body odour, genitals, oral hygiene, brushing teeth, cleaning eyes, ears and tongue, and caring for the belly button.

A baby with a beep

1. Baby Genital Care

Being parents can be a euphoric feeling! But tending to the needs and wants of your little one may not be that easy, to begin with, especially for new parents. Babies are unpredictable and vulnerable too. Only timely care and proper tending will ensure that your babies stay happy and healthy. One of the most significant aspects of baby care is attending to their genitals. Baby genitals are tender and exposed and it is only good if you keep it clean. Genital care differs for girls and boys. While attending to these delicate parts of your baby, always make sure to wash the area with mild soap and water and check regularly for rashes, bleeding or pus filled boils. Genital care is mandatory for good health. Follow these tips to minimise your worries for your tiny toddlers.

Tip for Genital Care

- ❑ Check your baby's diaper often and see if it is soiled from bowel movements. Clean the genital area thoroughly with wet cloth and diluted soap. You may buy disposable diapers or cloth diapers for your babies. This will cause more hygiene and comfort for your little ones.

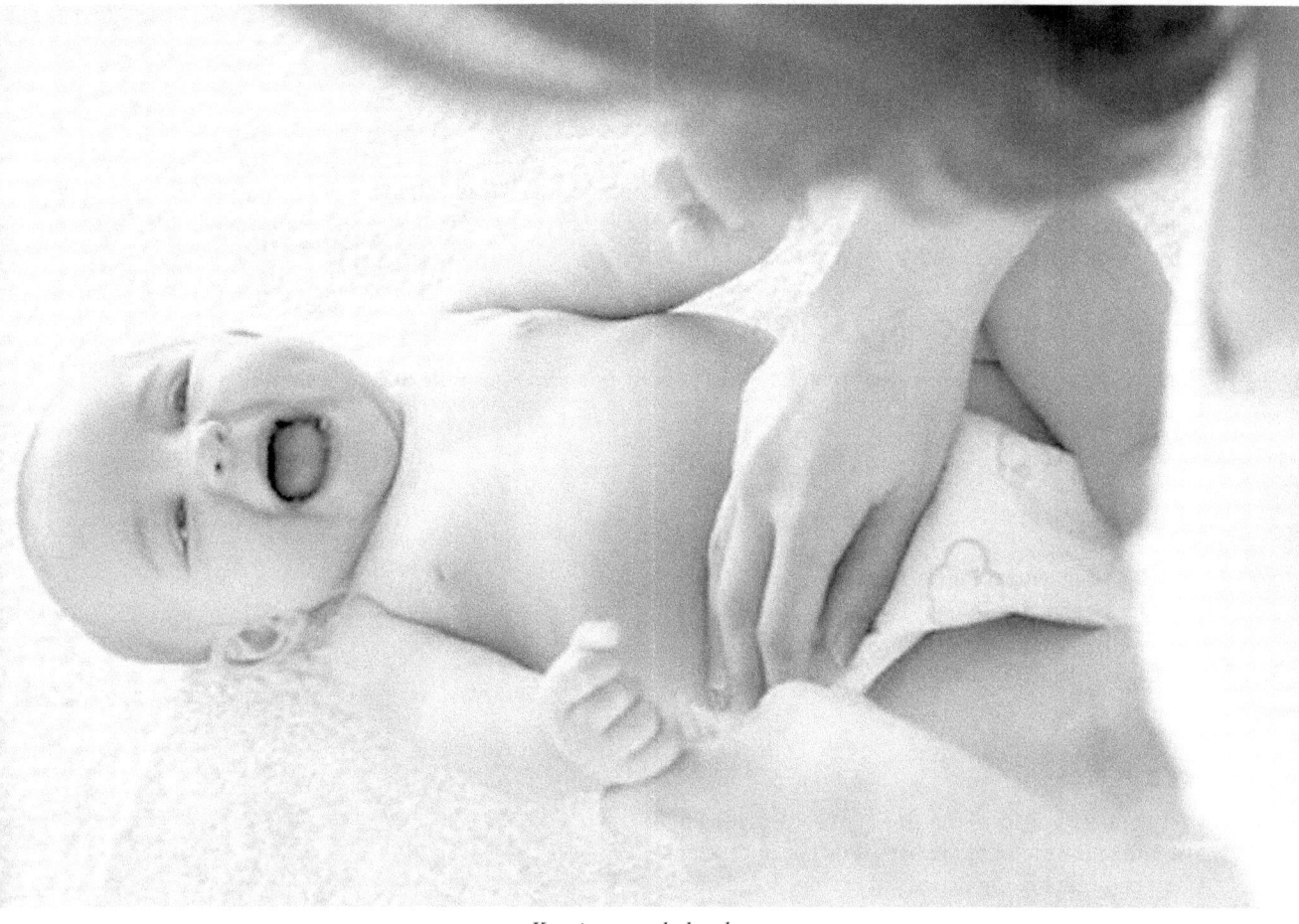

Keeping your baby clean

- Always wipe from front to back for baby girls and wipe under the genitals for boys. Also, take care to clean the buttocks and fat creases under the thighs of your child. Apply baby lotion in case of skin rashes. Maintaining regular hygiene is the key to care for your baby's genital area.
- Baby boys can suffer from circumcised or uncircumcised genital problems that need your special attention. In case of circumcised genitals, keep the area clean. Bathe the area every day with warm water and use a gentle baby cleanser to clean it.
- In case of uncircumcised genitals, wash the area with warm water and baby wash. Do not use any cotton swabs, cotton balls, astringents, or other harsh detergents on your baby. Keep the tip of the penis clean. Avoid pulling the foreskin back while cleaning. Gently hold the foreskin against the tip of the penis and wash it.
- It is never good to keep your babies on soiled diapers for longer periods. If your baby pees or poops at night, do take care to attend to it immediately. Properly clean and dry the area before putting on a new diaper.

2. Body Odour in Babies

Body odour is one of the most common problems in any individual; they can be kids, adults or even your little angels. It's a matter of wonder that even these little ones have problems like body odours. Although babies do not have a bad body odour, it is important enough to take notice of it and know the why's and how's of it. Generally, babies may have two kinds of body odours, one can be the milky odour and the other can be urine odour. Babies may also have occasional body odours like a sour smell, when they have split up or have sweated and there is dirt trapped around them. Even babies with thicker and shorter necks may face this problem more frequently, because dirt gets stuck on the neck and results in odour. Sometimes underarms are also affected by body odour, because it's one of the main areas to sweat and if it's more than normal, it can lead to bad irritation and even redness of the skin. In this situation, a baby skin specialist ought to be consulted for cures. Read on to know about the causes of body odour and the precautionary measures to avoid them.

Causes for Body Odour in Babies

Here are some of the major causes that may lead to body odour in your little one.

- Dirt and dust
- Milk
- Urine
- Clothes
- Saliva
- High temperature
- Heat and pollution
- Perspiration
- Dietary Imbalances

Remedies

Body odours in babies can be very problematic and also affect the mood of the baby. His/her unpleasant smell can lead to long periods of crying! Read on to know more about the remedies to body odour.

- **Baby Powders**
  Soft touch baby powders are available in the market and can be used to prevent the general body odours due to perspiration and can reduce sweat and resulting odours.
- **Fragrant Baby Wipes**
  Baby wipes have a sweet fragrant smell and after babies feed, can be used to wipe their mouths and other parts, which they playfully make dirty leaving a nice fragrance around them.
- **Rosemary Herb**
  Rosemary is a light herb and can be used with massaging oil of your babies, making them smell pleasant.
- **Clothing**
  Clothing is an area many people overlook. Loosely fitting clothes allow the body to breathe better than tight clothes. The perspiration escapes and doesn't become a breeding ground for bacteria. The type

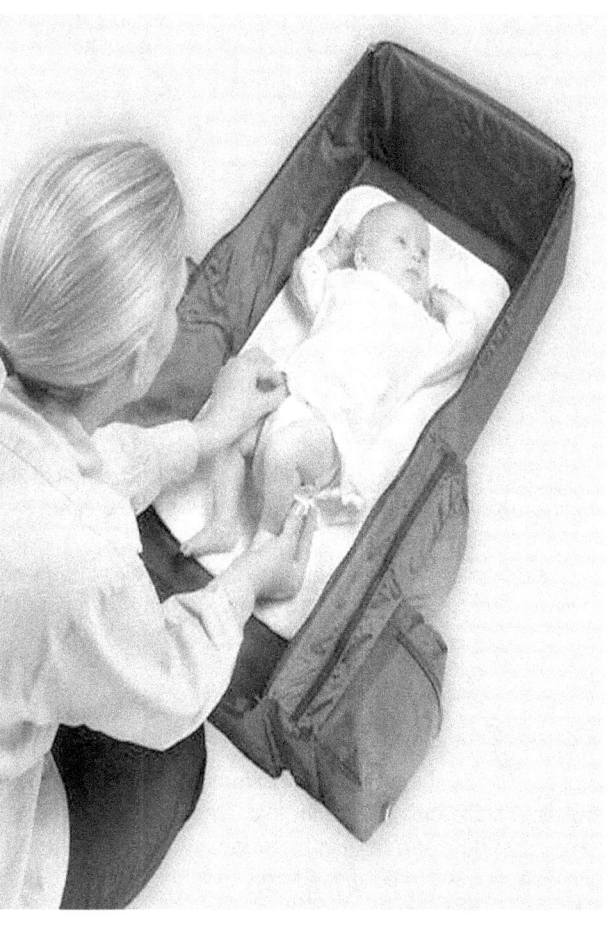

Mother changing baby's clothes

of fabric is also very important. Synthetic fabrics don't allow the body to breathe, so use only natural fabrics for babies.

3. Caring For Baby's Belly Button

Babies are just the perfect addition to your happy family. However, taking care of your little bundle of joy needs a whole lot of effort and a great level of awareness. New parents are often clueless and almost easily intimidated on how to attend to the personal, delicate, and little known body parts of their newborn. With little idea and loads of apprehensions, anxious parents often go to great lengths to make sure that their little ones get a hygienic upbringing. However, basic hygienic care may not be sufficient for your baby. What you really need to understand is that apart from the basic precautions of sterilizing your baby's bottle and using anti-bacterial soaps and cleaners, there are some other important things that you need to take care of. Baby's belly-button or navel care is one important aspect of your child care that should not be neglected. The navel is a delicate part of your child's body and after birth; care should be taken to ensure that the umbilical stump dries and falls off naturally. Baby belly buttons are susceptible to infections and other complications like blood emission, discharge of white smelly fluid, among other things.

Tips for Baby's Belly Button Care

You baby's belly button is something very special; it's that one thing that connects the baby to you and serves as a source of nourishment, while the baby is still inside you. However once the cord is snipped after the baby's birth, it is important to take care of the leftover part of the cord to protect it from infection and help it dry well.

❑ It is sensible to allow your baby's belly button heal naturally by always keeping it dry and clean as possible.

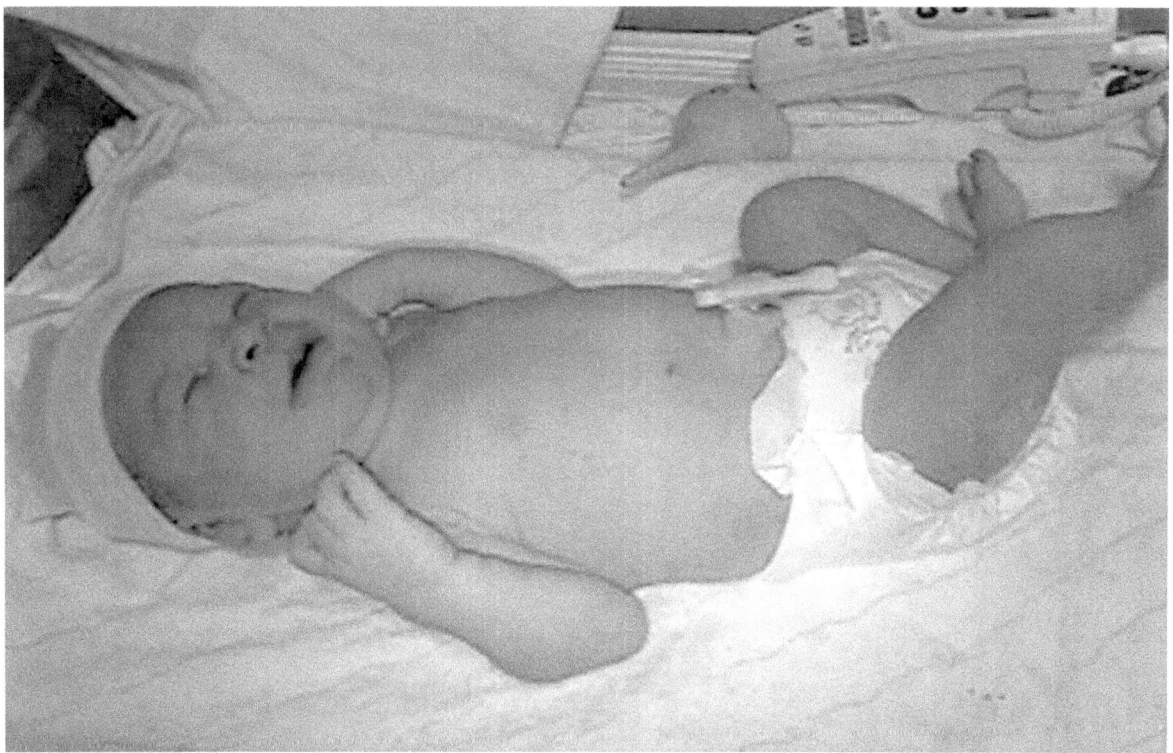

Baby's clamped belly button

- Always wash your hands before attending to your baby's cord. Unwashed hands can be potential carriers of harmful germs.
- Until the stump dries and falls off, it is advisable to keep the baby's diaper off her belly button and avoid anything from rubbing against it. Each time you put on a new diaper, fold the nappy at the top to ensure that there are no skin abrasions. Also, roll up the dress to allow free circulation of air.
- It is essential to keep the cord dry until it has fallen off. You can avoid giving a full bath to your baby or be careful not to drench the cord while bathing before the stump has fallen off and the area is healed.
- It is advisable to clean your baby's belly button area, at least once a day. To clean the cord gently use a cotton tip applicator dipped in cooled, boiled water and softly pat the area. This will help the cord to dry off fast and reduce any risk of infection. Repeat the process for a week after the stump has fallen off.
- Do not forget to dry the area with a cotton swab after cleaning it. Also avoid using cotton balls as fibers from it can get stuck to the cord and cause complications.
- Never use lotion, oil or powders on or around your baby's cord.
- After 1-3 weeks, the cord will dry and fall off naturally. However, if there is recurrent bleeding or infection, or abnormality of any kind, please consult your pediatrician.
- When falling off, it is sometimes normal for the stump to bleed and this should not make the parents anxious. It might take 5 to 10 days for the area to heal after the stump has fallen off. No special care is needed after this.

Watch out

- If baby's belly button gives off a fluid which is thick and smelly.
- If the belly button releases any bad odour.

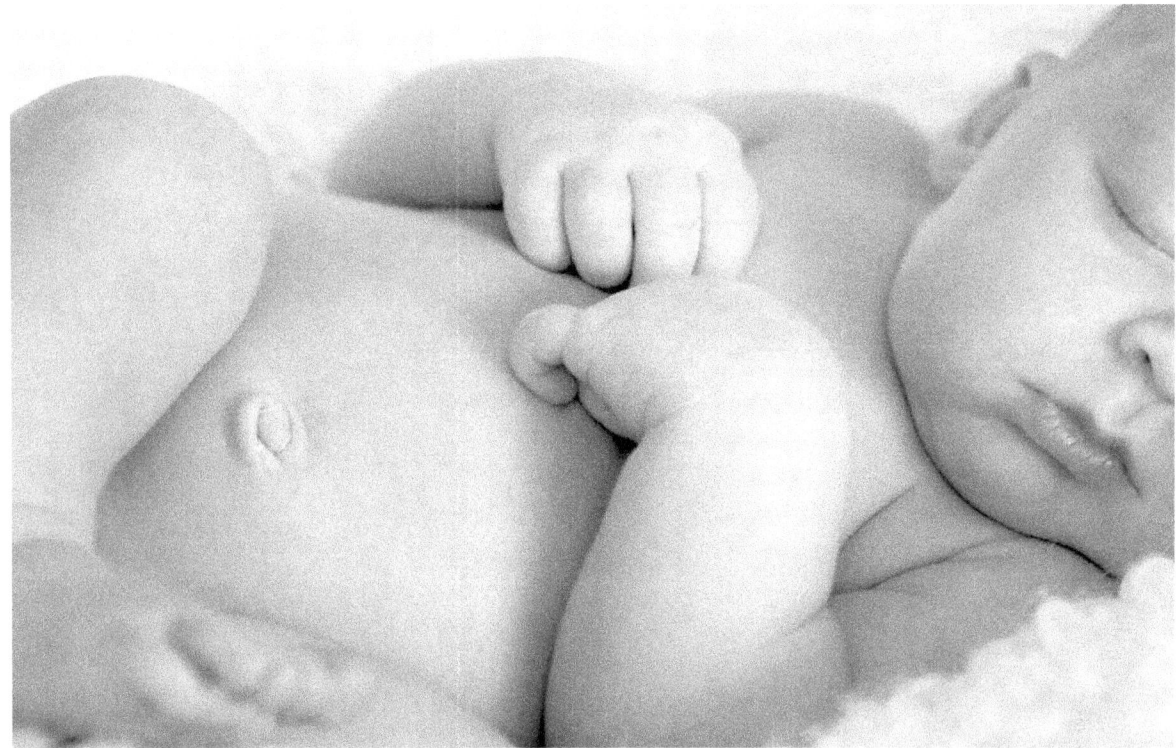

Baby's normal belly button

- ❑ If the skin around the belly button area is inflamed.
- ❑ If your baby has got fever.

4. Cleaning Baby's Eyes

Eyes are said to be the mirror to the soul. In the case of babies, their eyes truly mirror what they are inside - innocent and pure. Their eyes gaze out in wonder at the colourful new world around them. These precious organs need proper care and good hygiene. It does not take much effort to clean your baby's eyes. All that is needed is a regular cleaning routine and periodical clinical check of your baby's eyes. Clinical experiences and research have shown that at six months, the average child has reached the critical development milestone, making it the age for the first medical assistance. Visual abilities are fully working by the age of six months. So at this age, no risk should be taken with regard to the baby's eyes and it should be cleaned and examined at regular intervals.

Tips to Clean Baby's Eyes

- ❑ Wash your hands properly with soap before going to deal with the baby.
- ❑ Dip a clean, soft baby washcloth or cotton ball into warm water and squeeze it to remove any excess water.
- ❑ Baby's skin is very sensitive, so avoid using soap or any other face wash on the face.
- ❑ Sing or talk to the baby while cleaning to distract his/her attention, so that you don't face any difficulty while cleaning.
- ❑ Use the cloth or cotton ball to clean the corners of your baby's eyes, wiping gently from the inside corner to the outside edge of each eye.
- ❑ Use a different clean, moist cotton ball for each eye to avoid potential cross-infection.
- ❑ Some babies don't like their eyes to be cleaned, make sure the water is comfortably warm. Clean quickly and move it.
- ❑ If your child has an infection, it will clear up quickly with regular cleaning of eyes.
- ❑ While cleaning a sore or infected eyes, make sure that you use clean cotton balls and that you use them only once. Wipe from the inside to the outside. Use a separate cleaning ball, if you need to continue cleaning the same eye.
- ❑ Do not clean inside the eyelids; wipe the eyes only when it is closed. You may risk damaging the cornea if you try to clean inside the eyelid.
- ❑ Use warm and not hot water. Be firm while cleaning to ensure you dislodge any sticky discharge or pus.
- ❑ Ensure that your baby takes a well balanced diet. A diet rich in proteins, vitamins is very essential for a baby's eyes.
- ❑ Regular medical examination by your pediatrician or an eye doctor is very important.

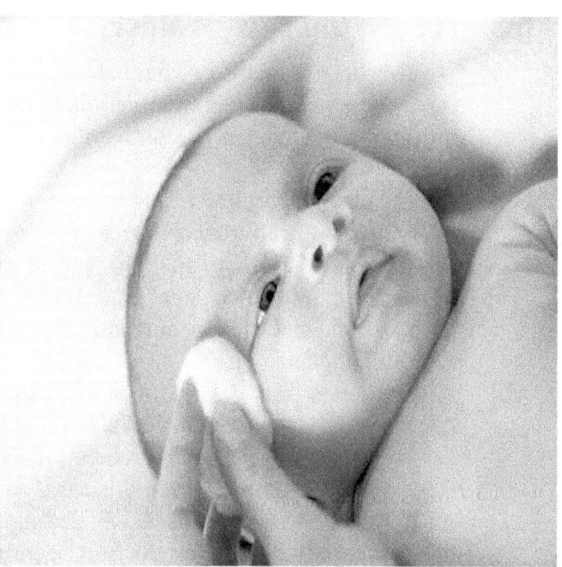

Cleaning baby's eyes

Watch Out

Some babies are born with *blocked tear ducts*. It causes tears to form in eyes and roll down the cheeks. Blocked tear ducts should be evaluated by a pediatrician, as it may require treatment if any infection develops.

5. Cleaning Baby's Nose

Babies commonly have clogged and dirty noses, especially due to the lack the ability to clean themselves the way adults do. This can be rather harmful to the child with regard to hygiene and health care. Babies with stuffy noses suffer from difficulty breathing, noisy breathing, difficulty sleeping and infections, just to name a few. The responsibility to clean your baby's nose frequently and properly lies with you, the parent. While there are some who might find it cumbersome to keep cleaning the baby's nose, remember that your baby depends on you. If you fail your baby on the hygiene care front, you will be harming your child much more than you can imagine. Health and hygiene are as important for babies as they are for adults. Therefore, you will need to take extra care for ensuring that every part of your baby is kept clean. A clean baby is a healthy baby. A healthy baby is a happy baby. While it might seem a cumbersome and complicated task to clean a restless baby's nose, the task is not as tough as you might think.

Tips to Clean the Baby's Nose

- Use a vaporiser to moisten your baby's nasal mucus, vaporizer can be kept near the crib to avail it fully and make sure you do not put very hot water in it as it can burn the nose itself. Clean the vaporizers properly before the next use so that it is germ free.
- You can also go for nose drops if the mucus is too thick and can't come out easily. Nose drops contain a saline solution and it is available at any medical store. It will loosen the mucus and make it flow outwards with the help of a handkerchief.
- Usually babies can get rid of stuffy noses over a period of one or two weeks, but if still they are stuck with the same problem, it can become difficult to manage. In this case, you can go for an alternative solution by getting a rubber suction bulb. To use the bulb, gently stick the rubber bulb in a nostril and release the bulb. In this way, the bulb will suck out all the mucus from the baby's nose. You can use the same bulb for the other nostril and flush out the mucus into the sink, wash it and then repeat the same process.

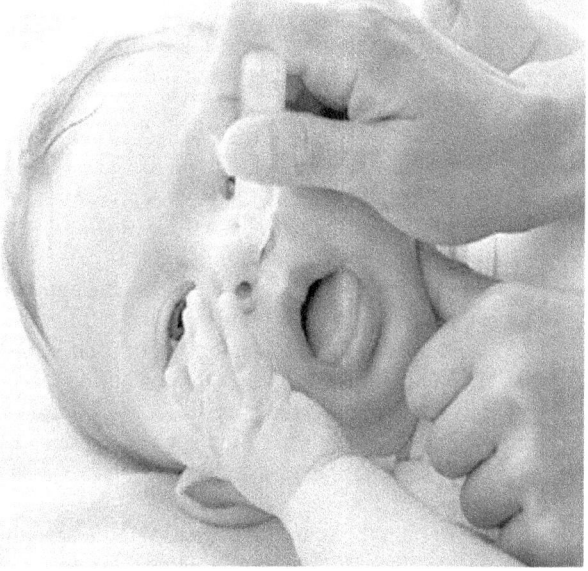

Cleaning baby's nose

- Another simple way to clean your baby's nose is to apply some balm on the nose and neck area. Also, rub a small amount of balm on the foot and cover it with socks. In the morning, the blocked mucus will come out in the form of running nose.

6. Cleaning Baby's Tongue

It's not as easy to clean the tongue of a baby as it may sound - after all babies make a big hue and cry for even thing smallest thing that seems to trouble them. Some parents might want to make babies laugh and clean the tongue with a finger. However, your playful baby might bite your finger and nothing will come out of the attempt. Even if you try to use the back of a toothbrush, your baby will begin to feel nauseated. Therefore, it is very vital to know how to clean your baby's tongue effectively, so that she/he doesn't have any oral hygiene issues to be faced in future. In case you are not giving much attention to tongue cleaning and focussing only on the gums and teeth, it can prove detrimental to your baby's overall oral hygiene and care. The baby's mouth can give a bad nauseating smell which can become permanent over a period of time and accumulation of germs and bacteria can produce plaque and oral problems in future.

Tips for Cleaning Baby's Tongue

- Take a clean soft cotton cloth and pour some warm water on it, make sure the water is not too hot as it will irritate baby's tongue and make it hard to eat or take any other thing into mouth.
- Encourage your baby to open his/her mouth by lowering the tip of lips, while you hold him/her.
- Now, wrap the wet cloth in your index finger and take it into the mouth and start rubbing the tongue gently in circular motions to clear the build-up.
- In some babies, tongue particles stick into it very badly. In this case, apply pea sized toothpaste on the tongue and rub it with a cloth to remove the solidified particles.
- Make sure you wash baby's mouth properly, so that toothpaste doesn't remain in the mouth and your little ones don't swallow it.
- When you clean the tongue remember to clean the gums, cheeks and teeth too, as your baby may not give you a chance to do that again.
- Some babies may not get their tongues cleaned properly by this process. In that case, you need to visit a child specialist for oral queries and the doctor will take care of it by giving some treatment.

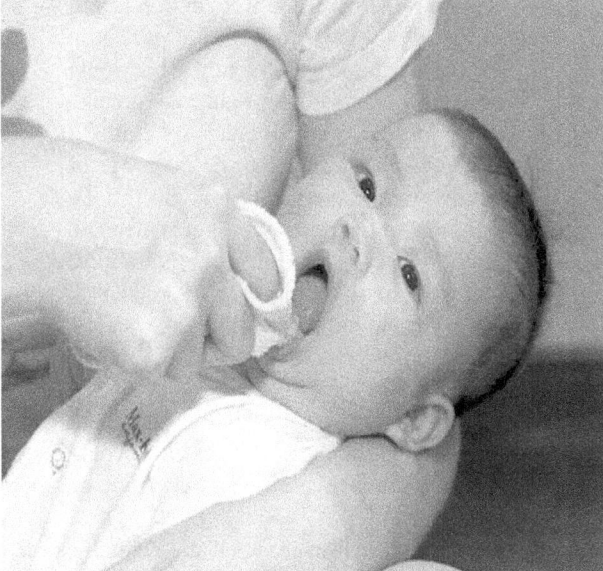

Cleaning baby's tongue

7. Cleaning Baby's Ears

Nothing can be more daunting for a mother than having to deal with those delicate parts of her little one. Understanding your limits and finding the right approach to look after your baby in a way that you find comfortable, is very important. Cleaning the ears of your young ones is something that must never be taken lightly. An old medical saying goes, "Never put anything on your ears smaller than your elbow" and that applies to your child as well. You should use extreme caution while dealing with this aspect of baby care. Most often, ears are neglected and less cared for in regard to other body organs. It is important to realize that ears, like all other body parts, go through same hygienic complications, and extra care must be employed when addressing these problems. Cleaning a baby's ears involves a multi-step process. Here are some pointers on how to clean baby's ears.

Tips for cleaning the Baby's Ears

- After bathing your baby with tepid water, you can use a delicate cloth to clean the ears while holding your baby securely by balancing him/her on your hand.
- If the ear is dirty, then use a wet cloth to wipe the ears. Do not use soap. You can use the cloth to gently scrub the ears, reaching out for the gap behind the ears, which is one common place for wax buildup.

- ❑ Damp the cloth again and use it gently to wipe the outer parts of the ears as some babies tend to have buildup in the outer areas as well. The external air contains small folds which can trap dirt. Gently wipe those folds to get rid of excess dirt.
- ❑ Now, twirl the tip of the wet cloth. Squeeze out the extra water, if any. Gently tuck it in the baby's ear and roll it gently. This would remove any debris from the outer ear canals.
- ❑ Pat the baby's ear with a clean dry cloth.
- ❑ In case you wish to clean the inner ear of your baby, it is advisable for you to take your baby to the doctor and get it cleaned. Doctor's use special instrumentation to clean your baby's ears that avoids the risk of puncturing or scratching your baby's delicate eardrums.
- ❑ While cleaning the ears, don't forget to keep your child warm. Drape him/her in a hand towel to prevent him/her from catching cold.

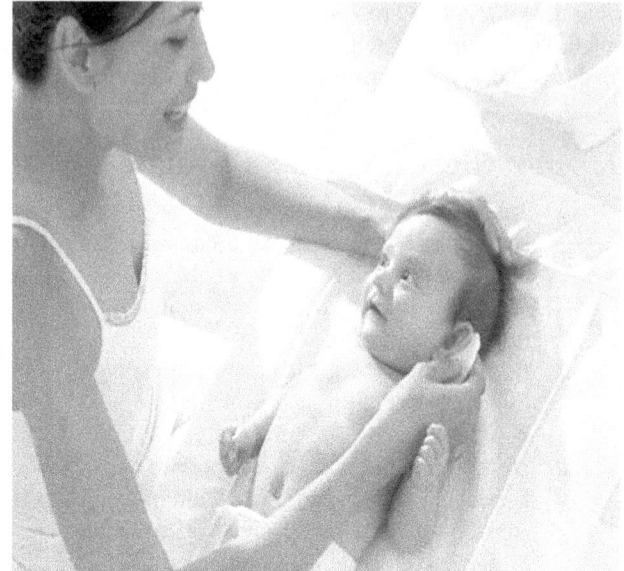

Cleaning baby's ears

- ❑ Some babies have more wax buildup than others. If the problem persists, don't forget to consult your pediatrician.
- ❑ Do not use cotton swabs to clean your baby's ear. Instead of cleaning the wax, they push the debris inside which can cause major harm to their soft eardrums.
- ❑ Avoid using ear cleaning kit on babies. If there is excessive wax in their ears, get them cleaned only by a pediatrician.

8. Trimming Baby's Nails

Have you come across babies with numerous scratches on their faces? The source of these scratches, in most cases, would not be the family pet, but rather the baby himself! Since babies lack muscle control, flailing of limbs is very common. Uncut or improperly cut nails can cause them to scratch their delicate skin and lead to a whole lot of discomfort for the little one. If you have a little bundle of joy at home, you might find that trimming his/her nails is a virtual nightmare. Clipping the nails of a squirming, inquisitive baby can often be very challenging. You just might end up cutting your baby's delicate skin or cutting the nails in such a way that they might re-grow inside the child's skin. Well, trimming a baby's nails does not have to be such a terrifying experience, after all. If you are equipped with the knowledge of how to trim nails correctly, and if you have the right tools to do so, you will find that cutting your baby's nails is just another pleasant part of baby care.

Tools You Need

- ❑ Baby Nail Scissors
- ❑ Nail File/Emery Board
- ❑ Sterile Gauze Pads
- ❑ Mild Antiseptics

Tips for Trimming Your Baby's Nails

- ❏ It is best to trim your baby's nails just after you give the baby a bath, so that the nails will be soft. Try to put your baby to sleep. If your baby refuses to sleep, distract him/her with a favourite toy.
- ❏ Incline the baby's nail and gently press the finger or toe pad away from the nail, so that you will not clip the skin in the process.
- ❏ Trim the nails along the curve of the finger. In the case of toenails, cut the nails straight across. If you are hesitant about clipping your baby's nails, you can choose to file them instead. This will rule out the chances of accidental cuts.
- ❏ Ensure that while you trim the baby's nails, there are no rough edges. Use an emery board or a filer to smooth out any rough edges.
- ❏ If your baby is overactive, get someone to hold him/her, while clipping the nails. After all, you would want to minimise the chances of hurting your baby as much as you can.
- ❏ If you happen to accidently clip a bit of the baby's skin, apply pressure to stop the bleeding. Once the bleeding stops use sterile gauze pad to dab some mild antiseptic onto the cut.
- ❏ Never bite your baby's nails instead of trimming them. While this might reduce the chances of accidently cutting the baby's skin, you just might be encouraging the spread of germs.

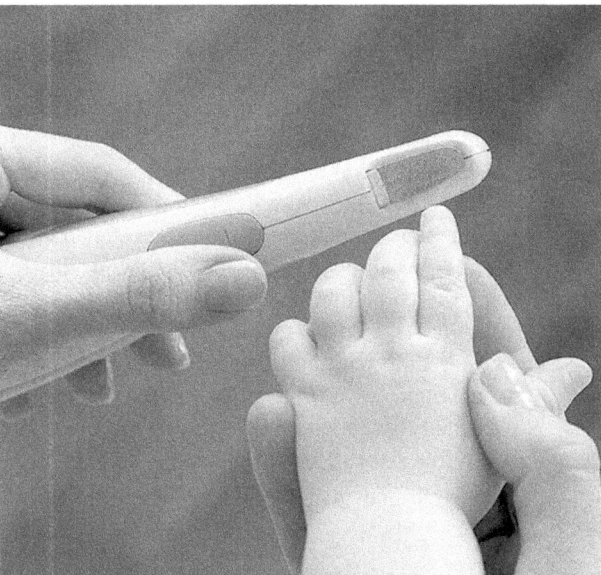

Trimming your baby's nails

9. Baby's Oral Hygiene

A baby's oral hygiene is a very important part of his/her overall hygiene. As parents, your apprehension over your baby's oral health is likely. Ensuring healthy oral habits in babies should be done at the stage of infancy to help teeth grow faster with healthy gums. Concerns about oral health care pop up, for the most parents, when the first tooth erupts. With the occurrence of the first teeth, you should become very careful about maintaining your baby's oral hygiene. Oral health complications in your baby may be due to a host of common problems like tooth decay, thumb sucking, lip sucking tongue thrusting, and early tooth loss. Although a baby's teeth are sooner or later replaced with permanent teeth, you must observe the necessary oral hygiene so that oral problems are kept at an arm's distance of your baby.

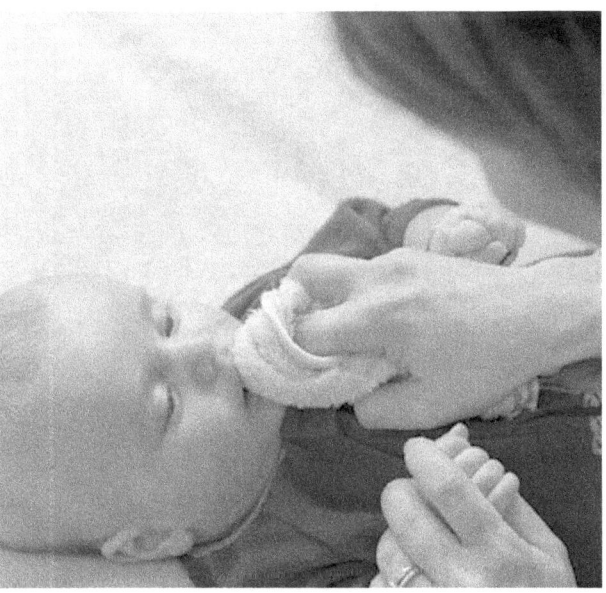

Oral hygiene of your baby

Tips for Baby's Oral Hygiene

- When you feed your baby, do not forget to wipe his/her mouth and gums with a wet cotton cloth. If your baby has already begun teething, you can use a soft-bristled toothbrush to clean the teeth. This will help eliminate any bacteria-forming plaque and excess sugar that have built up on the teeth and gums.
- There are times when brown or white spots may appear on your baby's gums. Make a habit to check your child's mouth regularly. Also, keep a tab on the formation of any smelly tartar collection in their mouth.
- See a dentist if your baby suffers from persistent bad teeth odour. Timely medical advice will help and reduce any further chances of tooth decay.
- If your baby is extremely fond of sweetened milk or cerelac, try cutting down on sugar content and avoid creating sweet pools in the mouth of your tiny tots.
- Make sure you thoroughly clean your baby's milk bottles and the pacifier with hot water and sterilize it with water for some time to remove germs from entering the mouth.
- If your little ones are teething, they would want to chew something to relieve the pressure. In order to maintain good oral health, give them teethers and toys made of nontoxic materials and specially designed for teething babies. Some are made of firm rubber; others are filled with water and chilled in the refrigerator. Don't freeze these types of rings or teethers, because they become too hard and may harm your baby's gums.

10. Brushing Baby's Teeth

Proper oral care and hygiene starts from the very first time your baby begins to drink milk and you clean his/her gums with a damp cotton cloth to remove milk residues from the gums. It is very important to induce these habits in your babies as they will become used to them over time. When teeth erupts into the mouth, you should start cleaning the baby's teeth twice in a day, because bacteria occurs in mouth naturally and tend to convert sugars in food into acid, which can attack the tooth enamel. Brushing the teeth from an early age is important as the primary baby teeth are responsible for making spaces for permanent teeth to grow afterwards and even your baby needs primary teeth for speaking correctly, chewing and biting. Choosing a small brush having soft bristle with a small head is as important as it is to confirm the quality of the brush because if your baby bites on it, he/she may swallow some bristles too!

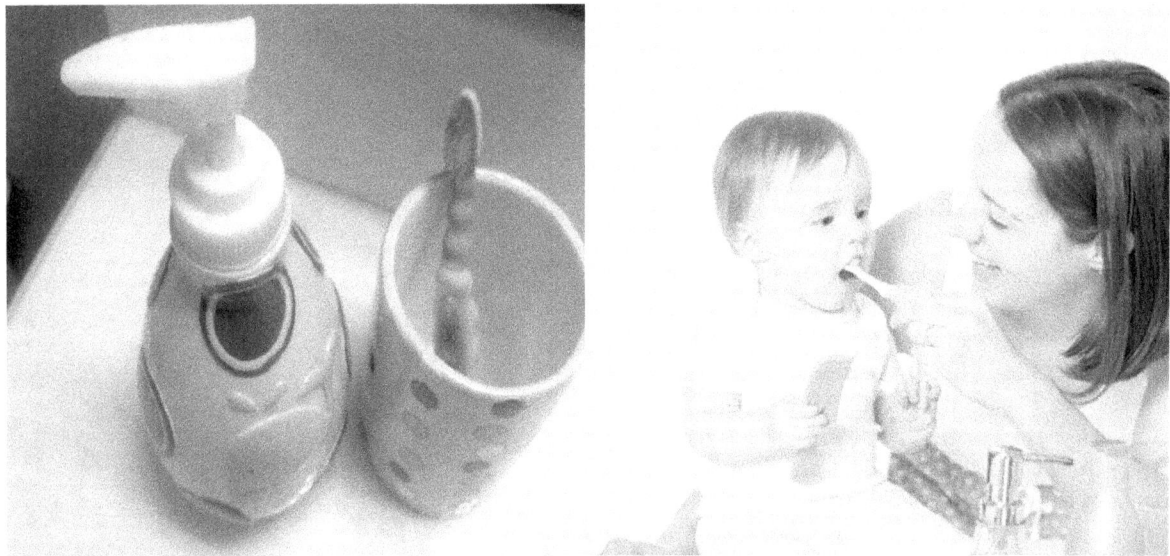

Brushing baby's teeth

	Primary	Permanent
Upper Teeth	Erupt	Erupt
Central Incisor	8-12 mos.	7-8 yrs.
Lateral Incisor	9-13 mos.	8-9 yrs.
Canine (cuspid)	16-22 mos.	11-12 yrs.
First Premolar		10-11 yrs.
Second Premolar		10-12 yrs.
First Molar	13-19 mos.	6-7 yrs.
Second Molar	25-33 mos.	12-13 yrs.
Third Molar		17-21 yrs.
Lower Teeth		
Third Molar		17-21 yrs.
Second Molar	23-31 mos.	11-13 yrs.
First Molar	14-18 mos.	6-7 yrs.
Second Premolar		11-12 yrs.
First Premolar		10-12 yrs.
Canine (cuspid)	17-23 mos.	9-10 yrs.
Lateral Incisor	10-16 mos.	7-8 yrs.
Central Incisor	6-10 mos.	6-7 yrs.

Tips to Brush Baby's Teeth

❑ Make the baby to open the mouth a bit wide, may be you have to act so to make him/her imitate you. Make the baby sit on a slab to help you fully reach all the portions of the mouth.

❑ Gently brush his/her teeth with a small headed toothbrush containing pea-sized less fluoride content paste as your babies may swallow it at times. In case he/she swallows the paste, make them drink a glass of water to dilute it, repeat it before he/she goes to bed at night.

❑ Remember to wash the mouth of your baby with lukewarm water and make him/her spit out the water 4 or 5 times.

Preventing Dental Caries

❑ You can find a white spot on the front teeth, which is termed as lesion. It is a white chalky area close to the gum line. It develops as a result of bacterial action which produces acid. It affects the enamel of the tooth. One can induce good oral habits to prevent it and seek dentist's opinion. Fluoride can solve the problem if it is diagnosed long before.

❑ A golden white cavity like structure can be found in the inner most teeth and it is very important to get it cured by a child dental specialist as soon as possible, because it may hamper the growth of permanent teeth and may infect other teeth as well.

❑ Bad breath can be another indication for tooth decays. In such a condition, sweetened liquid diet should be avoided for some time and proper brushing should be done regularly.

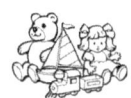

FAQs

Q-1. What is wet eye?

Ans. In some babies there is an inborn narrowing or obstruction of the tear passage, tear gland from which tears normally flow. In such cases, the eyes of the baby look constantly wet or full of tears. In severe cases, the skin around the eyelids may become red and cracked. This problem can be managed by doing a light massage over the inner angle of the eye near its junction with the nose three or four times a day. Clean the eyelids frequently with warm water. Normally, this problem settles down within a few weeks. If it persists then blocked duct may be opened by a small surgical process.

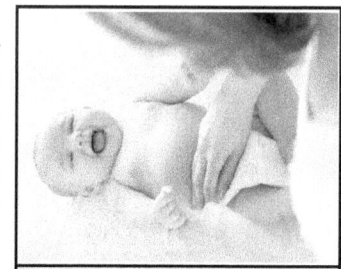

Q-2. My baby has large bluish spot on his shoulder. What should I do?

Ans. Some babies have quite large bluish patches of skin discolouration. These areas of pigmentation are called 'mongolian spots'. They require no treatment and disappear on their own with time.

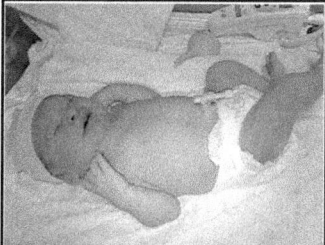

Q-3. My baby is about a month old. She has lost all her hair at the back of her head. What should I do?

Ans. There is nothing to worry about. It is common with small babies. This hair will grow back with time.

Q-4. My daughter has hair all over her body. My mother-in-law wants me to rub them vigorously with bran and oil. But this rubbing brings rashes on her skin. What should I do? I am really worried.

Ans. The skin of babies is very soft and sensitive. Do no such thing like vigorously rubbing it with harsh things. Just give her a simple light oil massge. Do not worry about these hair. They will go away with time.

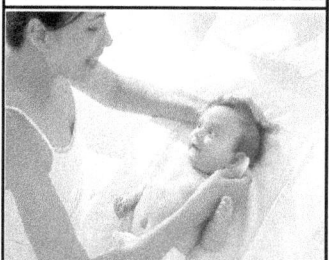

Q-5. My baby has four front teeth. Whenever I try to brush them with paste, she swallows the paste. I am worried that this will affect her health. How do I keep her teeth clean?

Ans. Do not use paste till the time your baby is old enough to understand the correct process of brushing the teeth. Take a soft cloth, wet with clean water and wipe your baby's teeth with it each time you feed her. This way her teeth will remain clean and she will not swallow the paste either.

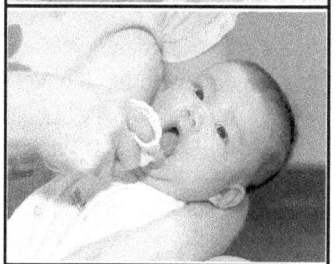

Q-6. My daughter drinks milk from the bottle and most often she goes off to sleep with bottle in her mouth. I am worried that she might develop cavities in her teeth because of sugar in the milk which remains in her mouth throughout the night. I can't clean her teeth because then she wakes up and demands bottle again. What should I do?

Ans. Keep a bottle with plain water handy. Give her this bottle for a while so that the water from the bottle may rinse her mouth and she does not develop cavities. Remember, it is important to take care of your child's teeth right from the start.

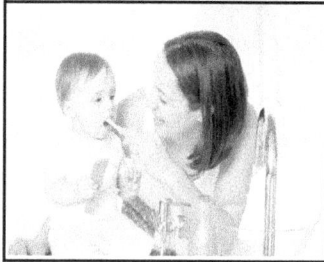

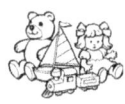

III
Baby Skin Care

From being couples to being parents, parenthood is a blissful journey that demands constant attention and commitment. Both first time parents and experienced ones need to understand that successful parenting is not easy and can only be attained by taking some proactive steps. Talking about the initial phase of parenthood, new born babies need a lot of care and concern. Right from the time they wake up in the morning till the time they go off to sleep and sometimes even during the night; parents need to be on toes to ensure their little one's sound health and wellbeing. However, most parents would complain that even after taking all the due precautions and measures, some way or the other their baby incorporates a problem.

A simple answer to the above mentioned problem is that babies are constantly growing. What may be good for your baby today can be bad tomorrow! Talking about baby skin care, it demands a lot of attention and care. Almost all of you would agree that there is nothing as lovely as the soft, delicate skin of the baby, but nothing as irritating as a cranky baby who cries all day due to rashes, cradle cap or any other skin condition. The delicate skin of your baby needs utmost care and attention. A small rash can be extremely annoying for the baby and if not treated in due time, chances are it might take bigger shape in days to come. If like most new parents, you too are confused about how to maintain the proper skin care of your baby to keep him/her happy and comfortable; then read on to know more about baby skin care.

1. Baby Acne Treatment

Baby's acne is a common occurrence in infants. These little red rough rashes are generally non-toxic and usually appear on the cheeks, nose, back and even tummy. It is basically transient in nature and painless, though the condition can aggravate if the baby comes in touch with saline water. However, to see your baby in distress is never a good feeling. A multiple number of reasons that are attributed to the occurrence of acne are hormonal causes (transmission of mother's left over hormones in the baby's body), bad bowel movement, unsuitable weather conditions, sticking of milk and saliva on the face, germs etc. Parents need to take it as nature's course, but if the acne persists for a longer period of time, it is advisable to consult a dermatologist. Parents should make sure that baby does not scratch his/her face as acne would get worse in that case. Treatment for baby acne is rather simple. All you need to do is take certain precautions to avoid aggravating the skin condition.

Treatment for Baby Acne

- Always use a mild baby soap on the acnes and do not rub the skin much, make sure your own hands are clean enough before you treat your baby's face and have a clean towel to pat it dry in order to reduce further complications.
- To ease out your baby's discomfort, dress him/her up in cool, comfortable cotton clothes that are not harsh against your baby's skin. Use soft natural detergents to wash their clothes.
- Do not use any lotions or creams on the acne site, as it will exacerbate the condition and make it difficult for the toddler or you to deal with it.

- ❏ Take advice from your dermatologist about using some diluted vinegar solution on the face of your baby. It is known to have some curable properties and can be helpful to treat your baby's rashes.
- ❏ Remember, never expose your babies to direct sunrays as it will harm them and may cause the skin to inflame further.
- ❏ Overall hygiene is crucial to your baby's health. Dirty and unhygienic conditions will only add to your bundle of worries. Keep your baby's body clean and germ free.
- ❏ Just keeping your baby in hygienic condition is not enough. Remember to wipe your baby's face with clean cotton wipes after every few hours. Also, regularly apply prescribed medication to the affected areas to heal the acnes as soon as possible.

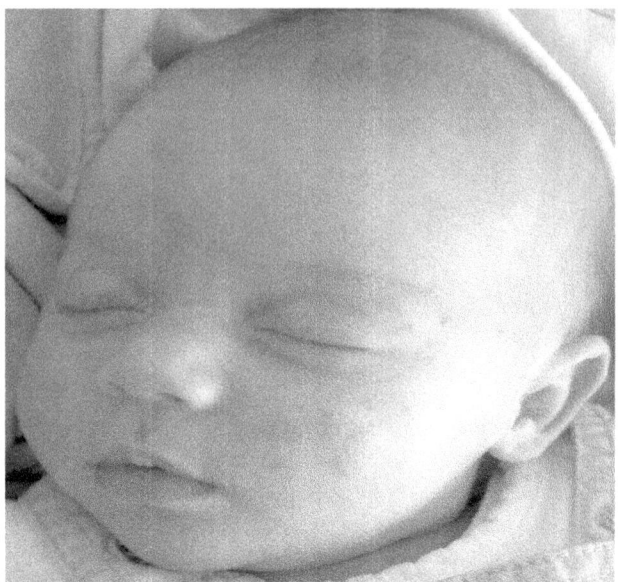

Treating baby acne

2. Cradle Cap in Infants

Cradle cap, also known as 'Crusta Lactea', is a yellowish, patchy, greasy and crusty skin rash that occurs on the scalp of new born babies. It is something quite common among the newborns and begins in the first 3 months of the baby's birth. It is usually not itchy and doesn't bother babies much. But, if it starts getting thicker and starts spreading, it becomes a matter of concern. The rash is prominent around the ear, the eyebrows or the eyelids. It can also spread and appear at other places also, where it is called 'Seborrhoeic dermatitis'. Almost half of the babies have a mild version of cradle cap. Since it is quite common among the babies, it is not taken seriously by the parents. Parents usually resort to homely remedies to deal with the problem, but, it is advisable to refer to the doctor. The earlier it is taken care of, the better it is for the baby.

Causes

The causes of cradle cap are not clearly defined. It is not caused by any infection, allergy or from poor hygiene. It is possibly caused because of the *sebaceous glands in the skin of newborn babies*, which is due to the mother's hormones still in the baby's circulation. These glands release a greasy substance that makes the old skin cells attach to the scalp instead of falling off after drying. Practitioners and physicians have also speculated that this disorder is caused because of baby's immature digestive system being unable to absorb sufficient 'biotin' and other vitamins of B complex.

Symptoms

- ❏ Thick and crusty yellow-brownish patches can be found on the scalp of the babies suffering from cradle cap disorder.
- ❏ The skin on the scalp of the baby becomes quite oily and greasy. An oily and shiny skin is a clear indication of the disorder.
- ❏ Babies suffering with cradle cap disorder may also experience hair loss.
- ❏ White and yellow flakes of skin form on the scalp.
- ❏ The skin of the scalp might even turn red in the worst scenarios. This is a rare happening, but if the problem increases, it might lead to a red itchy scalp.
- ❏ Sores can also get formed on the scalp, if the problem goes unattended for long.

Diagnosis

There is no well defined diagnostic test for cradle cap. The diagnosis is based on a thorough medical history and physical examination of the child. Examination of medical history includes family history of any skin problems, allergies or anything else that might have contributed to the problem. A physical examination, on other hand, includes the examination of any signs of cradle cap in the baby and its location. Also, any other rashes on the baby's body are also checked in for. If the doctor tracks any allergic reaction, then the baby is recommended to an allergist.

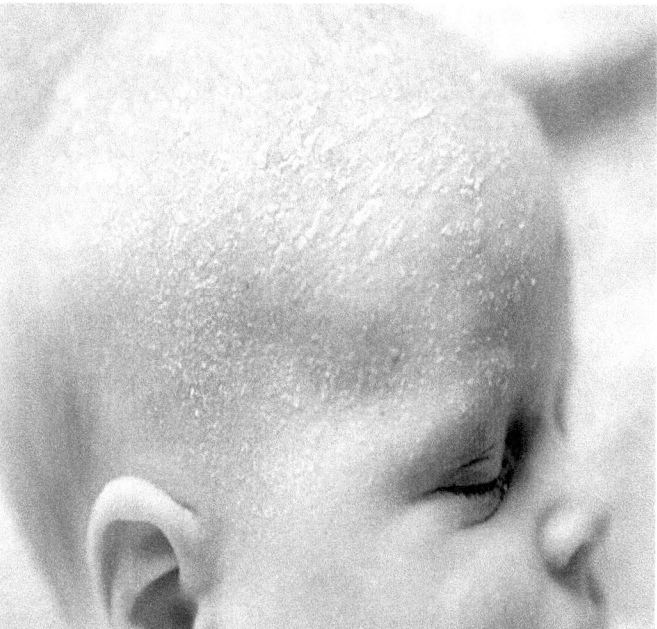

Cradle cap in babies

Treatment

- Oil can be gently applied to the scalp if it is very hard. Applying mineral oil or any baby oil before shampooing can help soften crusty patches of skin on the scalp. After applying oil, wrap it with warm cloth for an hour. Do not apply oil after shampooing, as it may stick the flakes to the scalp, which can worsen the condition.
- You can apply petroleum jelly like Vaseline liberally and leave it for overnight. The jelly will help the scales to soften and either fall off during night, or it can be brushed off in the morning.
- Brush the scalp gently with a soft brush or with your fingers. This will help loosen the flaky skin and will improve the circulation in the area. This should be done before shampooing. This will help clean the dead skin cells.
- Shampoo your baby's scalp every other day with a mild baby shampoo or soap. You can reduce the use of shampoo to twice a week once the skin flakes are no longer present on the scalp. The shampoo should not be used for more than once in a day as too much of cleaning of the area may cause dryness, thus worsening the condition.
- A paste can be made from sodium bicarbonate which can be applied on the affected area for 10 minutes. This is an effective method to get rid of the scales.
- Ketoconazole shampoos and creams are proving to be very effective in the treatment of moderate and serious cradle cap cases. Research indicates that this anti-fungal medication is not absorbed in the bloodstream.

3. Baby Skin Care in Winter

Everyone is concerned about their skin care, especially in winters and of course, the most delicate creatures among us are babies, who deserve it the most. Humidity starts to vanish from air and you start battling against cold waves that dampen your baby's skin badly. Cold waves in winters may result in chapping, redness and irritation on your baby's skin. A proper balance has to be maintained between clothing and skin care because even after ensuring proper skin care, wrong selection of clothes can hamper the care part. Spending long hours only on baby skin care can be worthless without knowing the right way to do it.

Tips for Winter Skin Care

- It's advisable not to make your baby take bath daily as there is less humidity in air and daily exposure to water can make the skin more rough and dry. Even if you daily do it, restrict the bathing time to just two or three minutes.
- Use baby lotions containing greasier contents and massage it on their body immediately after bath and try to maintain a cozy temperature in your room, especially at that time.
- Don't over dress your baby with woolens, as he/she may sweat internally, clogging their sweat pores and develops red rashes. Just try to cuddle them in soft fur like clothes for a soft touch to their skin.
- Your baby's skin can be oily or dry. For dry skin, give a massage of warm unscented oils and for babies having oily skin, a moisturiser massage is sufficient as more oil will give rise to acne.
- Use mittens and head covers like hats, caps and hoods for your baby's winter wear. These will help protect the delicate skin on hands, face and head. Consider using accessories, including stroller that has covers or blankets to shield against wind.
- During winter time, go for creams in place of baby powders in the baby's diapers. Creams form a protective layer that protects the skin against friction, moisture and discomfort.

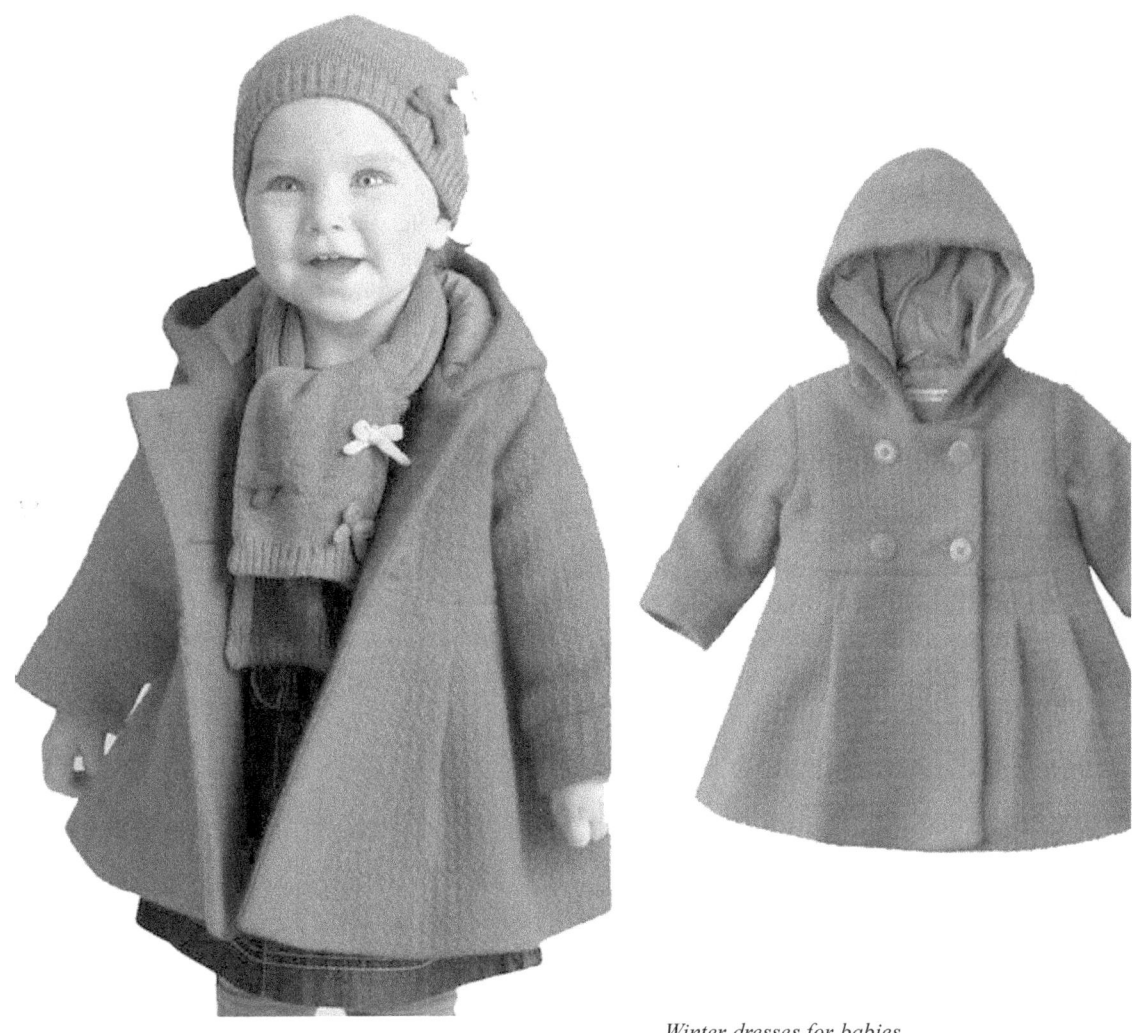

Winter dresses for babies

- Babies are vulnerable to frostbite as they rapidly lose heat in cold temperature and their lips tend to dry badly developing into painful sores. To prevent it, always apply lip care jelly for babies within a period of two to three hours.
- Also apply a light coat of petroleum jelly inside baby's nose, as harsh cold air can induce dryness in the nose and can result in bleeding at times. Check that your baby doesn't rub his or her nose.
- Make your baby drink an average amount of lukewarm water to keep the skin hydrated from within.

4. Baby Sun Protection

Wiggling toes, chubby little fingers, petal skin and glazing faces are the most prominent physical features of babies. However, they are also the most sensitive among all of us and can be badly affected by sunrays, if exposed to them without taking proper precautions and care. Their skin doesn't produce enough melanin, which acts as a shield to harmful sun rays. At the same time, if babies are inappropriately exposed to sun rays and get a sun burn, they can develop malignant melanoma later in life. It is a common belief that a couple of hours of sun exposure in a day helps babies to absorb vitamin D and all the metabolic functions in the body can be very well regulated by it. However, what matters is the time when you expose your baby to the sun. When the sun rays are the harshest, they can burn your baby's skin badly.

Tips for Sun Safety

- Set a time to expose your baby in the sun, preferably not between 11 to 3 as run rays are the harshest at this time and will harm your baby's skin, instead of benefiting it.
- If you are exposing your baby to sunlight, cover him/her with light coloured fabric, such as light blue or white, covering the head as well, as these colours do not absorb fully the sunlight but reflect it back. Always place the baby in such a position that his/her back is facing the sun. In this way, he/she will only get the healthy sunlight energy.
- If your baby is more than six months old, you can also buy some non-alcoholic, milky sun creams for them and apply it all over the exposed parts to seek more protection.

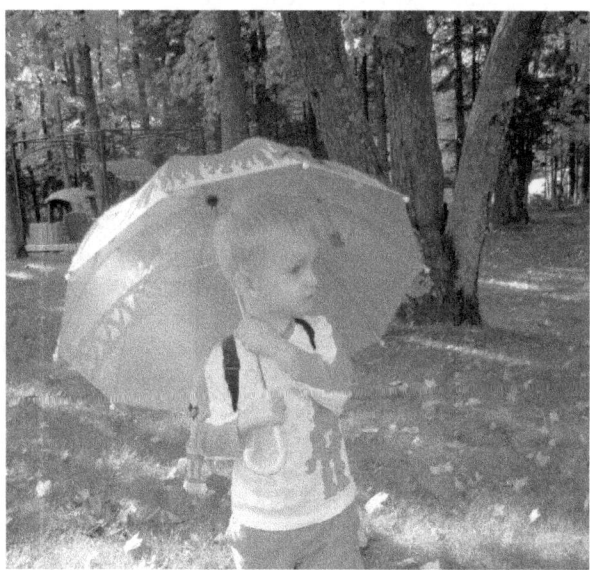

A baby boy with an umbrella

- You need to ensure that after you expose the baby to sunlight, he/she doesn't get any rashes on the skin, as it a sign of allergy and need not be overlooked.
- Look for toy sunglasses which have 100 percent protection from sun rays as pupil in their eyes absorb more light in the sun, which is not safe for your baby.
- Get a nice thick cloth cover for your baby, in case you are going outside and need to take your baby with you.
- Your baby's lips are also very sensitive. Always use petroleum jelly to shield lips from sun even on cloudy days, as most of the sunrays penetrate through clouds and can be harmful.
- If despite all possible efforts your baby does get sunburns, seek treatment for it and give your baby lots of fluids.

5. Daily Skin Care

The delicate and sensitive skin of your baby needs proper care. The air doesn't seem to be so much pure and crisp as before and the pollution in the air and surroundings can irritate the skin resulting into more sensitiveness. Special attention and care has to be given to your tiny tots, and their skin should be taken care of everyday, apart from daily body massages. Baby's skin is very delicate and much different from the adult's and can become extra sensitive to sunrays as enough melanin is not produced in babies. Parents are often seen to expose their babies directly to sunlight; however it is not a very healthy practice. Apart from taking certain precautions, use and application of baby skincare products is extremely relevant and proper guidance should be taken from dermatologists to serve the purpose.

Tips for Daily Skin Care

- Skin care for babies starts from their very first bath and parents should make sure that bath water is lukewarm in summers and a little bit warmer in winters, so that skin doesn't become dry or rash. Diluted soap should be applied to the skin for keeping it moisured. A mild moisturising lotion should be applied in good quantities on the skin to make it supple and soft.
- Babies often suffer from acne problems, but most of the time it is a temporary thing and disappears on its own, the reason being there are left over hormones in the baby's system from the mother. For the treatment part, make sure you never prick the acne, as it would result into scarring. Try some specially made natural baby skin products for acne prone skin or just make sure you often clean the acne area with damp cotton to make it dirt-free.
- Mineral-based oils can be avoided as they tend to dry the skin when absorbed, rather go for organic and natural oil like coconut, lavender, chamomile, rose, etc as they soothe the skin more and impart it more moisture.
- The soap used for baby's bath should be low alkaline baby soap. Harsh soap may hurt the baby's soft skin.
- Apply good amount of baby cream to the baby's skin especially during winters. Apply it soon after bath when the skin is moist. This will keep the baby's skin soft and supply throughout the day.
- Talcum powders for babies can contain bleach like substances that are harmful for your baby's skin and can darken portions of baby's body if accumulate on any area.
- Babies are always put into diapers and irritation starts to develop due to that, so make sure that you free your babies of diapers for two or three times in a day and apply some diaper rash cream on the parts in case of rashes, before fixing the diapers.
- Always use dye-free or fragrance-free detergents for washing baby clothes as usual family detergents may irritate the baby's skin and rashes can appear due to that.
- Selection of clothes is also very important as per the season, make sure you use linen or cotton clothes in summer as these fabrics make the air pass through quickly and rashes will not develop. In winters, clothes should be warm enough and loose-fitted, as skin can get red at some parts if tightly tied.

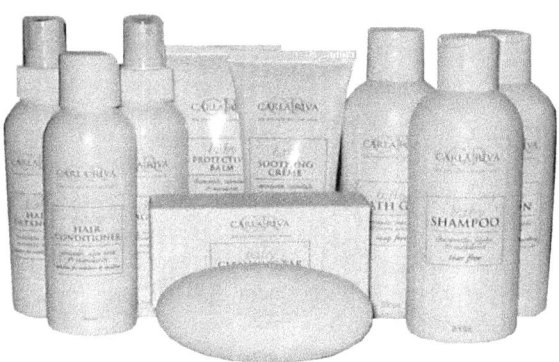 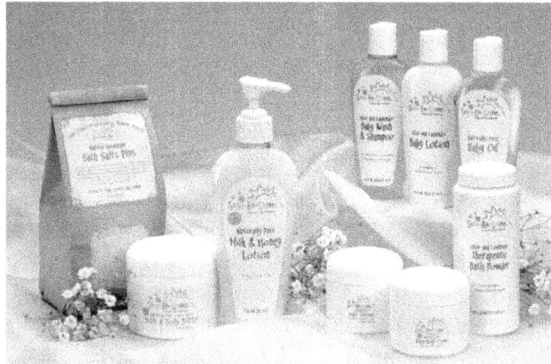

Skin care for babies

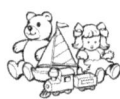

FAQs

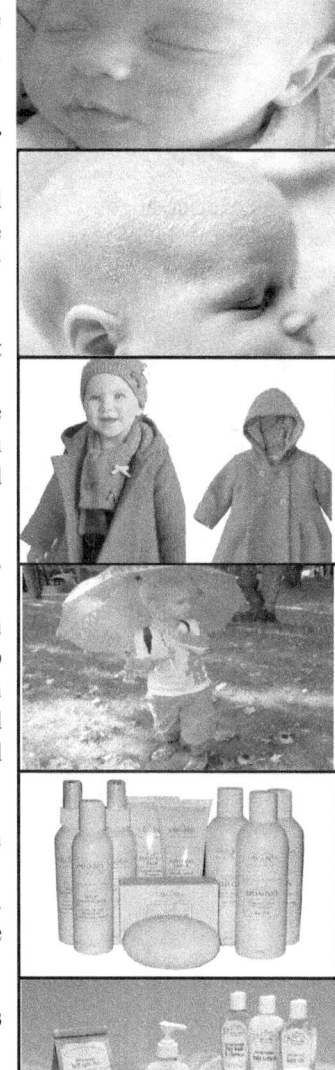

Q-1. What is cradle crap? How should I remove it?
Ans. Cradle cap is a type of dandruff of the scalp. It may be found as thick white or yellowish crusts and scales on the scalp. You should wash the baby's head regularly. If the rash persists or spreads to the face, ears, neck, armpits, etc, you should consult the doctor.

Q-2. My daughter has tiny pearly-white raised spots scattered over her face. How do I deal with them?
Ans. Often babies have 1-2 mm sized, pearly-white raised spots scattered over the nose, chin and forehead. They are called milia. They occur due to blocked sebaceous glands. Do not try to squeeze them.. they usually disappear without any treatment on their own.

Q-3. My son has little white, raised spots near the roof of his mouth. What are they and will they hurt him while feeding?
Ans. These little white, raised spots near the midline of the baby's palate are harmless cysts. In medical terms they are called Epstein pearls. If you look closely, they may be seen on gums as well. They are harmless and go away on their own. No treatment is needed.

Q-4. During winter, my baby's cheeks and chin become dry and chapped. What should I do?
Ans. The skin of the babies is very sensitive. Even a little rubbing with woollens can cause rashes. Make sure that his woollens do not rub on his chin and cheeks. Keep him away from cold winds as they can take away the natural moisture from the skin. Give an oil massage and moisturiser massage to the baby throughout the winter to avoid dry and chapped skin.

Q-5. How do I make sure that my son gets enough vitamin D from the sun but does not get sun burn?
Ans. While exposing your son to sunlight cover him in light coloured clothes. Do not let him face the sun directly. Allow his hands and feet to absorb the nutrition from the sunlight. Avoid harsh rays of the sun for too long.

Q-6. Should I sprinkle talcum powder on my baby during summer months to prevent prickly heat?
Ans. Use of talcum powder should be avoided as it tends to collect in the skin creases and may cause skin irritation and rashes. It may also enter the baby's eyes and nose and irritate him. To avoid prickly heat, keep the baby in a cool place and in cotton clothes.

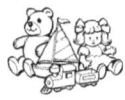

IV
Common Health Problems

Parents often worry that they will not be able to tell when their baby is unwell. After a few weeks, as you get to know your baby and understand his/her feeding-routine, sleeping and waking, you will be able to tell if the baby is behaving differently. It won't be long before you are able to judge your baby's health perfectly, once you understand his/her temperament and behaviour. The common health problems faced by all the babies can be dealt with at home, unless the case is not extreme. New parents often worry that they will not be able to tell when their baby is unwell. Once you get accustomed to the routine of your baby, you will be able to notice any change in behaviour or routine. Sometimes, you may not realise that your baby is ill. Here are a few signs that will help you detect that the baby is ill:

- ❑ Lack of energy
- ❑ Doesn't pass urine for over eight hours
- ❑ Stools are yellow-green in colour

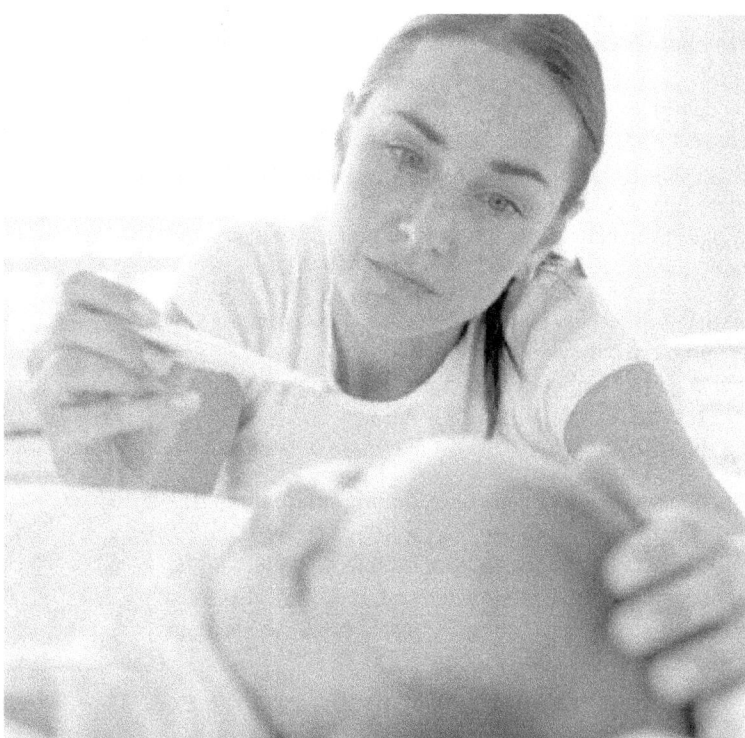

Child suffering from fever

- ❑ Not feeding normally
- ❑ Cries and is irritated when carried
- ❑ Is vomiting
- ❑ Feels hot and sweaty or hot and dry

However, a physician is to be immediately consulted if a particular condition is specific to your baby. Issues of sleeping, infancy problems and skin conditions are some of the general health related problems in babies. Vomiting is also a common problem that may occur due to some abdominal infection. Cough, cold and viral infection of the respiratory tract is also experienced by babies. However, with proper and regular care, these instances can be reduced significantly. It is important to keep in mind and follow some basic health guidelines that can go a long way in ensuring good health of your baby. A healthy baby will also keep active and display a pleasant disposition.

1. Body Temperature

Babies need to be comfortable at all times; their body temperature should neither be too hot nor too cold. No matter how healthy your baby keeps, fever among babies is a normal occurrence and though this is no cause to worry regarding your baby's safety, taking certain precautions can certainly help. If the body temperature constantly keeps high, you need to consult the doctor at the earliest and it may be an indicative of a deeper problem.

Ideal Sleeping Temperature for Babies

To sleep well, the baby doesn't need a specially heated room. Studies have found that a cool room allows both adults and babies to sleep well. The ideal temperature is around 18°C or 65°F. Babies, like adults, will need less clothing in summer. So, make sure you clothe your baby lightly, particularly while he or she is sleeping to ensure there is no overheating. If it is cold outside, you can wrap your baby with an extra blanket. However, once during the night, make sure you remove the extra layers of clothing to ensure that he/she doesn't get too hot.

Reading Baby's Temperature

People often tell you that you can find out whether your baby is hot or cold by feeling their palms and the sole of their feet. But these are not indicators of baby's body temperature. To find out the 'core temperature', place your hand flat against the skin of the baby's back or chest. If he/she feels pleasantly warm and not too hot or cold, it means his/her body temperature is normal. If the baby is very hot, he/she will feel sweaty, may have a heat rash around the neck and the face may be flushed. Reducing the number of clothes that the baby is wearing or the layers covering him/her will make him/her feel better. If the baby is feeling very cold, he/she will cry and even shiver. Sometimes, when the babies feel extremely cold, they will become motionless, as they want to safe energy to keep themselves warm. Adding clothing or covering will make them warm. You could hold them close to your body, so that they get warm as a result of your body heat.

Using an ear thermometer is the most accurate way of finding out the baby's temperature. You can find out the 'core temperature' by placing your hand flat against the skin of his chest or back. If he/she feels hot, it indicates that the baby has fever.

Dealing with Infant Fever

Put the baby in a cool room and dress him/her lightly. Sponging the baby with lukewarm water will reduce his/her temperature. Remove all his clothes except his nappy, dip the sponge in lukewarm water and gently rub all over his body. Allow this water to evaporate from the skin, thus lowering the temperature. When the baby has very high temperature, he/she may experience febrile convulsions or fits. This happens when the baby's temperature rises suddenly. Some children may face this before they are one year old. Consult the doctor if the body temperature doesn't come down even after sponging the baby.

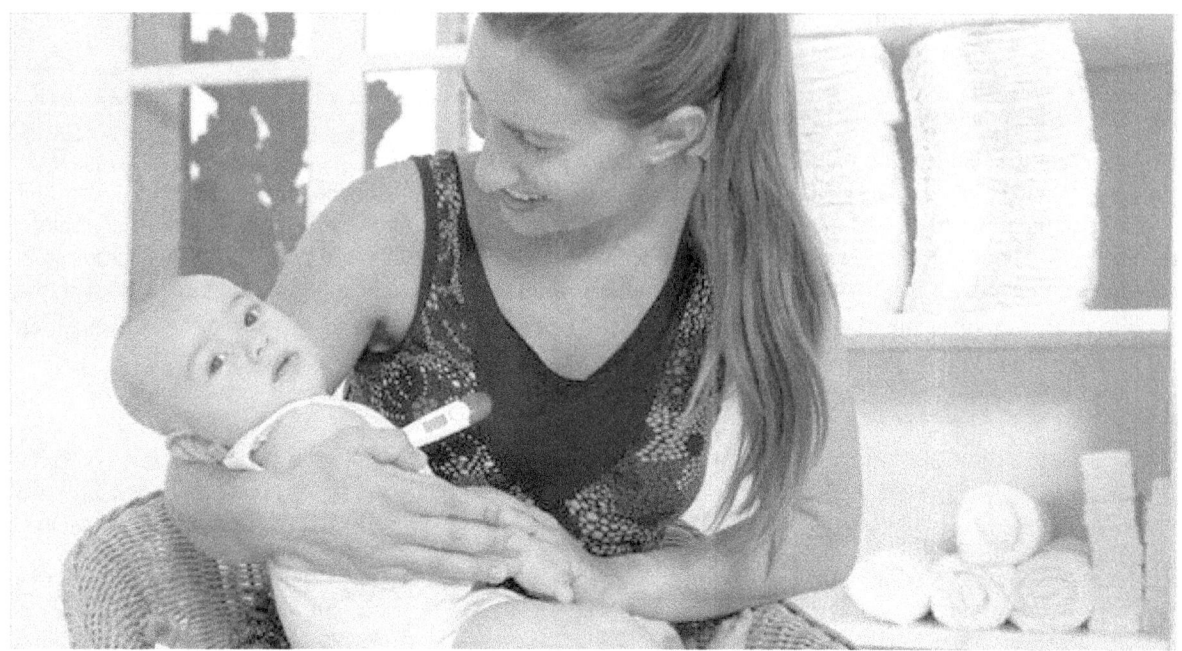
Dealing with infant fever

Tips to Maintain Temperature

- Baby's clothing should suit the weather and the heating within the house should suit the children and adults alike.
- If the house is centrally heated, your baby will be comfortable indoors in just a vest and a stretch suit.
- When the baby leaves the house, he/she may need more clothing depending on the temperature outside.
- At bedtime, cover the baby with as many blankets as you would use if you were sleeping in that room. Each folded blanket is equivalent to two blankets. You don't have to keep the central heating on through the night.

2. Teething Fever

Each baby has different teething patterns and symptoms, which can be generally recognised by fever, drooling, cranky behaviour and swollen gums. It takes a great deal of time in this process and involves much pain for them leading to discomfort and laziness. Babies generally do not have very high fever and the body temperature goes to a maximum of 100 degree Fahrenheit. In case it is more than that, parents should consult pediatricians for any medication advice. Most of the times, Pediatrics normally allow the baby to go through the teething process without any medication and gradually, they become fine. Teething also happens to be the root cause of ear infection due to the development of pressure on the infant's ear canal and sinus cavities by eruption of the new tooth. The process of teething can also follow hereditary patterns and will have almost similar patterns as per their parents.

Symptoms

- Fussiness is the initial and the main characteristic of fever from teething, as baby's mouth is painful due to sharp little tooth rising from the surface of the gums leading to soreness and discomfort.
- Drooling is caused by stimulation of teeth in the mouth and it can be excessive sometimes, so better pile a full lot of handkerchiefs around you!

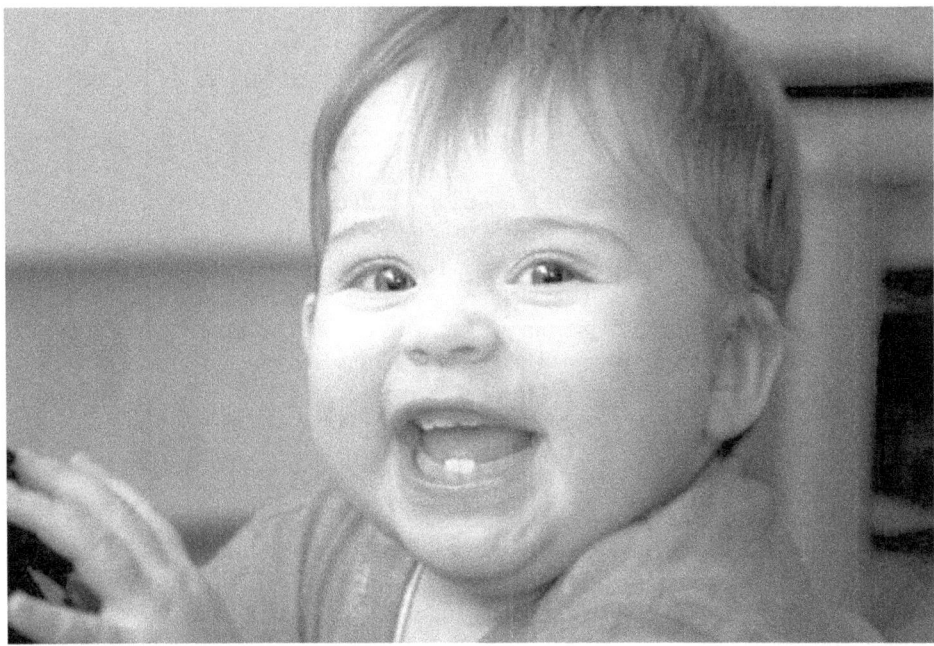
Baby with new teeth coming

- Fever is the most recognisable symptom of teething fever as it is a general indication to bulging out of teeth. The fever can be low or a bit high. In case of high fever, consult a pediatrician for prescription of medicines.
- Diarrhoea, running nose, lesser sleep, knowing, biting are common symptoms for teething fever in babies.

Treatment

- As the gums are painful and swollen, it is advisable to rub little pieces of ice on the gums which will help to relieve the pain and swelling.
- You can also gently rub frozen cloth or cold spoons on the gums of baby to soothe the pain relieving the heat in the body. This will also bring the fever down.
- With a prior consultation from pediatrician, take some gel or paste for gums and rub on the gums, with its disinfectant properties, it will kill the germs in the mouth and make your baby a little more less feverish.
- Getting a normal body temperature is purely natural, if the degree of fever is normal to 100 degrees. In case the temperature is above 100 degrees, you can keep some cold water cotton straps on the forehead of the baby. Try not to give medicines to babies and if required, consult a pediatrician for the same.

3. Flu

Your days were passing by happily with your baby. You were busy taking care of them and they were busy playing around and giving you more trouble. Suddenly one day, your baby gets uneasy and irritable. You take him/ her to the doctor and come to know that your little baby is suffering from some deadly flu. It is quite difficult to accept that suddenly your child has been attacked by some virus, isn't it? But, this uncertainty is always present with the growing babies. Their immune system is still developing and so weak. They are prone to get infected and attacked by any infection or virus if not taken care of. Flu of any kind is caused by a specific bug: the influenza virus.

Children under two years of age are more likely to get affected than the grownups, and the flu can prove to be quite dangerous for these young ones. Babies with flu require special care and full attention. The earlier the flu is detected, the better and easier it will be for you to provide medical attention to them. The symptoms of flu are quite common, which makes it difficult to diagnose. A baby with flu may simply be lethargic or may not eat as well, or they may have symptoms similar to that of cold. So because of the uncertainty and common symptoms and signs, it becomes important for the parents to be extra careful for their babies.

Causes

Influenza A and influenza B are potent pathogens flu viruses, which can easily spread through air. If your baby is near someone with the flu and is coughing and sneezing, they may breathe in infected droplets through their mouth and nose. The virus proliferates when people are in close contact. It travels easily through schools, playgroups, families and daycare centres. The victim will get sick one to four days after the exposure, making it difficult for diagnosing it. The severity of the virus differs from person to person, and because the symptoms are mild, many a time people mistake it to be just a simple cold. This unpredictability and invisible nature of the virus makes it a threat for the person affected and the ones around them.

Symptoms

- A child suffering from flu might show signs of sudden onset of fever, typically 101 degrees Fahrenheit.
- Congestion and normal coughing are also one of the symptoms of the flu, which are taken lightly and left unattended.
- The child may also suffer from fatigue and chills, followed by respiratory symptoms like running nose and dry cough.
- Your baby may also suffer with ear ache, which gets quite painful with time.
- Poor appetite, sore throat and swollen glands are few other signs of flu. The flu can also bring along abdominal pain, diarrhoea and vomiting making your baby irritable.
- The baby might also start wheezing or working harder for breathing than usual.
- A baby suffering with the flu might fall sick again and again, even after recovering back from the flu.

Treatment

- Nothing is better than giving your baby full rest and lots of fluids. Nurse your baby often and if they eat solid, try giving them frozen fruit bars to encourage them to get extra liquids along with soup or broth, this will ease their congestion.
- Do not pressurise your doctor to give antibiotics, which kill only bacteria, to your child. It is the virus not the bacteria that causes flu, so antibiotics won't be of any help. Antibiotics will only be useful if your baby develops any bacterial infection such as pneumonia, an ear infection as a result of having flu.
- If your baby is uncomfortable, ask your doctor whether you can give your baby a pain reliever like children's acetaminophen.
- Your baby may get better in three to five days. First the fever will break down and then their appetite will return. But, some children have cold and cough associated body aches that may hang on till two weeks or so.

Preventive Measures

Here are some ways to prevent flu in babies:

- **Vaccination**
  CDS or the Centre for Disease Control and Prevention, strictly recommends flu shots for all the people, children and adults. Even if your baby is too small for the shots, those who are in close contact should get vaccinated to reduce the risk of spreading the virus. This vaccine is more important for children in the high-risk group. Like if your baby is suffering with other diseases like diabetes, or a suppressed immune system, severe anaemia or a chronic heart, lung or kidney disease, they become more prone to get infected, so vaccination is a must for them.

But, this vaccination does not give a hundred percent guarantee. The effectiveness of the vaccine also depends on the health of your baby, and also how well the vaccine is matched to the virus that is circulating. If at all your baby gets flu even after getting vaccinated, there is a good chance that he/ she will get a milder case.

- **Be Hygienic**
  Hygiene is the best way to keep away from any kind of viruses or bacteria. Make sure that your baby's hands are always clean. Develop this habit in your baby and all other members of the family. This will prevent the germs from spreading. Keeping your baby away from the people who are sick will also help a great deal. No matter how clean and conscientious you are, your baby may get affected by the virus. So being hygienic is just a preventive step that you can take to help your baby stay away from the viral infections.

4. Common Cold

As parents, you can spend a long time distressing over your child's health and trying to figure out the exact reason behind that running nose or incessant coughing! Well, what you need to understand that babies being as delicate as they are, they are vulnerable victims to potent viruses. So it is normal for them to get frequent colds often. All you need to do is stop fretting and educating yourself more on the disease and ways of warding it off. A common cold is usually triggered by a viral infection that hits the upper respiratory tract of your baby, i.e., his nose and throat. Babies run a risk of catching cold because they are often surrounded by elders who don't always follow the basic hygiene of washing their hands. Also the chances of getting a cold increases during monsoons or cold weather. It is normal for your baby to get eight to ten colds in the first two years of his/ her life. Since common cold is quite common for babies, it is likely that one infection may linger on for several weeks. Also a cold can be an indication of some other infection too.

Causes

Common cold is nothing but a viral infection caused by rhinovirus, coronavirus, enterovirus and coxsackievirus. Once a baby has been infected with a certain kind of virus, it usually develops immunity against it. However, there are hundreds of other harmful viruses and your baby still runs the risk of catching cold every now and then. Some of the common causes of cold are listed below:

- Your baby can transmit cold by direct exposure with someone who is already infected.
- The virus can also spread if a sick person touches his mouth or nose and then touches your baby without washing his hands.
- Your baby may also catch cold by coming in contact with contaminated surfaces like toys, utensils, clothes, etc.
- Allergy and passive smoking can also speed up the intensity in which your child gets affected.
- Cold weather can instigate cold related problems. The air is usually dry during fall and winter and spending time outdoors can make your baby susceptible to cold.

Symptoms

Most colds are nothing less than an unnecessary trouble. However, it is important to note the signs of your baby when he/ she develop cold. Here are some common symptoms to check out for when your baby has cold.

- The first sign of cold is usually a runny nose followed by sneezing and coughing.
- Your baby may get fever due to infection.
- There may be congestion of nose which may in turn lead to breathing problems.
- Baby will refuse to nurse or show lack of appetite.
- The baby will become cranky, irritable and lethargic.

Complications

Frequent cold can lead to quite a few complications in your child. Though these complications are not very common, yet it is important to be careful and be aware of them. Some of the common complications that might show up soon after your baby have suffered a cold are:

- Babies suffering from common cold run a risk of developing ear infections. These infections can strike if the bacteria or virus creep into the space behind your baby's ear drum.
- Colds can lead to wheezing in your babies even if your child doesn't have asthma or other respiratory disorder.
- Colds can sometimes lead to sinusitis too. Inflammation and infection of the sinuses are common problems.
- Other serious complications generating out of common cold include pneumonia, bronchiolitis, croup and streptococcal pharyngitis.

Preventive Measures

A cold can be a miserable experience for your baby and the best way to combat cold is prevention. As they say "Prevention is better than cure", this saying especially stands true for cold since there is no perfect cure for it. You can avert the chances of your little one catching gold by following the below listed preventive measures:

- You can lower the chance of your baby getting infected by avoiding contact with any other person who is infected with cold. Keep a handkerchief handy to cover your baby's mouth to avoid all chances of droplet infections.
- Always keep your baby warm and avoid any exposure towards cold.
- If your child shows signs of cold, feed him with plenty of liquids as fluids are known to ease congestion and wash out all toxins from your body. You can also use saline drops to ease a baby's stuffy nose.
- Always wash your hands before feeding or attending to the needs of your child.
- Keep your baby's toys and pacifiers as much clean as possible.

Remedies

Sadly there is no known cure for common colds. Even the antibiotics don't help much when it comes to treating colds. The best way you can help ease your baby's discomfort is to keep him as warm as possible and consulting a doctor if your baby is below three years of age.

- If your child has fever, you can give him *Tylenol* or *Ibuprofen*. Never give aspirin to your babies as it can trigger other complications. Also avoid giving any medicines to your little one if he/ she is vomiting or dehydrated.
- It is important to keep your child hydrated when suffering from cold. Keep feeding him with fluids to avoid dehydration. If you are nursing, it is an added advantage since apart from keeping your child hydrated, breast milk is believed to offer extra resistance against cold causing viruses.
- Keep your baby's nasal passage clear to help him get over any breathing difficulty. You can use *nasal aspirator* with *saline nasal spray* to clean the passage and offer relief.

5. Asthma

Frequent cold and wheezing can indicate that your infant may be suffering from asthma. For that reason, it is always safe to check with your pediatrician and get your baby properly diagnosed. Asthma is a medical condition that causes airways and lungs to become aggravated and inflamed, thus making it difficult to breathe. It is difficult to determine if your baby has asthma until five years of age, as most other conditions in babies reveal similar symptoms. A baby's airways is usually small and a respiratory tract infection can cause the openings to swell and get congested with mucus leading to cough, wheezing and other related symptoms of asthma. A recurring wheeze is one of the initial signs of asthma. However, the presence of a cough alone does not specify that your baby is suffering from asthma. If you suspect that your baby is suffering from asthma, make sure to get it diagnosed as early as possible. Hence, early diagnosis and treatment is essential.

Diagnosis

It is difficult for a doctor to diagnose your baby with asthma before he/she is 12 months of age. Wheezing may not always indicate asthma as several other conditions can instigate this condition. Problems like bronchiolitis, respiratory viruses, cystic fibrosis, heart problems and milk aspiration can leave your baby gasping. Often, it is seen that babies with wheezing problem outgrow it when they grow old. It's important to understand that just one instance of wheezing cannot lead to asthma. Only if your child shows repeated signs of wheezing, you should take him to a pediatrician. Detailed observation and tests are required to confirm any signs of asthma in your baby. Doctors avoid making any early diagnosis as it might cause unnecessary anxiety to the parents and family. However, if the problem goes undiagnosed in your baby, it might lead to severe complications of lungs over time.

Causes

There are many things that might cause wheezing in infants. Any piece of food or alien object inhaled into the lungs might cause wheezing. Also, premature infants with underdeveloped airways may show signs of wheezing. Apart from these signs, any kind of physical exertion, too much crying or laughing, changes in weather, exposure to tobacco or cigarette, and allergens like pets, pollen and dust can trigger asthmatic attacks.

Symptoms

Asthma is generally the outcome of complex relationship between a baby's genes and his environment. The common symptoms of asthma include coughing, wheezing, tightening of chest, rapid breathing, fever, short of breath after any physical activity. The intensity of these symptoms may usually vary from child to child.

Consulting the Doctor

If your child shows repeated wheezing or suffers from bouts of coughing, especially in the night, you need to consult the doctor. Also check out for any kind of breathing problem in your child after any physical activity. Check if your child suffers from respiratory uneasiness in certain conditions like cold, or cold air allergens, or even pets or dust and smoke, etc. Also, don't forget to tell your doctor if you have a family medical history of allergies, asthma and sinus problems.

Treatment

Although it is difficult to say if your baby suffers from asthma before the first five years of his/her life, his/her wheezing can definitely be checked with proper medications. The doctor might even recommend asthma medications to see if the condition improves. As these medicines are meant for infants and babies, they usually outrun the risk of any probable side-effects. Most often, the doctor decides the medicines and its frequency is based on severity of breathing problems and the symptoms. Asthma medicines are often delivered using an inhaler with a spacer or through a nebulizer. It is important to teach everyone in the house how to use the inhaler and nebulizer, so that they can attend to the baby when in distress.

Misconceptions

Some common misconceptions regarding asthma are:
- ❏ It is said that breast-feeding can reduce the risk of asthma in your babies. Though there is no proper study to back this, it is believed that breast-feeding has many advantages and can thus help reduce the risk in your baby.

- Hydrolysed milk formulas or soy formulas are believed to be especially helpful in saving your babies from developing asthma. This belief is however very hypothetical.
- It is assumed that taking probiotics when pregnant can reduce the risk of asthma. But again, there is no concrete proof to support this theory.
- Skipping on potential allergens in the diet (e.g. eggs, milk, nuts and shellfish) during pregnancy or during breast-feeding does not appear to prevent asthma.
- Also avoiding house dust mites or not allowing pets inside the house does little to prevent asthma in babies as contrary to the popular belief.

6. Vomiting

Vomiting is actually a strong reflex action which involves an upward motion of all the contents in the stomach, from the body's digestive system to the mouth. At the time of vomiting, all the muscles of abdomen and chest contract together, causing pain and exhaustion. It is actually a symptom and not a disease. The episode is troublesome for all, but affects babies deeply as their body is not strong enough to take in the pressure caused. It is normal for babies to vomit during the initial weeks, because this is the time when their body adjusts to changes in feeding patterns. Usually, an episode of vomiting subsides after six to ten hours, without any treatment, except a minor change in the regular diet. However, if vomiting continues for the whole day or every time your little one binges on food and liquids, it is a cause of concern and should be immediately consulted, to find out the underlying cause and the treatment. There are numerous reason as to why vomiting in small babies occur and most of them can be treated by using simple measures. in the following lines, we have provided detailed information on the causes and treatments of vomiting in kids.

Causes

A common physiological problem, vomiting in infants is mainly due to the underdevelopment of the digestive system. The posture of the baby is yet another major factor which causes vomiting or queasiness. In an infant body, there are valves at various places of the digestive tract. These valves are underdeveloped and are mainly present to prevent the backflow of the content to the previous organs of the digestive tract. Since these valves are in an underdeveloped stage, they allow the contents of the stomach to travel back to the infant mouth, thereby causing vomiting.

Some of the underlying reasons as to why vomiting in kids occur are acidity, indigestion, worms and certain infectious diseases involving digestive systems like typhoid, cholera and enteritis. On rare occasions, dangerous situations in vomiting include bloody vomiting which suggest internal hemorrhage and tuberculosis. Dark greenish or some abnormal coloured vomitus implies ingestion of poison.

Treatment

The best treatment for avoiding vomiting in infants is *burping*. It is a method wherein the infant is gently patted on the back, from top to bottom, so that all the milk consumed goes down in the stomach and nothing remains in the food pipe. In case of vomiting in babies and children, the best treatment is to make them drink boiled water. This would prevent the infection which causes vomiting. Also, it is best advised not to over feed children. Leaving a small portion of the stomach empty is the best way to avoid vomiting or feeling of nausea.

The diet chart for kids should be such that it involves frequent eating of small meals rather than binging on large meals once or twice a day. Also, there should be a gap between two meals. This is mainly to ensure proper digestion of the food. However, if none of the above mentioned tips work, medications in the form of syrups, pills, tablets and injections that have anti-nauseant or anti-vomiting property is advised after proper consultation from a specialised doctor.

7. Nappy Rash

Nappy rash is a common problem faced by infants. It is characterised by the inflammation of the skin in the nappy area. Stale urine and faeces accumulated in the nappy make the baby's skin become sore. Irritation in the area surrounding the nappy is another indication of nappy rash. As a result, spots or blotches (red or pink in colour) may appear in the affected area, thereby, aggravating the problem. While most of the nappy rashes are mild and can be treated with simple skincare routine, the pain or discomfort experienced by the baby makes it a problem that needs to be fixed as soon as possible.

A baby with nappy rash

Causes

- When a nappy, with stale urine and faeces, is worn by a child for a long time, the waste products are converted into ammonia, a chemical that can irritate the infant's skin, making it become sore and inflamed.
- Fungal infection is another leading cause of nappy rash. In case your baby's skin is damp for a long time, it can lead to the growth of fungus known as *candida*. The baby's skin starts reacting to the production of ammonia. When it is exposed to the fungus, the problem is even more aggravated.
- Apart from the above causes, nappy rash can also be a problem due to *eczema*. If your child is already suffering from eczema, the skin around the nappy area can become dry and sore. Moreover, he/she will not be able to find relief from nappy rash even after frequent nappy changes.
- The red and scaly skin of the baby is caused by *seborrheic dermatitis*, which is another cause of nappy rash. This condition is commonly seen in baby aged between two weeks to six months.
- Bacterial infection is another prevalent cause of nappy rash. Check whether your baby's nappy is unhygienic, or infected with bacteria.
- Allergic reaction to a particular substance, such as grooming products including soap, fragrances, detergents, oils, and powders can trigger nappy rash. The condition may even lead to irritation and inflammation on the affected part of the body.

Baby Nappy Rash Treatment

- Change the nappy of your baby regularly. Be sure to replace the spoiled nappy with a new one, whenever your baby defecates. Even if a nappy can soak the urine for a long time, it is better to change it frequently.
- Leave your baby to play around without wearing a nappy, as long as possible. He/she would feel better without the nappy. Moreover, the rash will be healed quickly.
- Do not forget to follow a skincare routine for your baby. Clean the genital areas of the baby, every time after he/she defecates. Allow the area to dry completely, before putting on a new diaper.
- You may cover your baby's nappy area with a thin layer of protective ointment or a baby powder. Do this only after ensuring that your baby is not allergic to such products.
- Allow room for air to circulate in the nappy area. Therefore, do not tighten the diaper too much. Nappies should fit somewhat loosely, so that the area of the body is allowed to 'breathe'.
- A normal nappy rash may continue for two to three days. If the condition persists for more than five days, consult a doctor and get a medicine prescribed for the same.

8. Hypoglycemia and Colic

Hypoglycemia is a condition characterised by low levels of sugar in blood. We need a certain amount of sugar, in the form of glucose, for normal functioning of the body. When the level of glucose in the blood decreases, it affects the functioning of our brain. While in the womb, the baby feeds through the umbilical cord and the blood glucose levels are more or less constant. After childbirth, the umbilical cord is cut and the baby has to adjust to the resultant fall in blood glucose levels. Immediately after birth, it is normal for the glucose levels in the blood to drop for a day or two. The baby's brain will get the energy it requires from the glycogen that is stored in the liver and is a substitute for glucose. In certain babies this may not happen, thereby leading to *hypoglycemia*.

Causes of Hypoglycemia in Newborns

The baby may not feed well for the first few days. As long as he/she is healthy and normal, there is no cause to worry. If the baby is breast-feeding, there is no need to give him sugar water to increase his glucose level. Some causes of Hypoglycemia in Newborns are:

- Sickness in babies
- Premature birth
- Not developing well in the womb.
- Babies whose mothers are diabetic are also susceptible to Hypoglycemia.

Monitoring the Baby

In case the baby is suffering from Hypoglycemia, he/she is monitored in the above categories closely.

- Baby's body temperature
- Baby's respiratory function
- Baby's skin colour
- Watch whether the baby is restless

If the blood sugar levels are very low, the baby may be administered glucose drips intravenously.

Colic and its Symptoms

The word, 'colic' is used to describe a specific crying pattern. If the baby draws his knees to his stomach, clenches his fists and makes a disgusting face while crying, he/she has colic in all likeliness. Colic usually begins when the baby is three or four weeks old and is, at its worst, when the baby is about eight weeks old. Babies with colic cry for long spells, which can last a few hours, usually in the evening or night. Though the child can be consoled for sometime, he/she begins to cry again for no apparent reason. Normally, babies with colic are happy, in good health and well developed. It is in very rare cases that colic lasts beyond three months. Some babies may show signs of colic, till they are about five months old.

Causes

- An upset stomach
- Underdeveloped nervous system
- Fluid that flows back into the esophagus from the stomach.
- Air trapped in the stomach forming gas.

Tips to Help the Baby

- Bath the baby in lukewarm water.
- Wrap him/her in cotton covering so that he/she feels safe.
- Give him/her feet a massage.
- Give him/her a dummy to suck on.

- ❏ Give him/her gripe water or colic drops.
- ❏ Dissolve three tbsps of sugar in a cup of boiling water, cool it and then slowly give it to the baby using a teaspoon.

You can consult your doctor for more advice. Ask family members to help out in taking care of the baby if crying is a regular feature.

9. Irritable Bowel Syndrome

Babies often suffer many serious problems and they become more complex when you follow your own treatments and wait for the problems to vanish by itself over a period of time. Sometimes, parents seldom realise that some overlooked matters related to your child's health can subject to severe results detrimental to baby's health. One of the common health problems among your babies can be irritable bowel syndrome which is not a very dreadful disease but can lead to crampy pain, gassiness, bloating and change in bowel habits. Babies are more or less fragile beings and even any small infection can adversely affect their health.

Parents have to take notice about any bad health and should fully understand its affects on baby. Sometimes food can be the main culprit and when given occasionally, can trigger the stools to occur more often thus, adding to the syndrome. For the accurate diagnosis of the syndrome, parents need to take the baby to the doctor and get him examined for tests. Tests are mostly carried out by blood sample examinations. In other cases, *endoscopy* can also be carried out and better diagnosis can be stated for the right treatment.

Causes

- ❏ Ordinary activities like eating or distention of gas or other material in baby's colon can trigger to overact with irritable bowel syndrome.
- ❏ Spasms can be pulled out in babies if fed with milk or milk products very often.
- ❏ Heredity is also a predisposition to occur in babies as they can inherit this syndrome from the genes of parents or ancestors.
- ❏ Mostly large intestine is not able to absorb much salt or water from the food and leads to uncomfortable contraction of colon producing irritable and uncomfortable movements.

Symptoms

- ❏ Abnormal passage of stools creating a feeling of emptiness in the stomach
- ❏ Mucus passage
- ❏ Green stool
- ❏ Frequency is abnormal like 3 or 4 stools per day
- ❏ Bloating of abdomen

Treatment

- ❏ Initially babies with this syndrome shouldn't be given much food to eat, especially milk or sugar rich products as they develop intolerance to sugar and fat rich food. If the symptoms for the syndrome do not disappear over a day or so, the baby should be taken to the doctor.
- ❏ A baby suffering from this syndrome should be given water containing ORS which is available at any medical store and is suggested safe by doctors. ORS is given to replenish lost fluids in the baby's body and the quantity should vary between one to two glasses a day.
- ❏ If parents observe that there is lesser constipation than fibre rich food can be provided to them and in case you figure out that after having fibre food, baby is still in the same condition then do not provide supplements rich in fibre.
- ❏ It is advisable to consult a doctor in this condition as it is the question of a baby's health and they are far more delicate than adults. Thus, complete care and precautions should be taken in these cases.

10. Jaundice in Newborn Babies

A baby in the womb is totally dependent on his/her mother for food and oxygen, which reach the umbilical cord that connects him/her to the mother. The distribution of oxygen through the baby's body is aided by the additional red blood cells present in the baby's blood. After birth, the baby begins to breathe through his/her lungs and hence, does not need the additional red blood cells. His/her body will start disposing of the extra cells, soon after birth. These red blood cells are destroyed in spleen. A major by-product, thus produced, is bilirubin. The liver removes the bilirubin from the bloodstream and passes it on to the intestines of the baby.

Since the infant's liver is still in its developing stage, it is unable to manage the sudden increase in bilirubin, during the first few days post birth. As a result, large amounts of bilirubin mixes in the blood, thereby, making the baby's skin appear yellowish, which is a symptom of jaundice. Although it is natural to find newborns suffering from jaundice in the first few days post birth, a high concentration of bilirubin in the blood is considered a serious case. In such a situation, you should get the condition monitored by the doctor.

Treating Jaundice in Infants

- Breast-feeding is one of the most effective ways to reduce the amount of bilirubin in the blood of the newborn, because mother's milk contains some of the important nutrients required for the development of the baby's functional organs. Breastfeed your baby every two hours post birth. Frequent feeding can help the baby pass the excess bilirubin through his poop and thus, reduce the jaundice symptoms.
- Sunbath is an effective remedy to treat jaundice in newborns. Remove the clothes of your baby and place him/her under direct sunlight or in a warm room for about 10 minutes. Lay your baby on a blanket, under

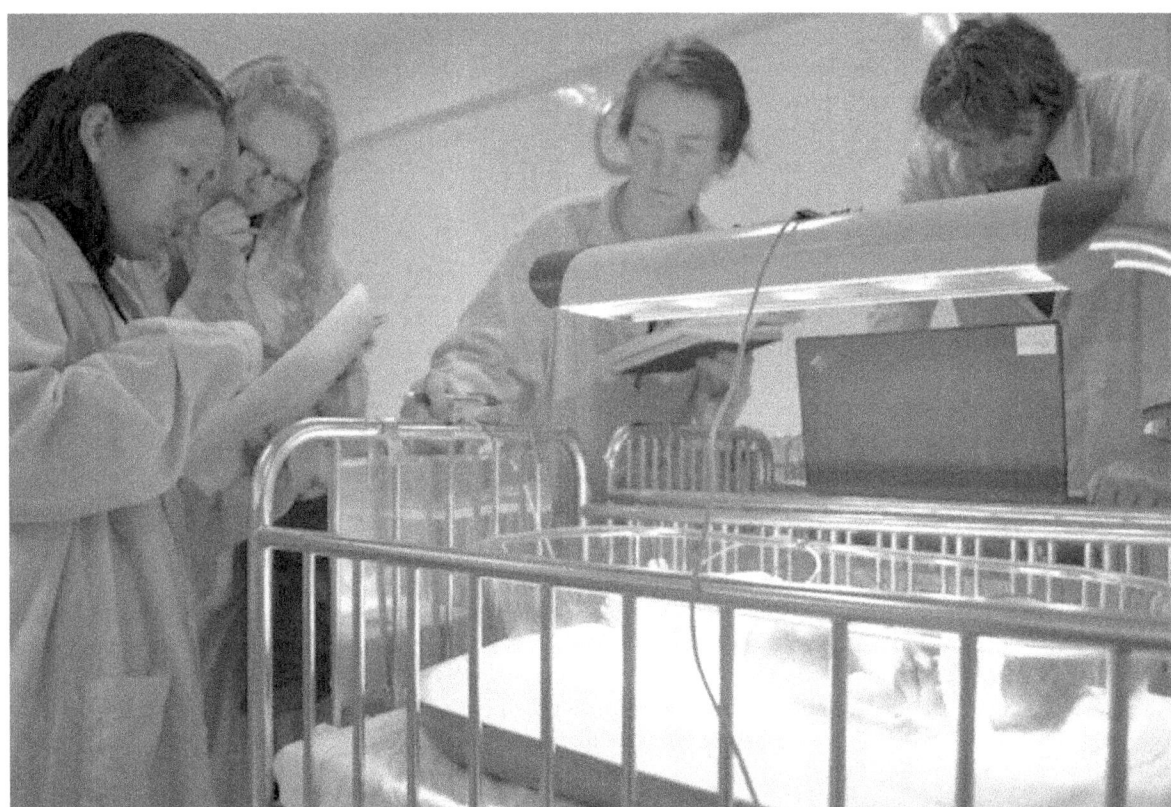

Treating jaundice in babies

the window, so that the sun's rays bathe his/her entire body. Be sure to block your newborns to avoid direct sunlight. The best time to sunbathe the baby is early morning hours, between 7 am and 8 am.
- In case the levels of bilirubin in your infant's blood are high, the doctor will administer phototherapy to treat the problem. During the treatment, your baby will be monitored under 'special lights' at the hospital, for 24 hours or 2 days. The special lights will eliminate jaundice by reducing the bilirubin levels.
- Another way to treat jaundice in newborn is to substitute breast-feeding with formula. Depending upon the level of bilirubin in the baby's blood, the doctor may suggest to feed the baby on a formula (similar to mother's milk), for about 48 hours. After the bilirubin levels are back to normal, the physician would suggest to switch back to breast-feeding.

11. Anaemia

Your active and playful child suddenly displays signs of tiredness, weakness, irritation and has a pale face. These are nothing, but signs of anaemia. Anaemia is a condition in which there is an abnormally low level of RBCs and haemoglobin in the body. Red blood cells are the oxygen carrying cells, so when they become less in number, the body has to work harder to generate enough oxygen. To identify anaemia in adults is not a difficult job, as they exhibit clear signs. However, tracking anaemia symptoms in newborns is rather difficult. Only a very observant and keen mother would be able to notice this in her baby. The most typical signs of anaemia in babies are tiredness, inactiveness and pale skin. It is important to know the cause of anaemia in your baby, to treat it at the earliest.

Causes

These are some causes of anaemia in babies :

- **Abnormality in Haemoglobin**
  The structure and function of the RBCs depend upon the quality and quantity of haemoglobin present in the body. Certain inherited disease may cause abnormality in the haemoglobin. This in turn, causes the life of RBC's to reduce and they get destroyed at a higher rate. When the bone marrow is not able to keep pace with the dying cells, anaemia occurs. One such example is the sickle-cell anaemia. However, this problem is not so common with the babies.

- **Abnormal Shape of RBCs**
  Blood vessels are little tubes which run throughout the body. Sometimes, these tubes are large, while sometimes, they are microscopic. The tubes may be so small that at times, only one RBC can fit in through. Normally, Red Blood Cells are in the shape of a doughnut, giving them enough flexibility to pass through these small passages. However, if the RBCs are of abnormal shape, they may get stuck in the tube, causing it to fleece and destroy, thus resulting in anaemia

- **Deformity in Bone Marrow**
  The bone marrow plays an important role in producing RBC's. If some deformity takes place in the body, it will hamper the functioning of the bone marrow. Certain viruses and medications may cause such a dysfunction. Leukemia or cancer of the bone marrow also leads to a decrease in the production of normal RBCs.

- **Lack Of Proper Nutrition**
  To make RBCs, the body needs adequate amount of iron, foliate and vitamin B12. A lack of iron and vitamins lead to inadequate RBC production in the body and thus, anaemia. However, this usually occurs in infants on whole cow's milk, prior to one year of age and premature babies. Breastfed infants hardly encounter this problem.

- **Other Causes**
  Many other chronic illnesses can also slow down the process of cell formation and reduce the RBC count.
  Lead poisoning can also cause *anaemia* in children.

12. Polio

In their early years, a child is exposed to the risk of developing serious ailments that can last for a lifetime and in certain cases prove fatal too. Educating yourself on the signs of possible illness in babies and the various vaccinations can outweigh all risks and ensure your baby has a healthy and happy childhood. Vaccinations today are considered as one of the safest and the easiest ways to deflect any possible threats to your child's health. Immunizing your baby can be a life saviour for your little one. Polio is certainly a big example on how immunization practice has helped to avert a grave disease among kids today. Polio has been wiped out of most countries with only a few developing nations facing its threat now. For this, babies are now being given routinely polio vaccines to ward off any possible threat to their health. However, due to polio being almost eliminated now, most parents often do not realise how important it is to vaccinate their little one against this disease. Polio is a serious life crippling ailment and if not taken care of, it may show up as an ultimate danger to your child's life.

Effects of Polio

Polio is a highly contagious viral illness that can induce graver health complications like paralysis, respiratory disorders and even death. A person exposed to polio may not reveal any serious symptoms initially. However, at times polio virus can show flu-like indications in non-paralytic form and a much graver symptom in paralytic polio. In paralytic polio, the polio virus attacks the central nervous system, crippling the entire system and at times proving fatal. Anybody suffering from paralytic polio may lose the ability to use one or both the limbs, and face complications while breathing. The rate of recovery depends from person to person, but people afflicted with polio will complain of weakness in their arm and leg for their entire life. Also the chance of recuperating from paralytic polio is quite low.

Symptoms

Given that polio can have life threatening complications, it is surprising to note that most people infected with the disease never realise that they are affected. People suffering from non-paralytic polio or abortive poliomyelitis may reveal the usual symptoms of viral illness like fever, sore throat, headache, vomiting, malaise, back pain, neck pain, pain or stiffness in limbs, muscle spasms and even meningitis. Paralytic polio, which is a more serious but rare form of this disease shows initial symptoms of fever and headache and other signs of non-paralytic polio in the beginning. However, later signs like loss of reflexes, severe muscle aches or spasms, loose and floppy limbs might show up as the infection progresses. Paralysis may hit all of a sudden.

Causes

- Polio is caused by a virus that lives in the throat and intestinal tract. It primarily spreads through human faces and thrives in areas with poor sanitation.
- It can also be transmitted through throat secretions.
- People with weak immune system and those who haven't been immunized are likely to catch poliovirus, if exposed to infected person or contaminated surroundings.
- Poliovirus spreads itself through contaminated water, food, or even through direct contact with the infected person.
- Due to the highly contagious nature of the virus, people infected with it can continue to spread the virus weeks on through their faces even after the disease has been detected.

Possible Threats

Anyone who has not been immunized against the disease has the maximum chances of acquiring it. Expecting mothers, young infants and children and adults with fragile immune systems living in unhygienic conditions and in areas without regular or non-existent immunization programs, are potent victims of poliovirus. If you have not been immunized against polio, here are some things to watch out for:

- ❑ Do not travel to areas where polio is common or has recently suffered an epidemic.
- ❑ Avoid being in direct contact with someone who is infected with poliovirus.
- ❑ Do not deal with lab specimens containing poliovirus.
- ❑ You need to be careful if you have undergone tonsillectomy.
- ❑ Stay away from doing any taxing physical activity once exposed to poliovirus as it might further depress your immune system.

Complications

Paralytic polio may have grave consequences like paralysis, disability, and deformities of the hips, ankles and feet in children. Although they may be corrected with surgeries or therapies, it may not be possible in areas where polio is still prevalent.

Diagnosis

Polio can be easily diagnosed by following symptoms like back stiffness, abnormal reflexes, and difficulty swallowing and breathing. A stool test or samples of throat secretions and cerebrospinal fluids may be checked to confirm the presence of poliovirus in the patient.

Treatment

- ❑ Polio is untreatable once infected and hence the prime focus of a treatment is usually aimed on offering comfort, quick recovery and averting further complications.
- ❑ The patient should be given complete bed rest.
- ❑ A nutritious diet is strictly advised.
- ❑ Antibiotics are usually prescribed to deal with secondary infections.
- ❑ Analgesics are advised to relive pains.
- ❑ Portable ventilators to help in comfortable breathing.
- ❑ Physiotherapy to avoid deformity and loss of muscle function.

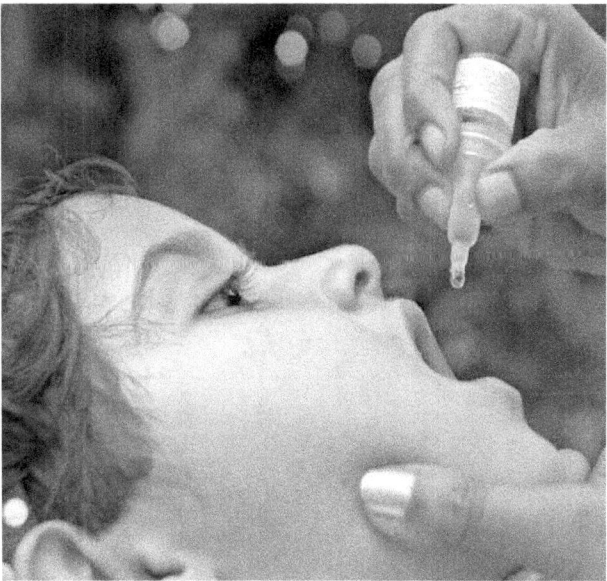

Polio vaccine being administered

Prevention

Apart from improving public sanitation and maintaining personal hygiene, another successful way to put a stop to this disease is through polio vaccine. The OPV (Oral Polio Vaccine) and the IPV (Inactivated Poliovirus) is effective against polio and offers resistance to people with weakened immune system. However, IPV is not recommended for anyone who is allergic to antibiotics, streptomycin, polymyxin B and neomycin. If you or your child experiences an allergic reaction after any shot, get medical help immediately. The common symptoms of allergy are high fever, breathing disorder, weakness, wheezing, skin rashes, rapid heart rate, swelling of the throat, dizziness and unusual paleness. Polio vaccine is normally given to your baby together with other vaccinations, including diphtheria, tetanus and acellular pertussis (DTaP); hepatitis B-Haemophilus influenzae type b (HBV-Hib); and Pneumococcal Conjugate Vaccine (PCV).

13. Malaria

It can be most disheartening for parents to see their little one down with sickness. Babies are more prone to infections during their early years of infancy. As parents, the best gift you can give your child is a healthy childhood. Nutritious diet and basic hygienic care may not be always enough to protect your baby from acquiring harmful diseases. What you need is a correct attitude and proper awareness towards your baby's health to combat all risks. Most parents often fancy thinking that their babies are less likely targets of diseases like tuberculosis and malaria. With the result they end up treating fever and flu as general signs of cold when at times it could indicate something graver. Educating yourself on some of the most common health threats of your child can help you fight all risks of infections. Malaria is one of the most common diseases to be found in children below five years of age. Malaria is a mosquito-borne parasitic infection generally characterized by fever, chills, and sweating. Malaria parasites contain the capacity to inflate in a short time thereby posing a risk of epidemic. A little care, proper diagnosis and timely medication can help save you a lot of trouble.

Causes

Malaria is more common in warm, tropical climate. A baby acquires malaria when smitten by an infected Anopheles mosquito and the parasites enter his/her bloodstream to his liver. Malaria can be treated with anti-malarial drugs. However, not all drugs are suitable for your baby.

Symptoms

- ❑ Babies suffering from malaria will show sudden behavioural changes like irritability, lethargy, drowsiness, loss of appetite and aversion towards food.
- ❑ Your baby is likely to get fever when suffering from malaria. In certain cases, the fever can rise with time while in some infants, the fever can shoot up immediately and go as high as 105 degrees.

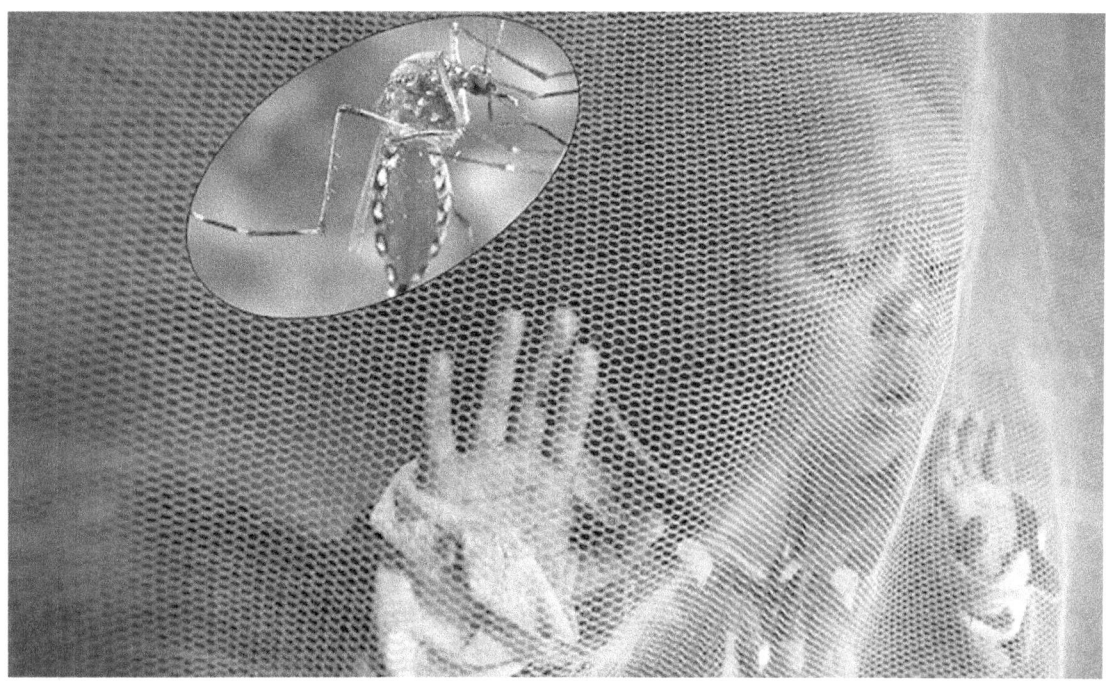

A baby in a mosquito net

- When your baby is down with malaria, he will show flu-like symptoms like chills, sweating, headaches and muscle aches.
- Your baby may also show some rare symptoms of nausea, vomiting and diarrhoea when suffering from malaria.
- If malaria affects your baby's brain, it might lead to serious and aggressive symptoms like seizures, convulsions and unconsciousness.
- Your baby might pass less urine or even suffer kidney damage or kidney failure if malaria affects the kidneys.

Diagnosis

Malaria can be diagnosed very easily. A blood test is all it takes to confirm if one is infected with malaria.

Treatment

Malaria can at times lead to severe complications. Therefore, prompt diagnosis and treatment is required to fight it. Anti-malarial medicines, such as *chloroquine* or *quinine*, given by mouth, by injection, or intravenously (into the veins) are used to treat malaria. The type of medicine prescribed, and the term of your treatment, will rest on a number of factors like the type of malaria, whether you are pregnant, your age, the place where you were infected and the severity of the symptoms. Doctors usually look out for signs of dehydration, convulsions, anaemia, and other complications that can affect the brain, kidneys, or spleen in the patient. Babies suffering from malaria should to be kept on fluids, blood transfusions, and breathing assistance.

Prevention

Malaria is a serious threat to underdeveloped nations, while health authorities are taking adequate measures to control it by using mosquito-control programs aimed at killing mosquitoes that carry the disease. If you travel to the vulnerable areas of the world that run a higher risk of malaria, be careful to use window screens, insect repellents, and place mosquito netting over beds.

14. Measles

Measles is a dangerous disease. It is a contagious infection that can spread from person to person. The virus of the disease present in the air makes it more dangerous and difficult for the people to take some precautions. It spreads like some flu in babies, causing many deaths also. Measles is also popularly known as 'Rubeola'. It is a disease of the respiratory system and spreads very quickly. A person suffering from measles lies down in a state of pity. The disease brings along shivering due to coldness and white spots which turn pink in a day or so all over the body. The patient gets rashes which grow quickly to the upper body, back and legs. There are not many treatments available for the disease because of it being an airborne disease. The best treatment is to prevent the disease, and you can prevent the disease only through vaccination. If the mother of the child is vaccinated then the chances for the kid to get affected is less, but it is better to get the kids also vaccinated. There are few vaccinations available in the market. The best and the most recommended among them is *MMR*.

Causes

Measles is caused due to the *paramyxo virus* present in the air, so it is also an *airborne disease*. The virus causes respiratory problems in infants. The babies suffering with rubeola may have high fever and rashes all over their body. This disease can spread if a child comes in direct contact with another child suffering from the disease. Secondly, the virus may be present in the saliva, sputum and phlegm of a child. So, there are chances of this virus to spread if that kid sneezes, coughs or spits.

Symptoms

The basic symptoms that a baby suffering from this disease will show is feeling cold, fever, rashes all over the body, cough and conjunctivitis. However, once the paramyxo virus hits a kid, it takes 10 to 12 days for it to show its full effect. Between these days, there will be certain symptoms shown by the kid which will appear in certain pattern.

Incubation Period

This is the time lag between the exposure to the virus and actual culmination of the disease. It may last for a period of 12 days and on the 14th day, rashes appear all over the body.

Prodrome

This succeeds the incubation period. This period projects a cold like symptom. Babies will have *running nose* and *watery eyes*. They can get *high fever*.

Appearance of Rashes

Rashes show out completely after 2 or 3 days of projection of cold symptoms. Rashes are pinkish in colour that grow dark in the later stages.

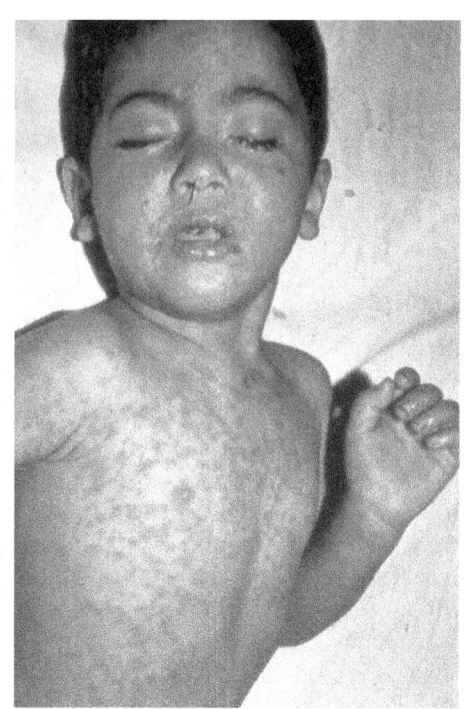

Measles

Disappearance of Rashes

The rashes begin to fade down after 3 to 4 days. Once the rashes disappear, the kid may or may not be running temperature.

Treatment

Though drugs like *Ibuprofen*, *Advil*, etc. are recommended for babies, home treatment is the best for this infection. It takes almost two weeks to recover from the disease. Doctors recommend bed rest in such cases. Measles reduces the level of vitamin A in the body which may complicate things. The best treatment is to immunize the person.

Prevention

It is a bit difficult to prevent rubeola as it is an airborne disease. However, there are few precautionary measures that when taken can help prevent the disease. The best among them is to provide vaccination to the patient suffering from the disease. There is a vaccine called MMR which stands for measles, mumps and rubella. This vaccine should be provided to all kids after fifteen months of their birth.

15. Chicken Pox

New parents cannot stop bubbling with excitement at the arrival of their little one. However, the initial joy is cut short when more serious concerns over health and hygiene take over your mind, leaving you jittery for a while. The road to parenthood is laid with challenges. And one of the toughest things that you face as parents is to battle against those malefic germs and diseases that pose a constant threat to your little one. As parents, your concern over the health of your baby is natural. Babies are more vulnerable to germs and your baby will have to deal

with common but dangerous diseases like typhoid, chicken pox, tetanus, polio and chicken pox, if not cared for. Chicken Pox is one of the most common occurrences among children. Though it is a rare thing among infants, who are generally defended by the antibodies generated in their mother's wombs until their first year, there may be some exceptional cases. Even if an infant is infected, it is likely to be mild and will be off in 5 to 10 days. Chicken Pox is contagious and you should take utmost care of your babies when infected.

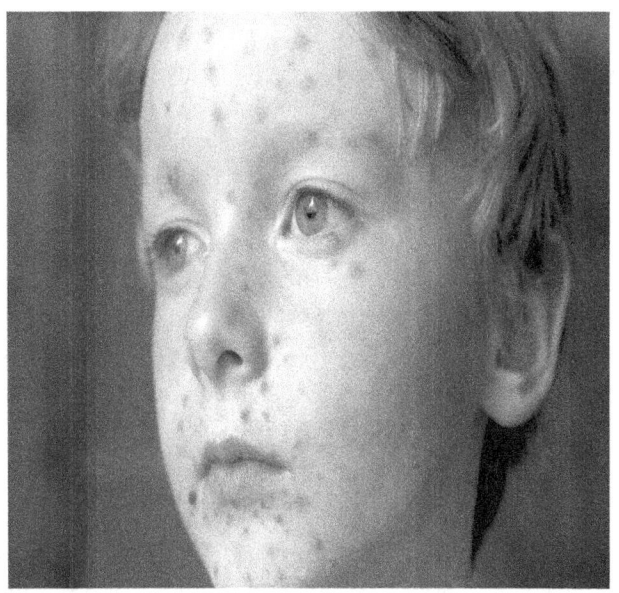
Chicken pox

Causes

Chicken Pox is caused by Varicella zoster virus, which spreads easily from one person to another. Any kind of direct contact with the infected person like touching, coughing or sneezing onto their hands or coming in contact with the infected air can expose your child to the risk of Chicken Pox.

Symptoms

Chicken Pox or Varicella initially pops up as tiny, red, prickly bumps that quickly change into fluid-filled pink blisters before crusting into dry brown flakes. The most common symptoms are fatigue, fever, loss of appetite, mild cough and running nose. It usually takes around 14 to 16 days for the pustules to appear, although they may show up anytime between 10 and 21 days. The bumps normally appear on the face, scalp, back and abdomen, but can show up on the entire body at times. A child can get as many as 200 to 250 blisters, although it is possible to have fewer bumps too.

Possible Threats

Although Chicken Pox itself isn't any serious threat to your baby, it may, at times, lead to serious complications like pneumonia, encephalitis, and bacterial skin infection and even swelling of the brain.

Prevention

You can prevent your baby from developing Chicken Pox by keeping him/her away from infected people. Also vaccinating your child against this disease is an absolute must. Vaccination doesn't immunize your child against the threat of Chicken Pox. Rather, it makes the disease a lot milder. However, it is not advisable for children below one year of age.

Vaccination

It is medically advised that your child should receive the vaccination at 12 to 15 months of age, followed by a second dose at the age of four. Vaccination has few side-effects. It is not advisable if your child has severe allergic reaction to gelatin. Again if your child has any kind of respiratory disorder or has undergone a blood transfusion, consult your pediatrician before taking your baby for vaccination.

Treatment

Prickly Chicken Pox can bring a lot of discomfort to your child. You can ease you baby's irritation with a cool bath after every three to four hours. You can add baking soda or colloidal oatmeal to the water for a cooling effect. Apply lactocalamine lotion to the itchy areas after bath to provide further relief. Also, keep your baby from picking and scratching his/her sores. You can help by trimming his/her nails. Unhealed sores can leave scars and even trigger skin infections, such as *impetigo*. Always keep your child indoors when down with chicken pox to avert spread of the virus. Give your baby complete time to recuperate before taking him/her out. If your baby has high temperature, try to bring down the fever by giving some medicines prescribed by the doctor. Avoid giving aspirin as it can trigger a rare but deadly syndrome, called the Reye's syndrome. If your baby's condition worsens, you can ask your pediatrician for over-the-counter children's antihistamine to help reduce the itching.

16. Conjunctivitis

Conjunctivitis is caused by an infection of the lining of the eyelids and of the outer protective layer of the eye called the *conjunctiva*. It can be caused because of a virus or any allergy and leads to sore, red and sticky eyes. Though it is not something serious, but is definitely uncomfortable. Some kinds of conjunctivitis may cause damage to the eyes if not attended on time. If it is due to an allergy, it will always come with other signs like fever including itchy nose and sneezing, while making the eyes feel itchy. But, if it is caused by some bacteria, both the eyes will always be infected with gritty feeling and pus. Conjunctivitis is notorious in nature and is a welcoming infection. It is welcoming in the sense it can get transmitted to anyone who comes in contact with the infected person. So a great deal of care and precaution need to be taken by parents whose babies are infected. They should keep the surroundings clean; keep themselves and their hands clean before coming near the infected child. There are other precautions and remedies that if followed can prove to be of great help to the mothers and their babies.

Treatment

- ❑ Consult your doctor at the earliest and get it diagnosed accurately. Use an ointment or drops, if necessary.
- ❑ Bathe your baby's eyes daily with warm water and clean up any debris. Use a separate clean cotton cloth for each eye to avoid cross-infection. Sweep gently from the inner to the outer part of the eye to remove any discharge.
- ❑ Give your baby his/ her own tweed and towel to use. This will prevent the infection from spreading.
- ❑ It is an infectious disease and has a notorious tendency to spread, so wash your hands before and after touching the baby's eyes.

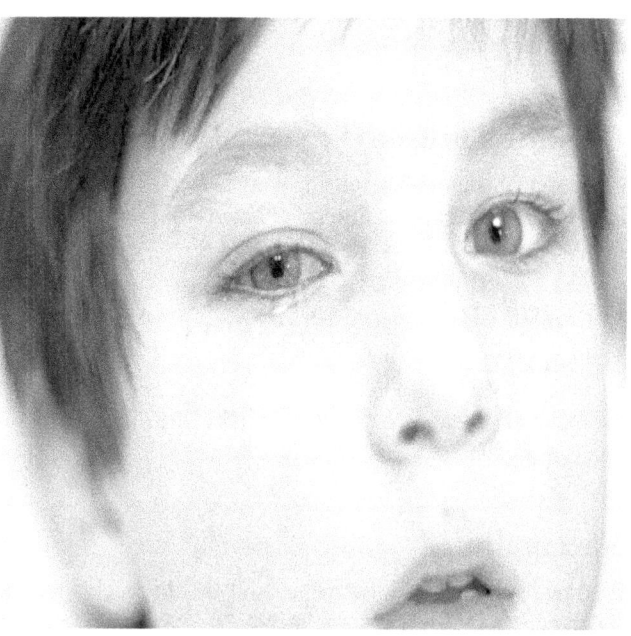

Conjunctivitis

- Bathing baby's eyes with a sea-salt solution will help the eyes remain free from discharge. It has a cleansing and mild antiseptic property which will help cure the infection.
- Eyebright is well reputed by herbalist to be the best herb for treating the eyes. It has both the cleansing and strengthening properties. Make a solution in a cup of boiled water. Let it cool down and strain, and then use a fresh cotton wool and apply gently on the eyes.
- Bacterial conjunctivitis may need antibiotic drop or ointment from the doctor.
- Viral conjunctivitis will get cured on its own. However, regular cleaning is required.
- Bathing babies in a little freshly expressed breast milk is also effective.
- Babies suffering from conjunctivitis may get sore eyes. In this case, regular cleaning away of pus is useful to make the child feel better. Eyes can be cleaned either from the outside inward or from inside outward, whichever is comfortable.

Precautions

- Careful hand washing is most important to stop the infection from spreading.
- Children and adults having conjunctivitis should stay away from schools and work places until the infection is cured.
- Disposal of tissues, cottons and towels after use is an important step to control the spread of infection.

17. Pneumonia

Pneumonia is a serious disease. It may become life-threatening if not treated on time. It is an inflammatory condition in which inflammation and solidification of air sacs in the baby's lungs takes place. This inflammation may be caused by a virus or bacteria or other organisms. Although pneumonia can develop at any age, but it is particularly serious in infants below one year.

Symptoms

During the normal process of breathing, purification of blood takes place. In the process, carbon dioxide is removed from the blood and oxygen is absorbed. This takes place by a process of diffusion within the air sacs or alveoli which are situated deep inside the lungs. In case of pneumonia, the air sacs become infected. Due to this, the baby's respiratory function gets disturbed. The baby's breathing becomes fast and shallow and he/she develops fever.

In small babies, a grunting noise can be heard during breathing and their chest heaves very fast and indrawing of the chest is clearly visible. The baby cannot take the feed properly and cries inconsolably. In severe cases, the baby's lips and face may turn greyish-blue due to the low level of oxygen in the blood. The baby may become drowsy or faint because of poor supply of oxygen to the brain.

Treatment

Pneumonia is a serious disease. It should not be treated lightly. This disease demands prompt and effective medical treatment. In severe cases, the baby will have to be hospitalised for the administration of oxygen. The effective control of infection is very important with appropriate antibiotics. Regular monitoring of the baby till the infection is cleared should be done under specialised care of the pediatrician. For immediate relief, nebulizers are used which help in dilating the respiratory passage and help the baby in easy breathing.

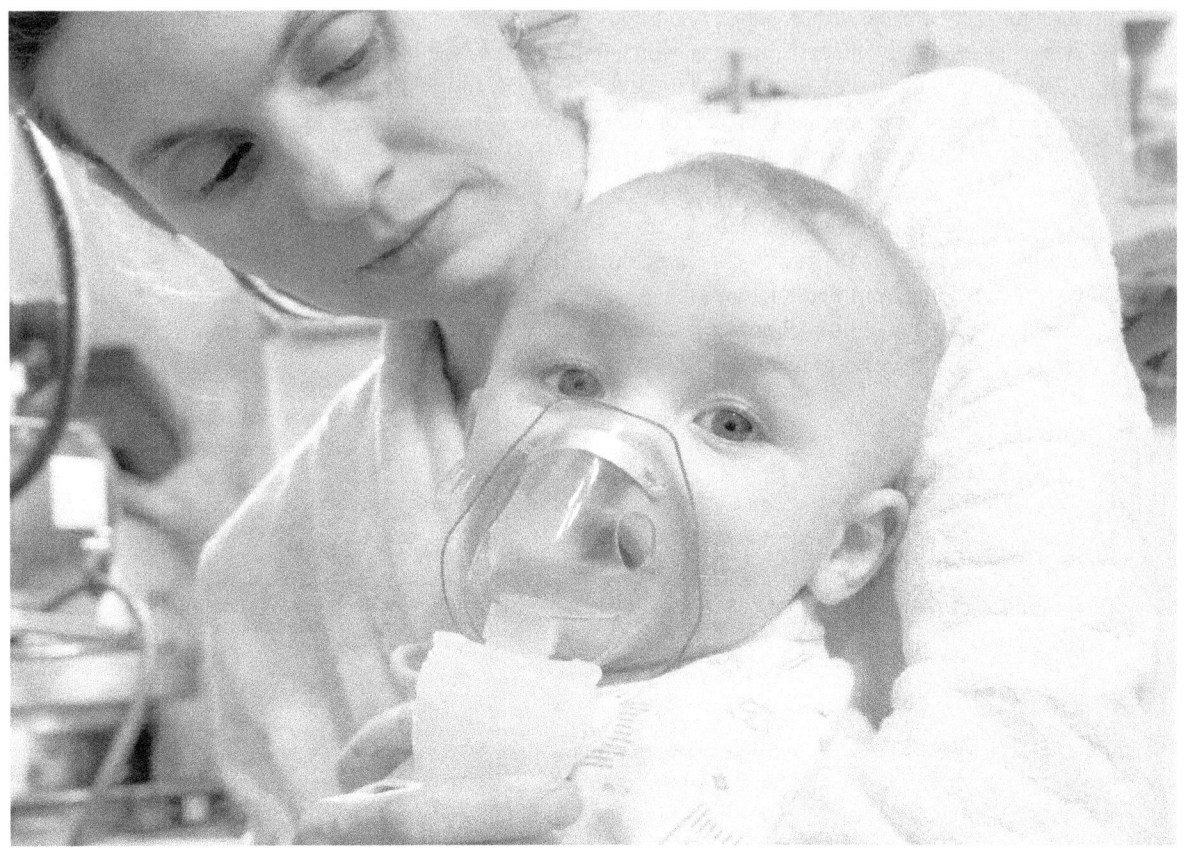

A baby with nebulizer for treatment of Pneumonia

18. Meningitis

Meninges is the sheet-like membranous lining of the brain. Meningitis is the inflammation of this lining and the spinal cord. Meningitis can occur at all ages starting from newborn babies. It is a serious disease. It occurs very abruptly sometime even in a matter of a few hours.

Causes

Meningitis is caused by different types of bacteria and viruses. Meningococcal meningitis and pneumococcal meningitis are two common types of bacterial meningitis in babies. In some cases, *tuberculosis can also cause meningitis.*

Symptoms

These are the symptoms of meningitis. A child suffering from meningitis may have some or all of these symptoms.
- ❏ Fever
- ❏ Headache
- ❏ Vomiting

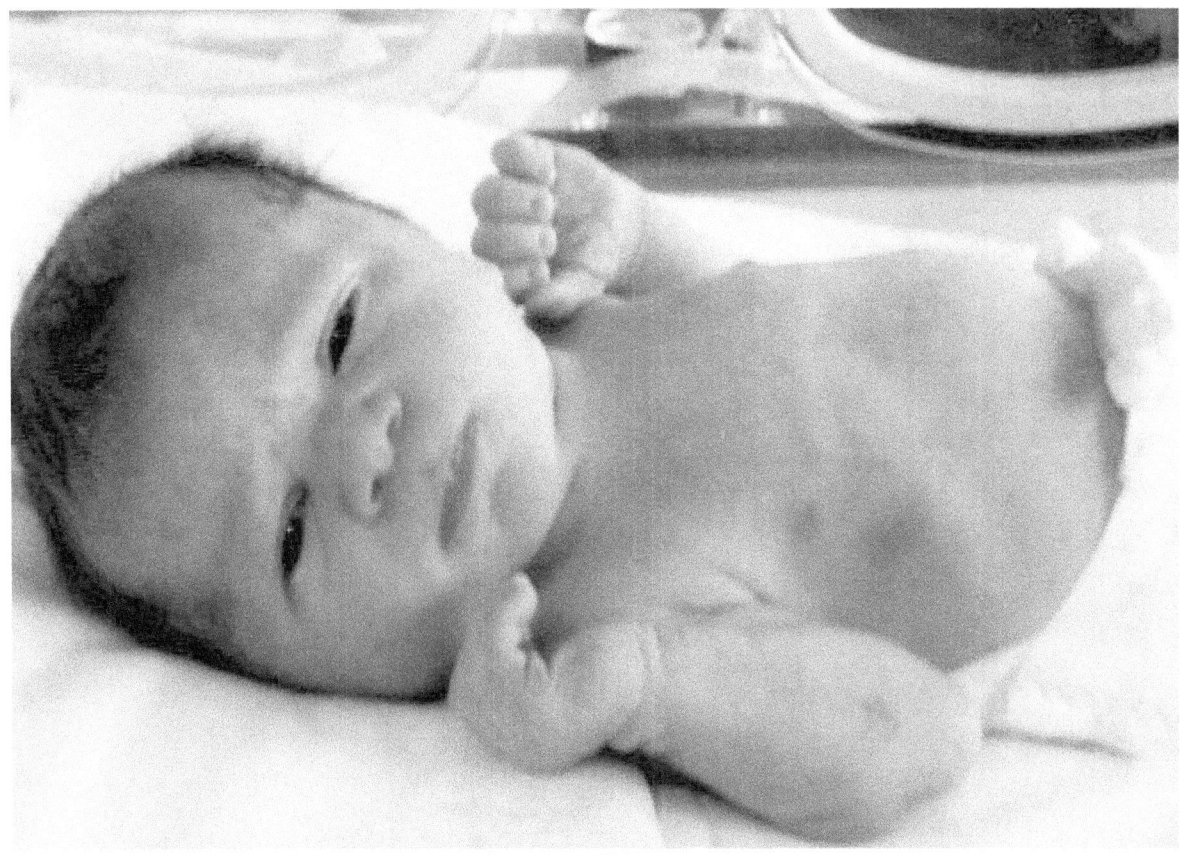
Symptoms of Meningitis

- ❏ Stiffness in the neck
- ❏ Pain on bending the neck
- ❏ Dislike of bright lights
- ❏ A desire to keep the eyes closed
- ❏ Drowsiness, irritability and confusion
- ❏ Tiny red and purple spots or bruise-like patches on the skin

In small babies, who cannot complain of their discomforts like headache, etc, these are the symptoms.

- ❏ Lethargy and feeling too sleepy
- ❏ Difficulty to wake up
- ❏ Vacant look
- ❏ Bulging fontanelle
- ❏ Blotchy skin
- ❏ Rash over the body

Treatment

A baby with meningitis needs to be hospitalised. The doctor would take a sample of the baby's spinal fluid and examine it before establishing the diagnosis of meningitis.

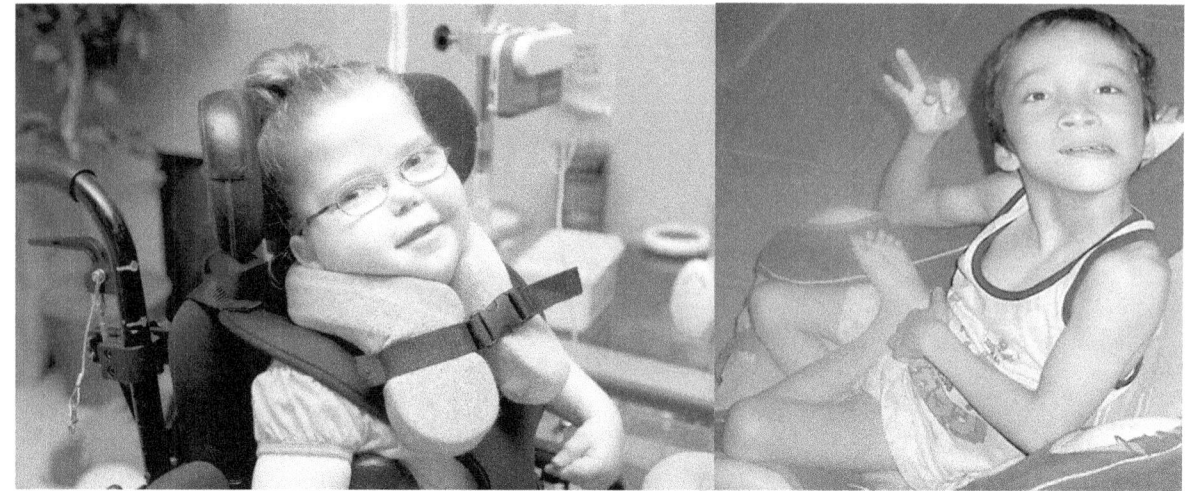

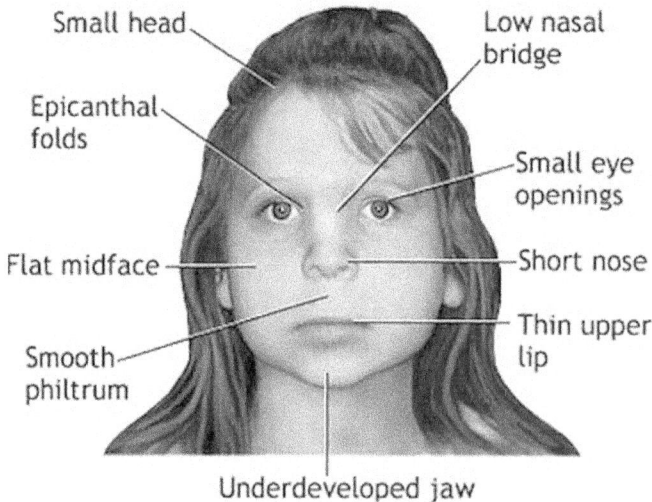

How Meningitis affects the brain

Regular and careful administration of antibiotics and careful supportive treatment is required for as long as the infection is not cleared.

Beware

If this disease is diagnosed early and treated quickly, then the chances of the baby to recover completely improve. But if the treatment is delayed, then the disease can result in permanent disabilities like deafness and brain damage. It may even prove fatal if prompt treatment is not given.

19. Hiccups in Babies

You are enjoying your food and suddenly you hear a 'hic' sound and it continues till you have some water. These are called *hiccups* and often come without any prior trigger. Hiccups happen when we do two things together, like laughing or talking while eating or drinking. Hiccups in babies happen while feeding. Like sneezing and snuffling, hiccups are also normal and very common in babies. Very rarely, hiccups happen due to any health problems.

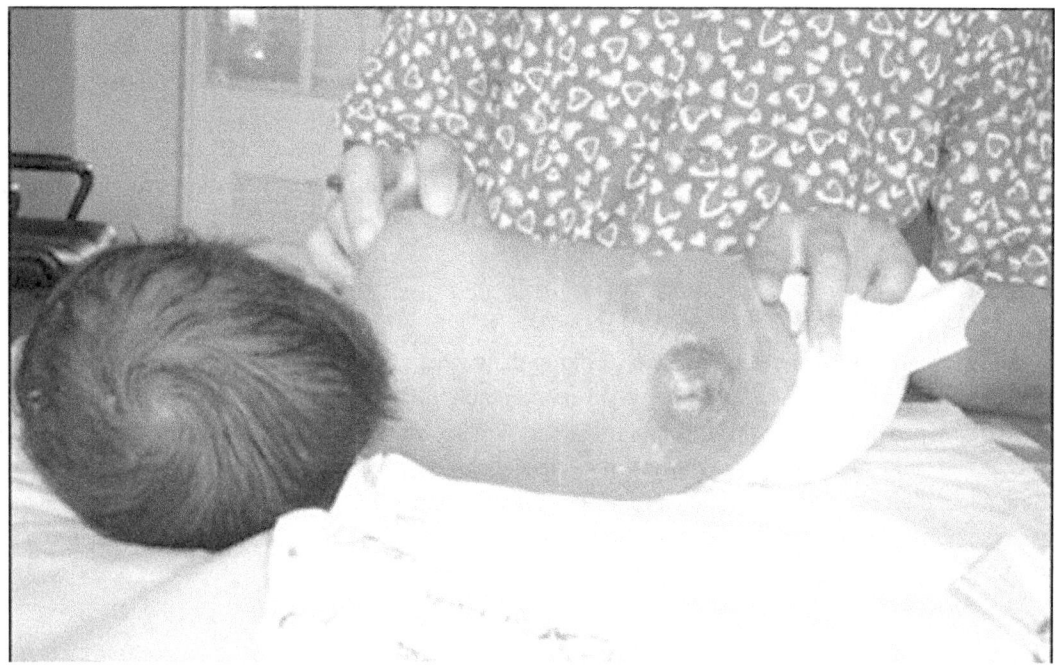
How Meningitis affects the spinal cord

Hiccups are definitely not a health emergency, but for some people, it may continue for months together. In such cases, medical assistance is necessary. Hiccups are caused by a sudden, unpredictable tightening of the diaphragm, i.e. the muscle at the bottom of the lungs that you use while breathing, sucking air into the lungs. Just after the muscle start moving, the epiglottis (a flap in the wind pipe which stops food and drinks going down the lungs) closes over the airway, causing the 'hic' sound. This is the scientific explanation for the cause of hiccups. In simple words, hiccups occur when we swallow in excess of air. Hiccups are very common with babies. They often get hiccups while being fed and also after meals. This so happens because the babies tend to swallow air when they are been fed, creating gas in their stomach leading to hiccups. This is not at all an alarming situation and does not call in for not feeding the baby. You can just follow simple steps and cure the hiccups of your babies even while feeding them. Here are tips as to how you can cure your baby's hiccups.

Remedies

- Hold the baby against your shoulder and pat his/her back. Some babies tend to swallow a lot of air during the feeding process and this distends the stomach which leads to hiccups. So some gentle pats on their back can stop these hiccups.
- A baby can take in a lot of air through the feeding bottle also if the hole in the nipple is too big. The hole should be such that there is drop by drop flow and not a continuous flow. This will not allow extra air to flow in for the babies to swallow, thus preventing hiccups.
- There is a myth stating that you should not feed your baby at the time of hiccups. This is not true and thus, you should do not delay your baby's eating process because of hiccups since hiccups will not create any problem while feeding your baby.
- Anise seeds for infants is also said to work. Add a teaspoon of anise seeds into a cup of boiling water and feed the baby two or three teaspoons. It often cures the hiccups immediately.

- If for the first few months your baby is continuously getting hiccups, then overfeeding can be one of the causes. Feed your baby in portions and with time intervals. If you have realised that you have been overfeeding your baby, then start feeding them only on demand rather than the schedule created by you. Also don't force them to eat more than what they want.
- This is a traditional European remedy. Gripe water contains safe, fast, effective and natural ingredients for curing colic discomforts. Gripe water is being used since centuries by mothers to cure their babies from hiccups, stomach cramps, gas and colic discomforts.

20. Nail-Biting in Toddlers

Toddlers and even grownups develop the habit of biting nails whenever they are in some trouble or are stressed out or simply when they are bored. Nail-biting is a very common habit that can develop in any person. It is a habit which gets developed without even the person himself knowing about it. Your child might be watching some horror movie and suddenly would have started biting his nails. Also when he/she is narrating you something new or different about their class or school, you might suddenly see them biting their nails. It is a very normal reaction by any person or a child. It helps them deal with the pressure of stress, anxiety, excitement or curiosity. It may become a matter of concern and worry when it becomes a routine for your child.

Causes

Here are few points on the causes and remedies for this unhealthy habit.

- **Boredom or Curiousness**
  Children tend to get bored very fast. They always want something new to happen around them. They are always curious to know and find out new things. This feeling of boredom and curiousness may also develop the habit of biting nails among them. In this case, there is nothing to get worried as the habit will disappear with time.
- **Nervousness**
  Nail-biting is a very common habit among the toddlers and falls in line of other habits like nose-picking, hair-twisting and tooth-grinding which kids develop to get rid of their nervousness and irritation. Almost all the kids develop such a habit before pre-school.
- **Tension and Anxiety**
  Nail-biting is often taken up by children to get rid of some tension or anxiety that they are living with. While taking the first steps towards the world outside, all kids tend to get scared and anxious. The first day of school, feeling shy in gatherings, learning something new in school are the common triggers. But, at times some serious problems at home or school may also be concerning them. Otherwise, there is no need to worry if your child is biting his/ her nail because it is just their way to get away from their small tensions.

Negative Effects of Nail-Biting

Nail-biting has negative effect on the physical and mental status of the baby.

- **Bleeding**
  Nail-biting can lead to red, painful fingertips. Your child may bite the nail so hard that it may swell up the fingertip which can turn out to be very painful and start bleeding.

- ❑ **Infection**
  Nail-biting transfers germs from the nails to the mouth and this can lead to various infections. Even bacteria from the mouth can get transferred to the skin through nails.
- ❑ **Deformed Nail Bed**
  Nail bed tends to get deformed due to continuous nail-biting. It may cause the newly grown nails to look odd and out of shape.
- ❑ **Chipped Teeth**
  Biting nails can result in broken or chipped front teeth. It may also transfer germs to the mouth which may cause cavities in the gums.
- ❑ **Cuticle Biting**
  Your child while biting his/ her nail may also pull off the skin from above the nail bed, called the cuticle. Cuticle damage may cause bleeding and painful nail bed.
- ❑ **Psychological Effects**
  Nail-biting may be a sign of great anxiety in a person. It can also cause self-consciousness and embarrassment in a person.

Remedies

Here are some pointers on ways to remedy this bad habit.

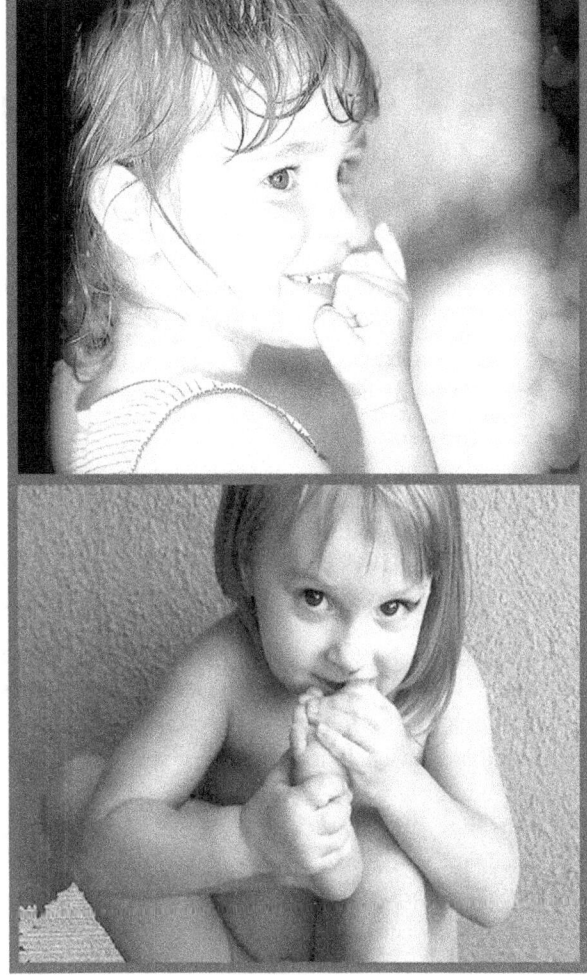

Nail biting habits

- ❑ **Provide Distraction**
  If you can determine and you know when your child will bite his/ her nails, while watching TV for example, find out something that will distract them from biting their nails. Give them some toys in hand or play with them so that their attention is diverted. This will prevent them from biting their nails.
- ❑ **Do Not Overreact**
  You are tired with your kid's habit and start inveigling and cajoling your kid. Offering them options like painting their nails, telling them every now and then that their habit is disgusting will only make the matters worse. Kids love attention, negative or positive, and they measure attention by quantity and not quality.
- ❑ **Take Advice from Your Pediatrician**
  Taking advice from your pediatrician is a good option. You may be told that the habit will fade away with time, but mention smallest details like if their finger bleeds and so on. This will help the pediatrician in judging the anxiety level in your child.
- ❑ **Make the Habit Less Tempting**
  Cut your baby's nails and keep them clean always. This will leave them with no option but to refrain from biting their nails. There are products available that if brushed on, leave a bitter taste which lasts for

days together. This discourages the little ones to opt for biting. However, parents are happy with such products but, experts consider them to be harmful for use.

- ❑ **Make Your Child Aware of Their Habit**
  Encourage your child to be aware of his/ her bad habit. Don't forget to give quite, secret reminders if they forget: a light pat on the arm, or some eye movement. This will make them conscious of what they are doing.
- ❑ **Be Patient**
  The first reaction from a parent, if they see their child biting his/ her nail is to scold or punish them. Nail biting like any other habit is unconsciously adapted. May be your child doesn't even know they are biting their nails. Nagging them or punishing them at that time will not serve any purpose. Speak to them in an understanding and compassionate way and make them understand that even though unconscious, biting nail is a bad habit and that you can't watch them doing so. This understanding gesture on your side will help them make an effort to get rid of their habits.
- ❑ **Praise Your Child**
  Praise your child if they are not biting their nails. Encourage them by rewarding them, if possible. Appreciate their efforts and make sure they continue to show such positive attitude towards you whenever asked for.

21. Restless Legs Syndrome in Babies

Is your baby not sleeping properly? Is he/ she quite restless? Is your baby throwing around their legs a lot? This may all sound very common a reaction from babies. But this is ironical when it comes to baby care. When you think it to be just nothing, it turns out to be a critical and complicated situation. When you notice any such symptoms in your baby, it means there is a need to consult a doctor. Your child might be suffering with *RLS*. *Restless Legs Syndrome (RLS)* is a neurological disorder, which gives creepy, crawly, itchy sensation accompanied by an uncontrollable urge to move the legs. The uneasiness aggravates as the day falls and it restricts the sufferer from sleeping. Therefore it is also known as 'sleep or evening disorder' and experts refer to it as "Ekbom's syndrome". In children, this disorder is associated with Attention-Deficit Hyperactivity Disorder that results due to inattention. We can also associate RLS with Periodic Limb Movement Disorder. This disorder can prove out to be too irritable for your baby if it is not attended at the earliest and cured.

Diagnosis

Diagnosis of the syndrome depends upon the manifestation of physical symptoms, child's description of what they feel and a polysomnogram showing typical limb movements.

Causes

RLS or Restless Legs Syndrome in adults could be due to many reasons. But in children, RLS is mostly due to the deficiency of iron content in the body. Genetic predisposition can also be a reason for children to suffer from the syndrome, and at times, it can be the combined affect that leads to the syndrome.

Symptoms

Being offensive, absentmindedness, inability to sleep at night, are few of the behavioural symptoms shown by children suffering from RLS. This all might be accompanied with pains and aches. These symptoms might be considered as a psychiatric disorder and might lead to misdiagnosis, increasing the risk. If your child is suffering from restlessness and agitations in the evening and fails to get sleep continuously, then it should be taken as an alarming situation. If the family has any history of RLS, then the babies are at larger risk of getting the syndrome.

Precaution and Treatment

There are several opinions regarding the treatment or precautions to be taken to curb the affect of the disorder. The uncertainty and cluelessness of this disease may lead to other complications. So it is always better to take precautions than opt for some cure. The iron content in infants should be regularly measured and taken care of. If required, food supplements and multivitamin tablets can be provided. There should be a routine life maintained for your child. There should be a time for everything, their sleep, food, play, etc. but the precaution and treatment of RLS is not at all a cakewalk. Firstly, detect the symptoms of the syndrome, which calls in for a lot of alertness and care on the part of the parents.

22. Shaken Baby Syndrome

A baby's body is immensely delicate and fragile as it has very soft muscles around the neck and contrary to that has a big head and big body. Violent shaking of its body can lead to unbelievable outcomes, especially in the brain portion, as a baby's brain is immature and needs room to grow in the small space between the brain and the skull. Violent shaking of the baby's body, although in a playful manner, can lead to internal bleeding, forming a clot inside the brain. Shaken body syndrome can also lead to bruising of brain tissue and tearing of blood vessels. None of the parents shake their babies intentionally but when a baby doesn't stop crying, parents do it angrily and shake babies violently. It is a result of intentional baby abuse most of the times, but can also be caused without any reasons, like playing with a baby while jogging. Parents should also take care of those guests who come to play with their babies which can also cause much trouble. You might have noticed that there are many small injuries which happen to your babies, but are all unexplained. The reason being is this particular syndrome that can happen over a twinkling of an eye can cause bruises, rib fractures and clotting of blood in the eyes.

Symptoms

- ❏ Symptoms are always non-specific and can remain unnoticed for sometime, but can have sudden vomits or fussiness caused by the internal pressures developed in the brain.
- ❏ Lethargy is also a characteristic feature of the syndrome and can be observed occasionally.
- ❏ Babies may also have some breathing difficulties and may show some signs of epilepsy.

Treatment

- ❏ Treatment depends upon the type of abuse and in case of rapid symptoms; the baby should be immediately taken to a hospital for close monitoring.
- ❏ Doctors watch for signs of brain swelling or bleeding, breathing difficulties and if these aspects are positive then the baby will be admitted in Intensive Care Unit (ICU) and treatment will be carried out accordingly.
- ❏ In case of less severe injuries, a cast is applied on the broken bones and cuts are stitched or bandaged.
- ❏ Those babies who are affected by epilepsy are further treated by neurologists and medication is provided by them, but epilepsy can lead to dangerous problems like physical disabilities or mental retardation also.

- If the baby is not much harmed by shaken baby syndrome then simple medications can also be followed by the parents and some prescribed pain gels can be applied on the baby's body.

23. Tourette Syndrome

Tourette Syndrome is often thought to be a type of mental illness, but it is not. It is an inherited neuropsychiatric disorder with onset in childhood. Individuals suffering with Tourette Syndrome feel an irresistible urge to make sounds and body movements, and these movements are beyond their control. These uncontrollable movements are called *tics*. Tourette is defined as a part of a spectrum of tic disorder which includes transient and chronic tics. For children suffering with Tourette's Syndrome, tics are very distressing, with they having no control over it. In few cases, patients might even blurt out obscenity in their behaviour, although this is very rare. People suffering with this syndrome get relief only when their tics are expressed out. Tics increase with tension or any worries,

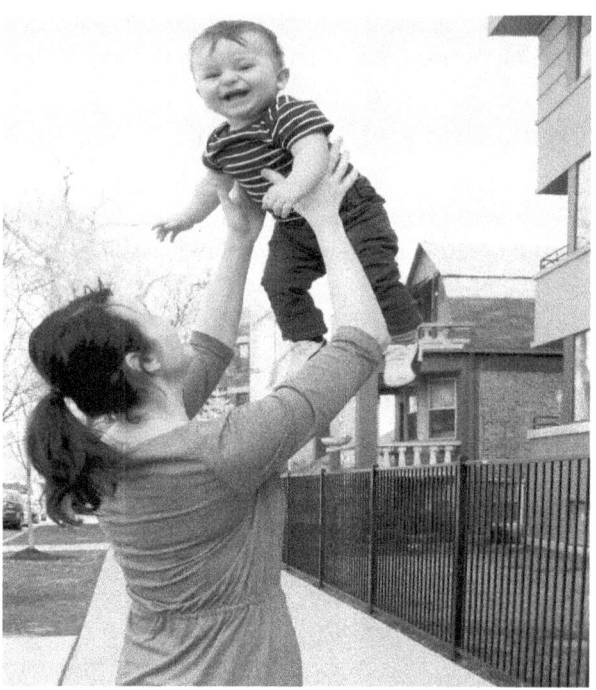

Mother shaking and throwing up baby playfully

and decrease with relaxation. So children suffering with this syndrome should always be kept calm and away from any kind of worry. Children suffering should be treated normally and should not be made fun of. You need to understand that the sudden actions or noises which they make are not under their control. These kids need extra care.

Diagnosis

It is important to diagnose the syndrome correctly. The moment you notice any unusual expression or movement in your kid, pay a visit to your healthcare professional. *Tics* are the first sign of the syndrome, though all tics signs might not be tourette. Few kids develop tics for few weeks after which it disappears. A treatment plan for the syndrome can only start with accurate and thorough diagnosis. There are no specific tests conducted for diagnosing Tourette Syndrome. Doctors just rely on the past history of the patient's symptoms. There is nothing as the perfect or a typical case of Tourette Syndrome. This condition follows a reliable course, in terms of the age of onset and history of severity of the symptoms.

Symptoms

The symptoms for Tourette Syndrome are the tics which the patient develops.

- **Simple Tics**
  These are a rapid, sudden and brief movement which involves a limited number of muscle groups. These include eye blinking, and other vision irregularities, facial grimacing, shoulder shrugging and head and shoulder jerking. Some vocal tics may include repetitive throat clearing, sniffing or grunting sounds.
- **Complex Tics**
  These are distinct coordinated pattern of movement and involve several muscle groups. Complex motor tics might include facial grimacing with a head twist and a shoulder shrug. Other complex tics might

appear purposeful, like sniffing or touching objects, hopping, jumping, bending or twisting. The vocal tics may include sniffing, throat clearing, grunting and snoring. There are few more complex vocal tics that might include words or phrases, like *coprolalia* or *echolalia*. These motor movements can also get dramatic and disabling and result in self-pain like punching oneself in the face. Some of the tics can also be preceded by an urge in the muscle group called the *premonitory urge*. People suffering from the syndrome will be relieved only after they complete a tic in a certain way or a certain number of times. Tics tend to increase with anxiety and reduce when the person is calm. Any physical experience can trigger a particular tic.

Causes of Tourette Syndrome

Here are some causes which lead to Tourette Syndrome:

- **Genetic Cause**
  Person suffering with the syndrome is most likely to pass it on to their children. Tourette is a condition of variable expression and incomplete penetrance, so not everyone who inherits genetic vulnerability will show symptoms. The genes may express a mild tic disorder or as obsessive compulsive symptoms without tics. Only a minority of children who inherit the infected genes show symptoms severe enough to require medical attention. Gender also plays a role; males are more likely to express tics than females.

- **Environmental Cause**
  Some infections and psychological factors may also cause the syndrome. In some cases, auto-immune processes may affect tic onset and exacerbation. The National Health of Mental Health in 1998 proposed a hypothesis that both obsessive compulsive disorder and tic disorder arise in children as a result of a post streptococcal auto-immune process. Children who meet five diagnostic criteria are classified according to the hypothesis as having pediatric auto-immune neuropsychiatric disorder associated with streptococcal infections.

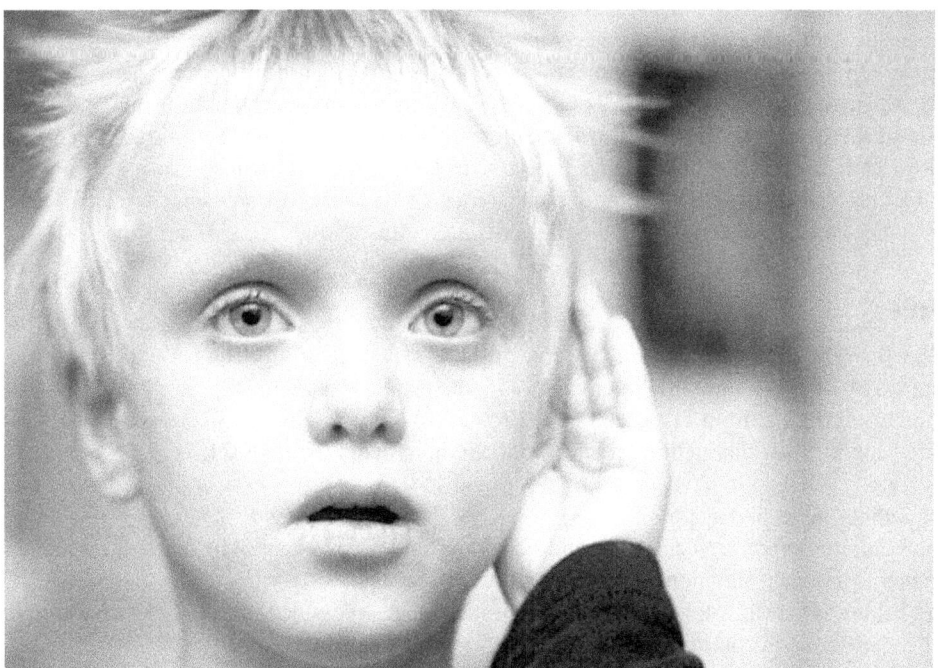

Tourette syndrome

Treatment

There is no specific treatment for the syndrome, so more attention is paid on controlling tics and helping the person to adjust and live with the disorder. Individuals should go through a thorough evaluation. Counselling, learning coping techniques, medication and natural remedies are few treatment options for the syndrome. Depending on the need of the person, the treatment options can be mixed and combined. This will all lead to assisting the person to cope up with the disorder. Parents of the newly diagnosed children should be careful and investigate all possible treatment avenues for their children.

24. Asperger's Syndrome

Self-centred behaviour, repetitive behavioural patterns and difficulty in social interaction – all these symptoms point to *Asperger's Syndrome* in your baby. Asperger's Syndrome is a part of the family of autism spectrum disorders. Those suffering from the syndrome show difficulties in social interaction, along with repetitive and restricted behaviour and interests. This syndrome differs from other autism disorders by its relative preservation of linguistic and cognitive development. Unlike other autism disorders, it is also very difficult to track and diagnose. The babies suffering from this syndrome might exhibit a few symptoms only and even they might be difficult to identify. Unlike the children suffering from autism, those with Asperger's Syndrome might show no delay in language development. They usually have a good control over grammar, but do exhibit a kind of language disorder. There are no delays in cognitive development or in age-appropriate self-help skills, such as feeding and dressing themselves. However, they may have problem with attention span and in organisation. Such children usually have average and, at times, above average intelligence.

Causes

The causes of Asperger's Syndrome are not very clear. Researchers are still investigating for the exact reasons behind this syndrome. It is believed that the pattern of behaviour that characterises Asperger's Syndrome may have many causes. The condition seems to have a hereditary factor or component in it. Studies indicate that Asperger's may be associated with other mental disorders as well, like depression and bipolar disorder. Researchers are also looking for any possibility of environmental factors affecting brain development. However, what needs to remembered is that Asperger's Syndrome is not caused by emotional deprivation or deficient upbringing of a person. Some of the behaviour may appear deliberate and intentionally rude, but people should not mistake it as the result of bad parenting or upbringing. It is a neurological disorder whose causes are not yet been fully understood. Currently, there is no treatment for the disorder, as the causes are so vague, so a child with Asperger's grows up with the same. However, it generally does not affect the normal living of a person.

Symptoms

- Babies suffering from Asperger's Syndrome usually stay away from other people. They are more of a shy nature and indulge in minimal interaction with the people around them.
- Children suffering from Asperger's Syndrome are often highly self-centred. From their talks and behaviour, it seems that nothing matters to them more than their own self.
- Such kids even tend to have a robot-like scripted speech or way of conversing. They keep repeating the same things again and again.
- The syndrome often projects some odd behaviour and mannerisms. The kids may behave in a strange manner to a certain situation, or just generally.
- The babies suffering from Asperger's might also lack in common sense. They may find it difficult to apply their brain in common situations.
- Such kids tend to show some kind of an obsession with any complex topic or situation, which does not even require the amount of attention they are giving.

- The children suffering from the syndrome may face some problem with regard to reading and writing. They may also have problem in subjects like maths, where reasoning is required.
- Patients may also face problems with regard to non-verbal cognitive abilities, which can be average or below average. The verbal ability remains average or above average.

Diagnosis

This syndrome is very difficult to diagnose as children suffering with Asperger's function well in most aspects of life. So, their strange behaviour can easily be attributed to them being different. According to mental health experts, the detection of the syndrome at the earliest is very important. Interventions involving educational and social training perform while a child's brain is still developing is highly recommended. Though the symptoms are not very clear, but if you are able to detect even few of them, it is advisable to recommend your child to a doctor. A complete psychosocial evaluation will be done while examining the baby. This will include careful examination of the history of symptoms, the language and motor skill development of the child and other aspects of personality and behaviour.

Treatment

These are the ways of treating Asperger's Syndrome (A.S.):

- **Parent 's Training**
  It is very important for the parents to be completely aware about all the aspects of the disorder. The parents whose child is suffering with the disorder should be well aware of the disorder and its affect, so that they can take proper care of their children, as prescribed by the specialist.
- **Social-Skill Training**
  Children suffering with this syndrome are self-centred. They don't mingle well with the society. It is important to give them some social-skill therapy. The parents or the family members can only help them by comforting them and granting confidence in them at social gatherings.
- **Language Therapy**
  Children suffering with Asperger's Syndrome show some difficulty in speaking and communicating, though they have good control over language. There is a need for them to go through a language therapy to make their expressing ability fluent.
- **Specialised Educational Interventions**
  Children suffering with A.S. can also face problems in educational field, so a special educational intervention is a must.
- **Sensory Integration Training**
  The sufferers of the syndrome might be highly sensitive to certain things or situations. So, a sensory integrated training can be conducted by a specialist, which will help decentralize the stimuli to which the children are highly sensitive.
- **Psychotherapy**
  Once a child grows up, they can also undergo *psychotherapy* or a *cognitive therapy* for better results.
- **Medications**
  There are no medications as such for Asperger's Syndrome. But some medications as prescribed by a specialist may improve some specific symptoms that might be complicating your baby's progress.

25. Thumb Sucking

As soon as the babies get control over their limbs, everything they can lay their hands on goes into their mouth. The same goes for their thumb. Babies around six months of age suck their thumbs as it gives them pleasure. This may continue for a few months and most babies outgrow it when they become toddlers. However, there are some babies who continue to suck their thumbs beyond that period.

Causes

The main causes of thumb sucking in a baby are :

- **Shyness**
  Some children are particularly shy. They contine to suck their thumb to overcome this feeling of shyness.

- **Feeling insecure**
  Some children resort to thumb sucking when they face unusual situations or new environment. This could be starting of a new kindergarten school or the arrival of unfamiliar guests in the house. All this makes them feel secure and they find comfort in thumb sucking.

- **Feeling frightened**
  When a child is feeling frightened, he/she sucks his/her thumb as it gives a soothing feeling. This is similar to holding tight the stuffed teddy bear.

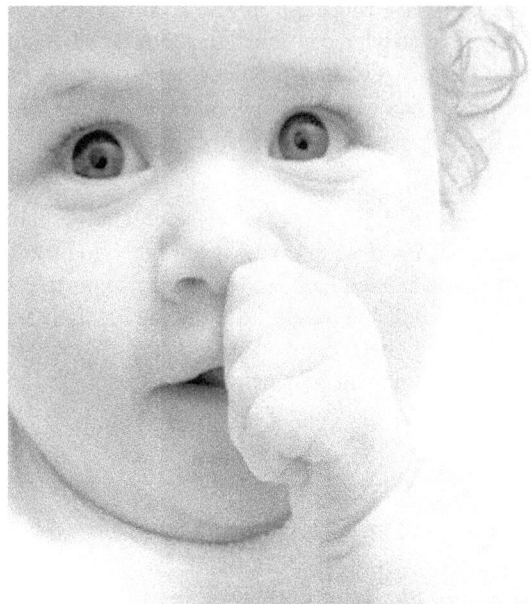

Thumb sucking habit

- **Seeking attention**
  A few children may return to thumb sucking which they had given up earlier when they are faced by some insecure situation like the birth of a sibling. In such a case when all the attention is bestowed on the new arrival, the older child seeks attention and picks up the habit of thumb sucking.

Treatment

There is no clinical treatment available for thumb sucking. You must understand that this habit signifies a growing sense of insecurity in the child. So be patient. Give more attention to your child. Do not try to punish him/her. Avoid scolding or making fun of the child in front of others. You may face some setbacks in his progress so be prepared for them. Slowly and gradually wean the baby from this habit.

Spina Bifida

In this condition, there is a raw swelling over a portion of the spine at birth. This results in *paralysis* of the legs (either partial or complete), inability to control bladder functioning and inability to feel anything below the spina bifida. In some cases, there is a build up and retention of water in the brain, which is known as *hydrocephalus*. This swelling can be closed by an operation by specialists.

Umbilical Hernia

In this condition, parts of the digestive system are lying outside the stomach cavity. This is because the

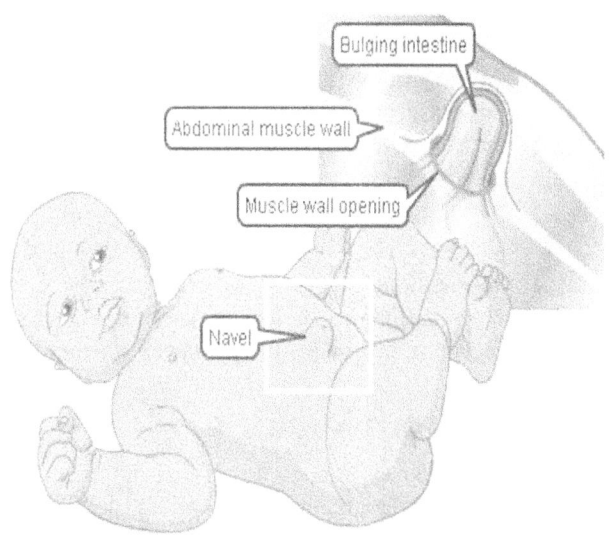

Umbilical Hernia

area around the navel is not very strong. Normally, cases of umbilical hernias around the navel heal on their own; if they don't, surgery is required.

Sickle Cell Disease

This is a hereditary condition that is most commonly found among people of West African or African Caribbean descent. The haemoglobin in the Red Blood Corpuscles disintegrates at a quicker rate than normal. Haemoglobin is important, as it carries oxygen to the different parts of the body. Reduction in haemoglobin causes anaemia and blocks blood vessels in the hands, legs and stomach. An attack can last for a few days and can be treated with painkillers. This is also known as Sickle Cell Disease.

Cystic Fibrosis

This is another hereditary illness, in which the tissues in the body produce unusually thick mucus. The commonly affected organs are the lungs, the intestines and the pancreas. If the lungs are affected, the air ducts are blocked and hence, vulnerable to infection. Children with this condition have an inability to digest food completely and have bad smelling bowel movements and constipation. They are well below the normal weight for their age. This illness has no cure, but if detected in the initial stages, lung damage can be reduced. These children are susceptible to chest infections and have to be treated with antibiotics. Chest physiotherapy is required regularly to remove thick phlegm.

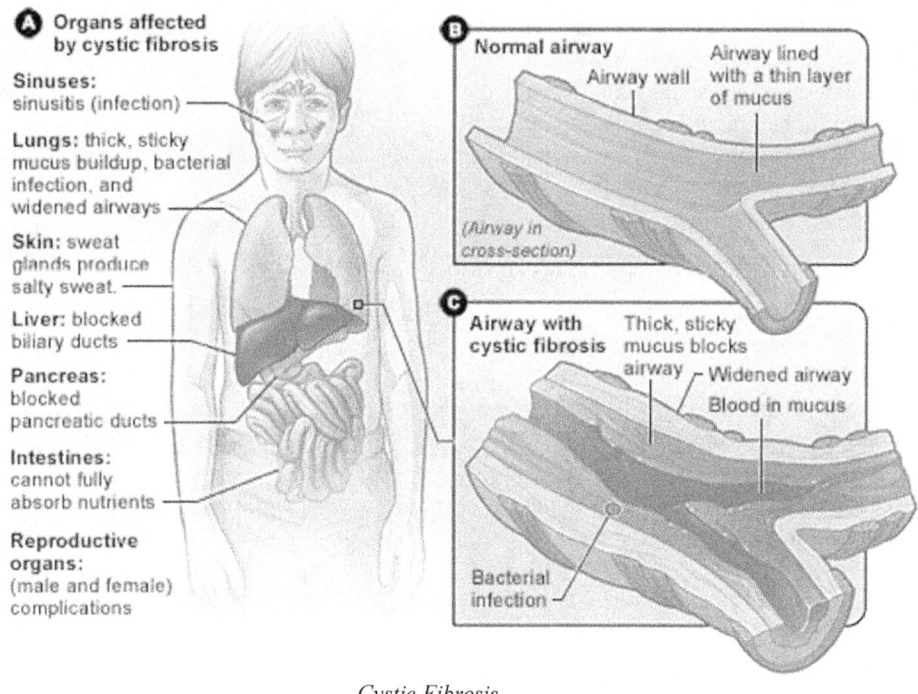

Cystic Fibrosis

Coeliac Disease

In this condition, the child's intestine reacts strongly to gluten, a protein found in wheat. These children have a severe case of diarrhoea, where the stools are fatty, pale and don't flush away. The child does not put on weight as required. The illness can be detected by a blood test. After being detected, the child will have to completely give up gluten containing food. Once this is done, stools return to normal and the child will put on weight.

Clubfoot

In this condition, the foot curves inwards or outwards. All babies are checked for this at birth, more so, if they were born in the breech position, as it occurs more frequently with these babies. Often, they can be manipulated into the proper position, with little or no treatment. Surgery may be required in severe cases. This condition is also known as *Talipes*.

Cleft Palate

In this condition, the cleft lip and the cleft palate are fused, thus the baby cannot be breastfed. Various support groups will help you deal with the situation and corrective plastic surgery is possible.

Congenital Dislocation of the Hip

All babies are screened for this condition *at birth* and when they *are eight weeks old*. If this condition goes undetected, walking can become a problem later in life. If diagnosed with this problem, the baby will have to wear a special splint for some time. Most recover without having to be operated on, but some do need an operation. This condition is prevalent more among girls and breech babies.

Cerebral Palsy

In this condition, the parts of the brain that control body movements are damaged. This can happen before birth, during birth, or in the first two years after birth. In some cases, damage may not be noticed at birth, but as the child grows, it becomes evident. It is difficult to pinpoint as to what causes this damage. There are a few tests that can be conducted when the baby is eight weeks old to screen him for cerebral palsy.

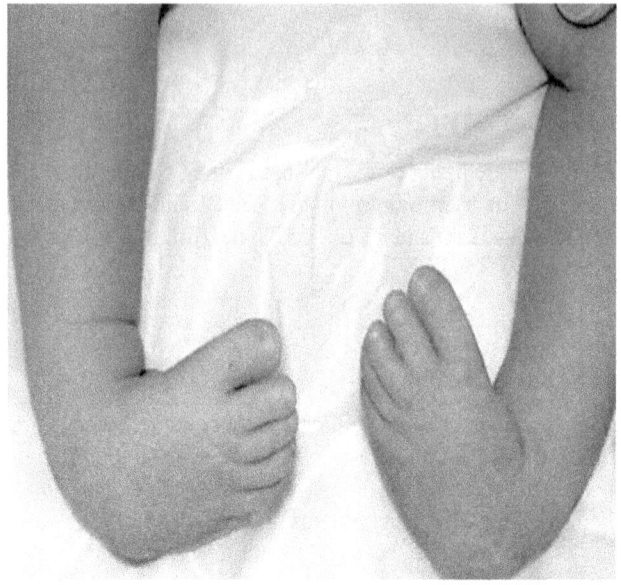

Clubfoot

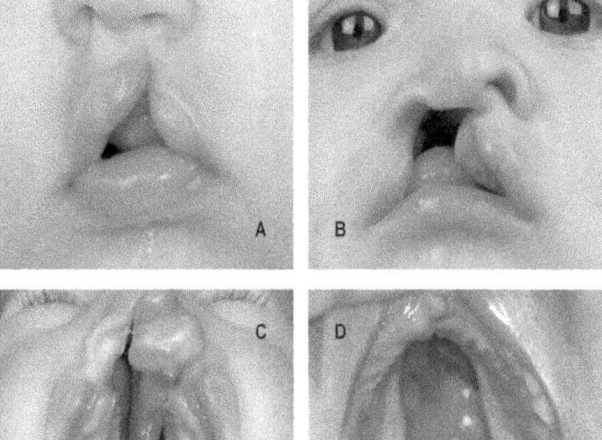

Cleft Palate

26. Autism

Having a baby calls in for a lot of alertness. Parents need to always be on their toes for any negligence on their part can make the baby suffer for the whole life. Babies are in a stage of development, but the process of their development can be hampered and slowed down by many diseases and disorders. One such disorder is 'Autism'. Autism is a complex brain disorder that affects many aspects of child development, including how a kid talks, plays and interacts. This is a disorder that appears in early childhood affecting their basic, expressive skills. The severity of the disease and its symptoms differ from one child to another. Some autistic children have only mild impairments, while some have more obstacles to overcome. To detect a child suffering with this disorder is not all that difficult, and the sooner the symptoms are detected, the better it is for the child. It is very important to sight the warning signs in toddlers, and the moment the signs are detected, help should be sought at the earliest.

Symptoms

Here are some common symptoms which indicate that your child is suffering from autism:

- **Communication Problems**
  Babies suffering from this disorder may suffer communication problems. They may face problems both in verbal and non-verbal communication. Spoken language is delayed in autistic babies and may even be absent. Even if they are able to speak, they might have difficulty in doing so freely and easily. Other symptoms involve odd or repetitive speech pattern, inappropriate facial expressions and gestures.

- **Impaired Social Skills**
  Children suffering from this disorder have impaired social interaction. They may lack in interest for their surroundings and people around. These children are always in their own world, not interacting or playing with others. They face trouble in sharing emotions, making friends and understanding the feelings and thinking of others.

- **Unresponsive**
  Babies are usually curious and playful. However, a baby suffering with autism will not be interested in human attention. They will not respond to any attention or any gesture made towards them. They will be least affected and bothered about what is happening around them.

- **Stereotypical Behaviour**
  Autistic children often depict stereotypical or repetitive and restricted behaviour and interests. They may show extreme restriction to change, obsession towards unusual objects, inflexible routines and schedules. They also are subject to repetitive body movements like hand flapping, rocking, etc.

- **Milestones**
  Lack of gestures and expressions is the sign of babies suffering with autism. When infants reach their first birthday, it is a stepping stone for them to a new world. They are curious and eager to use their limited communication skills to know about the world around. It is not the same with kids suffering with autism. They are least interested in knowing anything and might not perform typical gestures like babies of their age, such as waving hands, or pointing towards something.

- **Lack of Bonding**
  Babies suffering with this disorder might not bond with their parents, siblings or other members of the family. They may react the same way to their parents as they do with the strangers.

- **Lack of Interest**
  Autistic babies are very different from any other babies. They may not get attracted to popular play items like ball, stuffed toys, dolls, etc. They have their own way of passing time. They will perform repetitive actions like rotating their hands, turning the pages of books, etc.

Causes

The causes of autism are generally unknown, but experts label them as *genetic* and *environmental*.

- **Genetic Causes**
  Research has proved that genes inherited have a crucial role to play in getting autism along. However, no single gene is to be blamed. Scientists believe that atleast 5 to 20 major genes are involved in autism, with others contributing to the risk. The evidence that autism is hereditary comes from twin studies. Multiple twin stories show that when one identical twin develops the disorder, it is very likely for other to get affected

in 9 out of 10 cases. In fraternal twins, the ratio is 1 in 10. Studies have also proved that older parents are significantly at higher risk of having autistic babies. The age of father appears to be more important.

- **Environmental Causes**
  Genes alone do not explain the rising cases of autism, so scientists are also looking for answers in the environment. The idea is that toxic chemicals or other harmful elements in the environment may trigger autism, either by turning on or exasperating a genetic vulnerability, or independently disturbing brain development. Studies have suggested that autism can be triggered by exposure to viral infections, pesticides, insecticide at the time of pregnancy. Oxygen deprivation during delivery can also increase the risk of autism. Air pollution, food additives, flame retardants and certain chemicals used to make plastic and other synthetic materials can also cause autism. These toxins are more dangerous for young babies whose brains are more likely to absorb these toxins, but less effective in clearing them out.

- **Treatment**
  There is no best treatment package for those suffering with autism. However, experts believe that a well-structured specialised program can help. Early detection of the signs and early medical reference is very important. Before taking decision about child's treatment, parents must do as much research as possible. Parents should also ask questions like, how successful will be the program? Is the staff well trained? How are activities planned and organised? How is the progress measured? Asking these questions will not only make the doctors responsible, but will also provide you an insight of what is taking place with your baby.

27. Down Syndrome

Upward slanting eyes, unusual looking ears, broad hands with short fingers, sometimes pinkish in colour, small head are all characteristic features of Down syndrome. It sends waves of terror down your spine when you imagine the condition associated with down baby syndrome. Scientifically, it is the presence of an extra copy of chromosome 21 in the body. Down syndrome usually carries slow mental and physical growth. Even language also develops slowly and in the worst cases babies are born with heart problems and needs to be operated later. It is hard to believe that babies with Down syndrome are nothing but incomplete bodies marred with wrong functioning. It can also lead to hearing impairment and vision problems too, accompanied by intestinal infections. Babies can be treated over a period of time as they grow older and are resistant enough to bear pain involved in operations.

Causes

- If one of the parents is overaged at the time of conceiving, it can lead to Down Syndrome in some cases.
- Smoking by parents can be a prominent factor for a baby to get affected by Down Syndrome.
- It can be genetic in some cases and may pass from ancestors to next generations, but the probability is very low.

Treatment

It is really one of the most disheartening moments in one's life when one comes to know that the much awaited baby has arrived, but with Down Syndrome. The relief is that the treatment can help to alleviate the condition to a certain extent.

- A confirmed diagnosis of Down Syndrome requires a test. After your baby's birth, this test is performed on the blood samples and in 2 or 3 weeks time, the test displays results. This waiting period can be extremely difficult, especially if earlier test results were uncertain and your baby displays only subtle characteristics of Down Syndrome.
- Since it is a problem related to the chromosomes and nothing much can be done about these ingrained issues, it is important to, at least, reduce the syndromes symptoms as per the doctor's consultation.

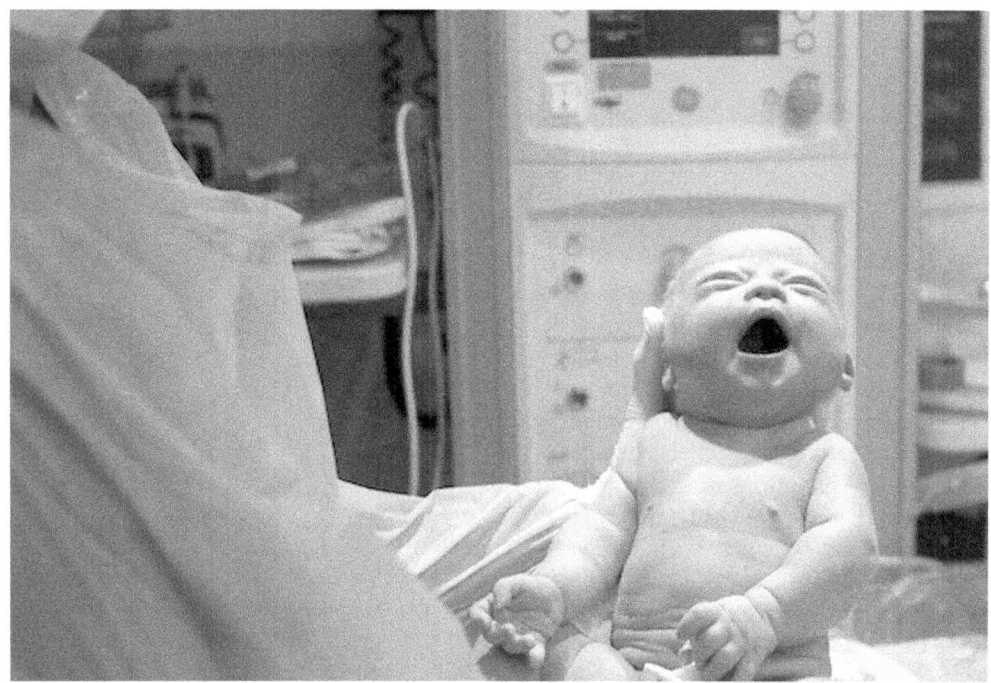
Down Symdrome in babies

- Doctors encourage several counselling sessions for parents and children to make them aware. Educating oneself on the syndrome will encourage parents to take corrective actions and consider the extent of mental retardation in babies and its influence in their child's life.
- Make sure your baby has regular checkups and tests and any symptoms and signs associated with it are diagnosed as early as possible, so that drugs and medicinal help can be given to the baby at the earliest.
- Apart from everything else, don't forget to lend moral support to your baby. Never give up on hope and try as much as you can to bring back your baby to the normal state.

28. Flat Head Syndrome

Babies are like newly published books that seem to reveal some new and astounding information every now and then. Babies are born with waxy and pliable organs and can develop some dramatic problems arising due to resting in the same position for longer times, may be in a car seat or their beds. This may lead to baby's head being flat at some spots. In such cases, you can always encourage the babies to rest their heads in alternative directions. You should take notice that they are not sleeping at one particular position and turn them whenever you can. You just have to make sure that the baby doesn't take pressure on a particular area of the head and even if the head has been flattened before, it can be resumed to normal shape again. Adding to your relief is the fact that flat head syndrome is purely a cosmetic issue and doesn't relate to the mental development of a baby. Yet it is a matter to be thought about.

Causes

- Apart from sleeping or resting postures, flat head syndrome can also be caused in the womb itself by mother's pelvis or pressure from a twin.
- 'Craniosynostosis' is a term characterised by a condition where the bones in the skull fuse together in a short time and can lead to the syndrome.

- ❑ Congenital disabilities can also add to the deformity of the head.

Treatment

- ❑ Babies are born with normal heads, but due to postures can be deformed easily; you can initially give the condition its own time to recover the flat head.
- ❑ If you are noticing the flat head of your baby for a longer period of time, you can take an appointment with your pediatrician and can check with his specifications and directions.
- ❑ Treatment starts with the recommended exercises by the doctor, which include sleeping more on tummy, using a U-shaped ring on the neck at the time of lying down, repositioning during sleeping can help, etc.
- ❑ All the recommended exercises should be beneficial but if it's not turning to be so, then you can again consult your pediatrician for more improvements and suggestions.
- ❑ Cranial moulding devices and helmets are also available under doctor's guidance at stores, which can be bought and used for the recovery purposes.
- ❑ Make sure you do not use the devices for a longer period of time as it may hinder the blood circulation in the head and may produce a numb feeling as well.

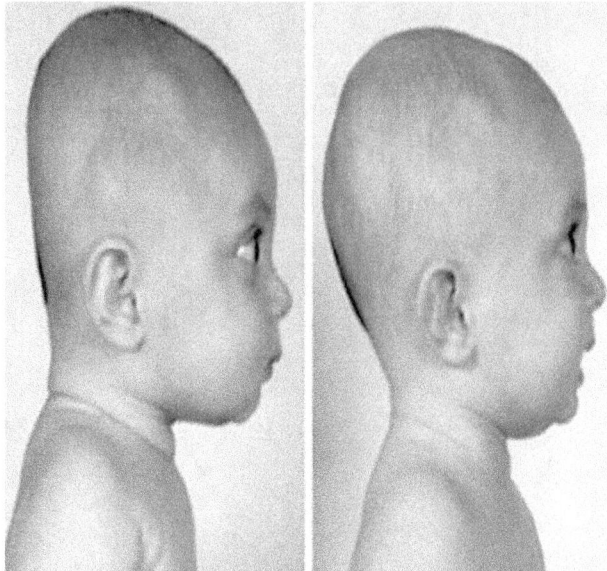

Flat head baby – before and after cure

29. Handicaps in Children

When any disability of body or mind interferes with the ability of the child to lead a normal life or to benefit from a normal education, then the child is considered to be handicapped. Most of these handicaps may be prevented by careful pre-pregnancy planning, regular checkups, care of the pregnant mother and supervised delivery of the baby. These are the various handicaps found in children.

Types of Handicaps

- ❑ Partial or total blindness
- ❑ Partial or total deafness
- ❑ Disorders of joint, bone or muscle
- ❑ Nervous system disorders like mental retardation, cerebral palsy, etc
- ❑ Organ diseases like lung, heart, kidney diseases

Early Detection

Timely detection of a handicap is very important. It helps to correct or limit disability and allow better chances of recovery with optimum results of rehabilitation therapy. Some defects are obvious and can be detected very early but some defects like mental retardation, visual and hearing defects, etc., may remain unrecognised for quite some time. Regular examination of the baby by the pediatrician helps in early detection of any handicap.

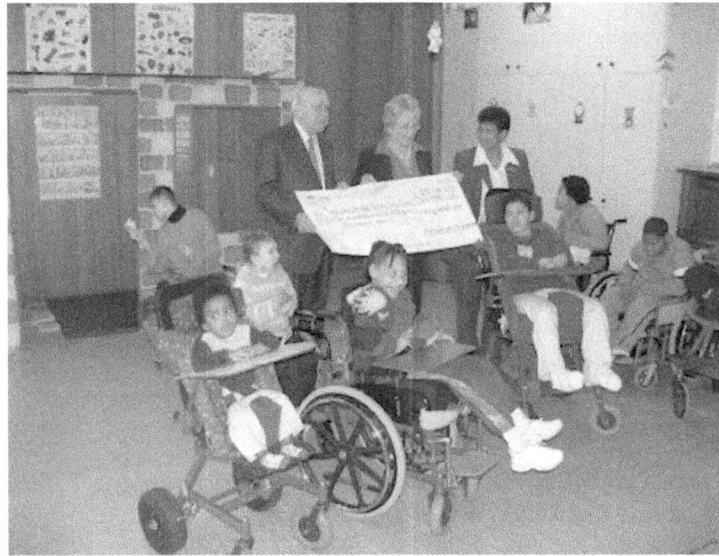
Handicapped children

Treatment

Depending upon the nature of disability, handicapped children require different kinds of treatment. Occupational therapies, speech therapy, psychotherapy, physiotherapy, etc., are some of the treatments which are given by specialists to the child according to the nature of handicap.

Handling of Handicapped Child by Parents

- ❏ Discuss the exact nature of your child's handicap and find out the underlying cause of the problem and its genetic implications. Also find out from the doctor the likely outcome of the handicap in the long run. You should learn the outline of the proposed management.
- ❏ Keep a positive outlook while remaining pragmatic and realistic in accepting the existence, nature and severity of the handicap.
- ❏ Do not harbour any sense of trauma, guilt or shame in association with the handicap.
- ❏ Avoid feeling embarrassed in public in the company of your disabled child. This mental approach will help you to look after the child properly.
- ❏ Give consideration and respect to your handicapped child like any other child.
- ❏ Help the child to retain his/her sense of self-esteem despite the disability and be strong enough to face the difficulties with confidence.
- ❏ Your love and security is important for the child but do not become overprotective.

30. Congenital Abnormalities

Some babies are born with certain abnormalities, which are present at the time of the birth of the baby. These are known *congenital abnormalities*. These abnormalities are a result of problems, while the baby was developing in the foetus or because of complications during labour. These may be hereditary abnormalities. The causes of more than half of the congenital abnormalities in human are unknown. They are referred to as sporadic, which implies an unknown cause in medical terms.

Given below are a few common congenital abnormalities that may be seen in babies.

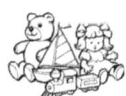

FAQs

Q-1. My two-year old son has worms in his stools. Is it true that this happened because he eats lots of sweet as he is very fond of sweets.

Ans. You will have to deworm your son by giving him the medicine prescribed by his pediatrician. Teach him the general rules of hygiene like washing hands properly after using the toilet and before and after eating food. Sweets can be responsible for tooth decay if the child does not practise oral hygiene but they are in no way responsible for worms in the stools.

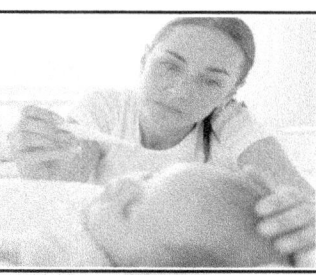

Q-2. My daughter's tonsils are enlarged due to frequent throat infections. Can I get them removed by an operation?

Ans. Tonsils are the glands which protect a child against infection. Giving proper and complete course of antibiotics can cure this problem. Improve immunity of your child by giving her good and nutritious diet. Removing tonsils should be the last resort and that too, in case they are obstructing the child's breathing.

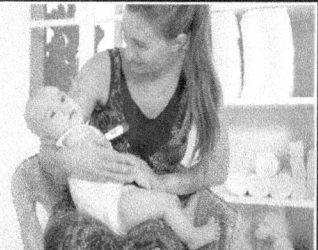

Q-3. My daughter has asthma. Her pediatrician has prescribed some steroid puffs to be taken every day. Are there any side-effects of these steroids?

Ans. There are no side-effects with steroid puffs so long as you make sure that the child rinses her mouth each time she takes the puff. This is done to avoid any possibility of developing a fungal infection or hoarseness of voice. Continue her treatment under the watchful eyes of a pediatrician and follow the doctor's advice properly.

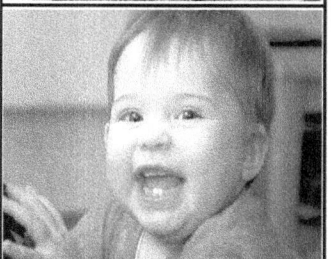

Q-4. My one and a half-year old daughter keeps getting urine infection often. What should be done?

Ans. Urine infection is more common among girls because urethra, the duct from which the urine comes out, is located closer to the anus as compared to boys. So the bacteria from the stools can reach the urethra easily and cause urine infection. Clean her genitae area from front to back after she passes stools so that chances of infection lessen. If she still gets frequent urine infection, consult her pediatrician. She may need to be investigated thoroughly.

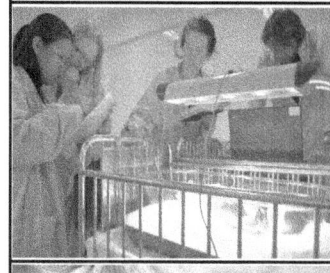

Q-5. In our family, no one eats curd and orange during winter season thinking they will catch cold. My son is very fond of these two things. Can I give him curd and orange during winter?

Ans. It is just a myth that curd and orange should not be eaten during winter. In fact, both these things contain vitamin C which is good to boost body's immunity and help in fighting infection. There is definitely no harm in giving both these things to your son so long as he does not have any allergic tendency towards them.

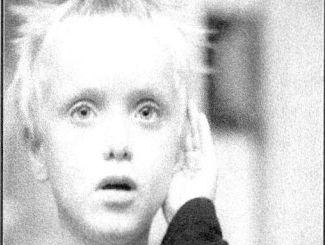

V
General Care

A child needs close loving care with due attention to food, clothes, hygiene and environment. While taking day-to-day care of your child, it is extremely important for you to be alert and to keep a close watch for any early signs of the disease or discomfort.

1. Caring for a Sick Child

Parents love to bestow love and care on their children, but when it comes to looking after their sick child, they find themselves at a loss about the correct way of handling the child. The daily chores for the child like feeding, bathing, clothing, personal hygiene, etc., become tedious chores for them as they feel unsure about their abilities to make simple observations accurately.

Tips for Caring for a Sick Child

- Keep the child's room at a comfortable temperature. Provide proper ventilation by keeping the windows slightly open.
- Use clean cotton sheets on the bed which should be changed periodically.
- Dress the child in loose comfortable clothes.
- Cleanliness and hygiene are very important but do not insist on giving full body baths to the sick child. However, in hot and humid weather, a quick bath would induce a general feeling of freshness.
- When sick, most children have a poor appetite. Do not try to force-feed the child. Let the child eat as much as he/she wants. Avoid fatty and spicy foods. Milk, fruit juices, thin soups, etc., may be given as they are light and nutritious.
- It is not necessary for the child to always lie in bed. Take the child in another room for a while. This change will make him/her feel better. When not in bed, provide the child with a comfortable chair with soft cushions to lean on.
- During illness, most children tend to cling to their mothers. They cry for no particular reason and want to be fed more frequently. So stay calm and give your time and patience to the child. Remember sick child needs your love, company and a sense of security besides your care.

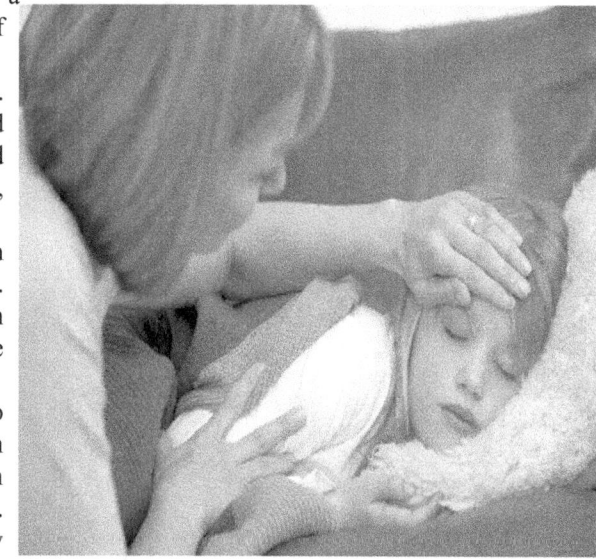

A child with mother attending to her lovingly

2. Safeguards Against Accidents

By nature, children are inquisitive. They love to explore everything within their reach. In the process, they get hurt. Every year, accidents cause a large number of serious injuries to children. It is, therefore, very important for parents to understand the cause of accident and prevent them. Constant vigil and adherence to basic safety precautions should be strictly followed by parents. Here are some tips to safeguard your child from possible hazards:

- Keep anything hot like teapots, tea cups, etc., out of the reach of the child. Do not drink anything hot with the child on your lap.
- Remove tablecloths hanging at the edge, which, if pulled by the child, may bring things down on the child.
- Do not leave the baby unattended on a table or in high chair. Carefully watch the child in baby walker as they can trip over steps or get caught in other things.
- When the baby begins to crawl, make sure he/she does not have the access to staircase, balcony or open verandah.
- Cover all unused electric sockets and keep all electric appliances out of their reach.
- Small objects like coins, beads, safety pins, etc., should be kept away from small children so that they do not put them in their mouth and choke.
- Store all the medicines, phenol, kerosene oil, batteries etc away from children.
- Always keep the bathroom doors bolted.
- Clean any spilled water or oil from the floor immediately.
- Remove carpets and mats which are torn or folded.
- Keep glass objects out of the reach of children. Preferably do not use glass furniture or crockery till your child is small.
- Do not let children play with stray animals like dogs. Do not leave small children alone with pets.
- Always put safety belt while taking the child out in the pram. Also lock the wheels when it is not being moved around.
- While travelling by car, keep the children secure with belts. A special baby seat with belt may be fitted in the car.

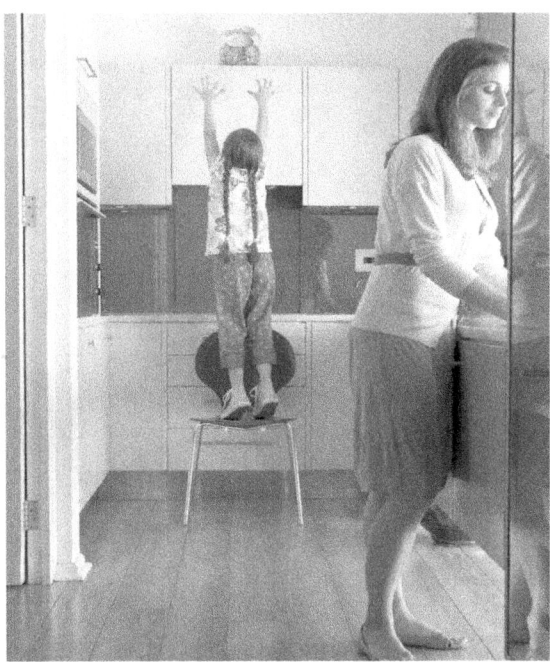

Do not leave the baby unattended on a table or in high chair

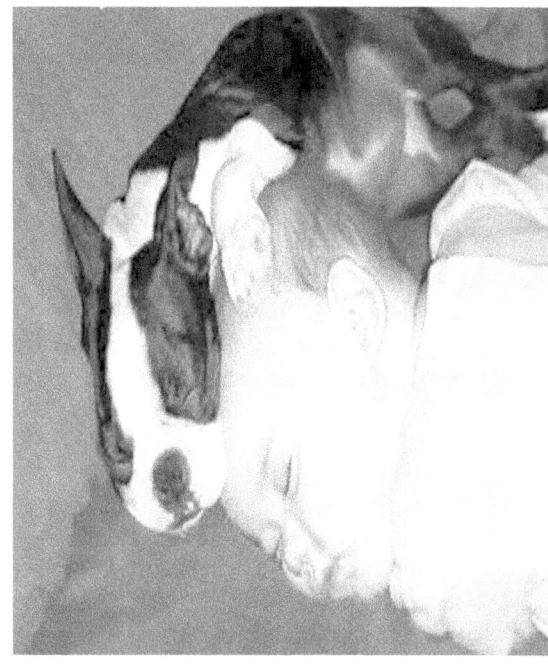

Do not let children play with stray or pet animals like dogs

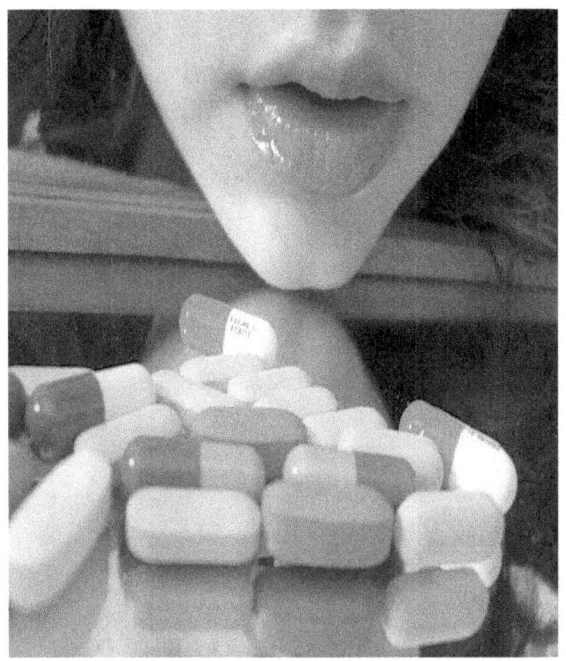
Store all the medicines away from children

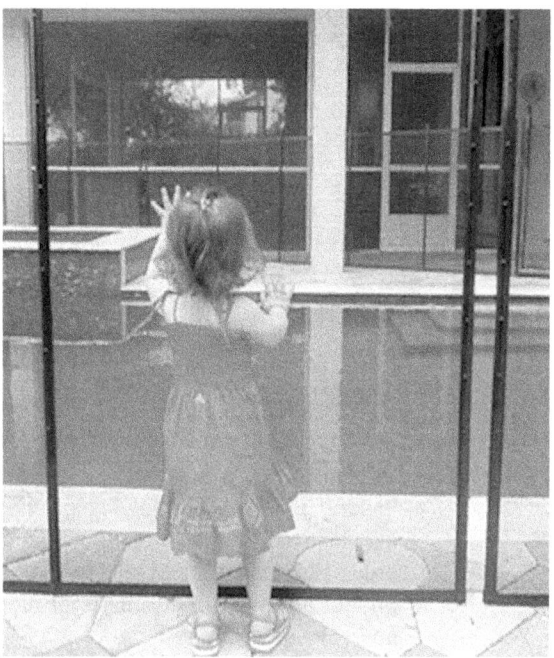
Open verandah should not be accessible for small children

- ❏ Discourage the children to laugh or play with food in their mouth.
- ❏ Do not allow them to play with polythene bags else they may suffocate because of being unable to remove the bag from their heads.
- ❏ Ensure that the children's fingers do not get jammed while closing the doors of your house or car.

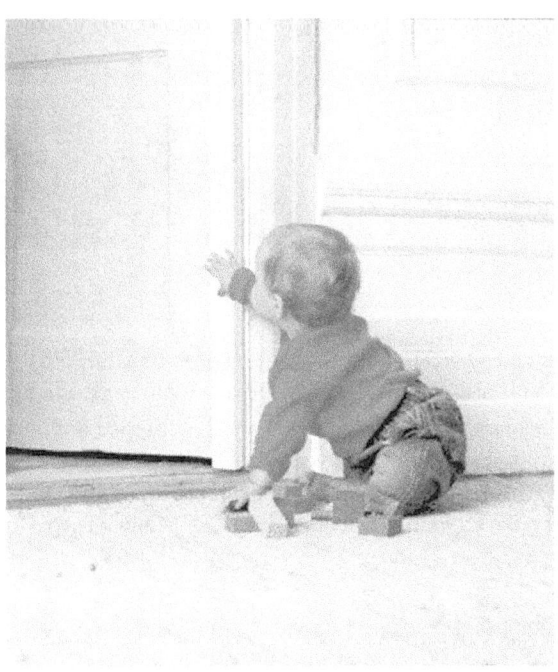
Always keep the bathroom doors bolted

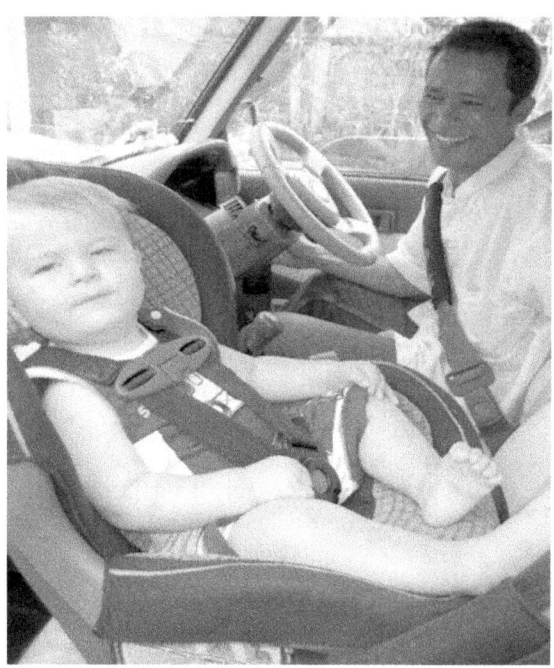
While travelling by car, keep the children secure with belts

General Care

3. Dealing with Medical Emergencies at Home

In every household with small children, emergency situations like burns, choking or swallowing a poisonous thing or accident take place. The life of the child depends upon the quality of emergency aid given immediately before a doctor can be reached. Here are some basic rules for handling emergencies.

- ❑ Be calm in an emergency situation.
- ❑ Act logically and firmly after assessing the problem carefully and quickly.
- ❑ Reassure the child that all would be well if he/she cooperates.
- ❑ Do not cry or let others cry in front of the child.
- ❑ Assess the nature and severity of the problem.
- ❑ Take the child to the doctor as early as possible.

Managing Emergencies

Here are some tips to manage some common emergencies which you may have to face sometimes:

- ❑ **Bleeding Nose**
  - ➤ Picking the nose or blowing or sneezing may lead to bleeding nose. Some blood disorders also lead to nosebleed.
  - ➤ First of all establish the cause for bleeding nose. Bend the child
  - ➤ S head over a basin and grip his/her nose between your thumb and fingers over the soft part of the nose just below where the bone ends applying firm pressure to both nostrils to stop the bleeding. Do not allow the child to put the head back during nose bleed because the blood is then likely to drip down the child's throat to his/her stomach causing vomiting later.

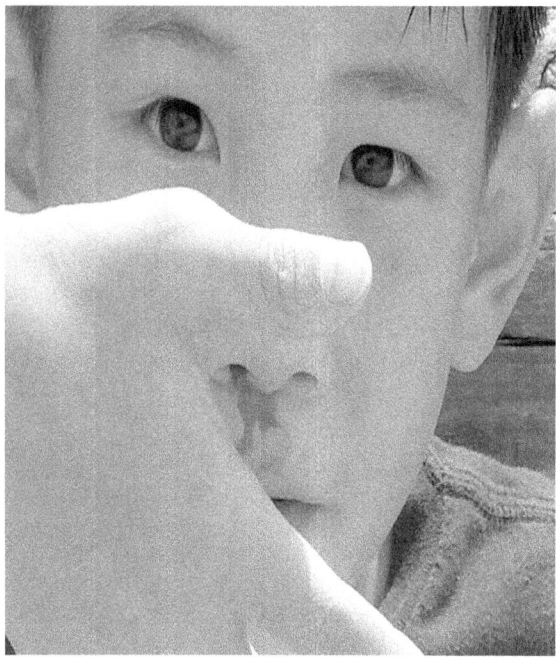

Bleeding nose

- ❑ **Burns**
  In case of burns, immerse the affected body part in a bucket of cold water or in running cold water. Ice packs may also be applied locally to cool the small area of burn on the parts which cannot be immersed in water like neck, face etc. When the burning subsides, put some burnol or toothpaste on the burnt part.

- ❑ **Foreign Body in the Nose or Ear**
  If your child has pushed something up his/her nose, then DO NOT attempt to take it out yourself. Keep the child quiet and ask him/her to breathe through the mouth.rush to the nearest hospital casualty department.

  If the child has pushed something int hear or an insect has crawled into the ear and got trapped in there, then ask your child to set down and tilt his/her head to one side so that you can see inside the ear with the foreign body. Gently flood the ear with mildly warm water so the foreign body or the insect may float on it and come out on its own. If it does not then take the child to the doctor. DO NOT in any case try to remove it with a pointed implement.

- ❑ **Head injury**
  If a child gets a minor head injury while playing, then observe the child for some time. If he/she resumes normal activities and shows no signs of distress even for 24 hours after the injury, then heave a sigh of relief. But if you find any of the following symptoms then rush the child to the doctor immediately:

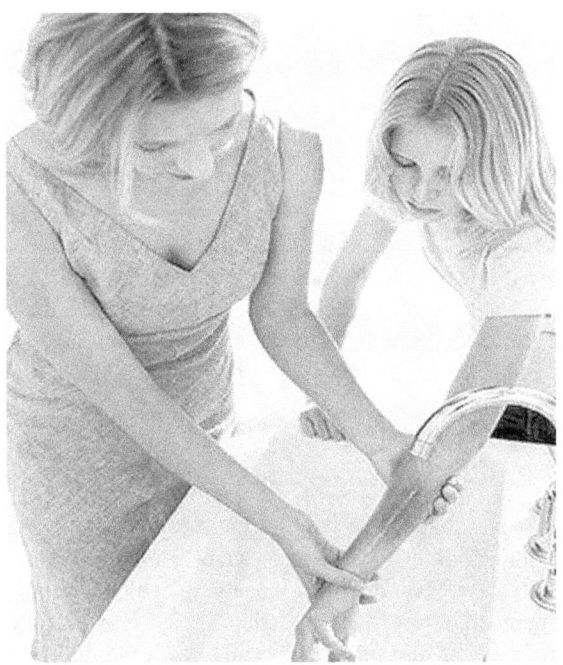
Child burn

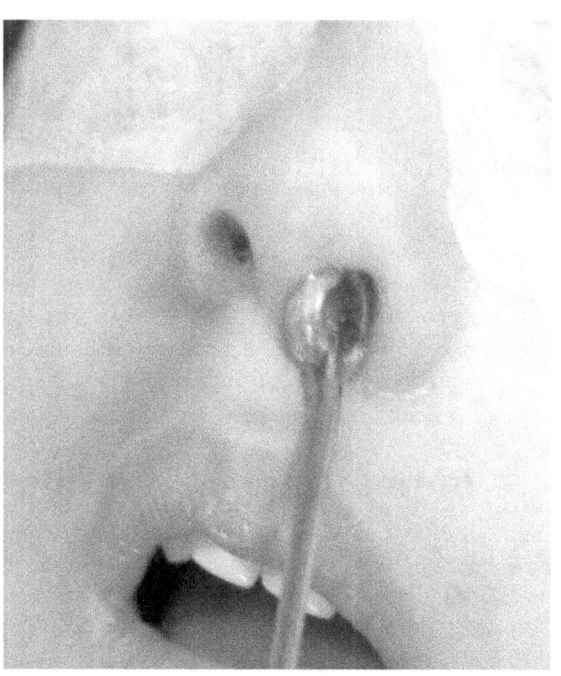
Foreign body in the nose

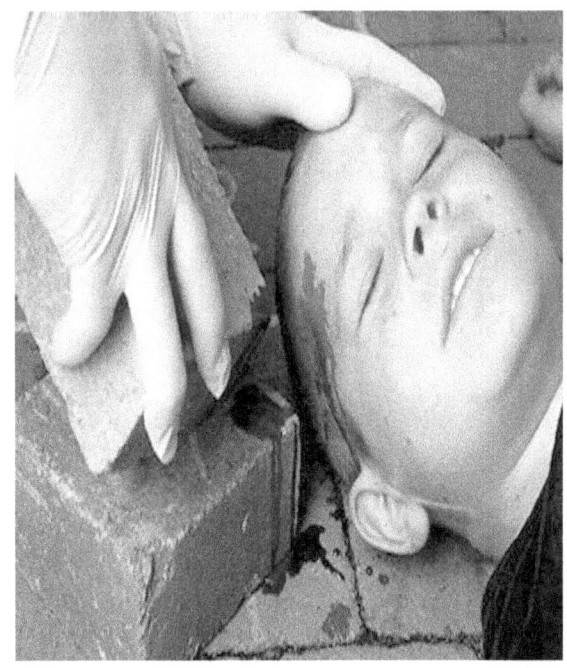
Head injury

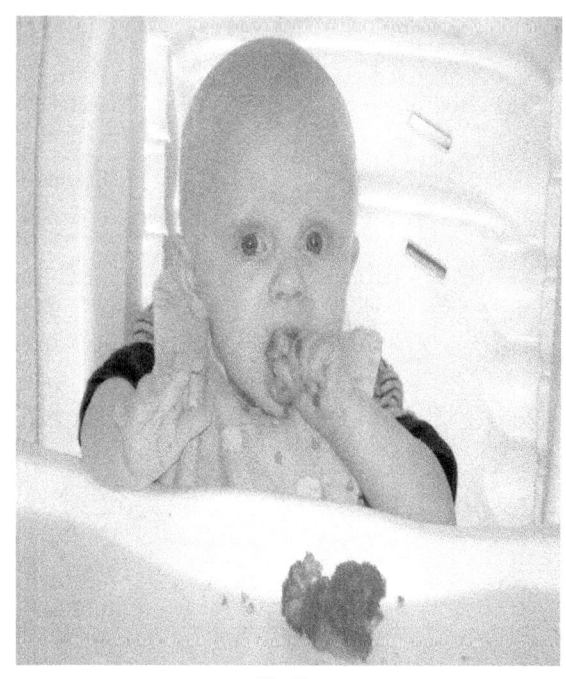
Choking

General Care

- Unconsciousness
- Dizziness
- Vomiting
- Persisting headache
- Drowsiness
- Bleeding from ears or nose

❑ **Choking**

If your child has swallowed a foreign object like coin, button pin and it has suddenly slipped into the back of his throat, then this may either block the throat or cause acute contraction of muscles around it and cause choking. The child may not be able to speak and breathe. In such a case, act immediately. Hold the child firmly by his/her legs with one hand and turn him/her upside down. With the child hanging upside down with his/her head facing the ground, slap his/her back firmly with your other hand. All this should be done quickly to save the child's life.

4. Immunization Schedule

Immunization is important to protect your baby from those diseases that can be fatal for him/her. It is one of the most important things you can do to guarantee your baby's health. Childhood diseases, such as whooping cough, measles, diphtheria, chicken pox, small pox, poliomyelitis and yellow fever are common among babies. Through immunization, a chemical substance that has the causative organism of any given infection/disease is injected to the baby to reduce the possibility of catching the disease. Oral doses can also be given as in the case of Polio. Over the years, immunization has greatly reduced the mortality rate among infants.

Some infectious diseases have the potential to cause long-lasting health problems that are permanent in nature. Immunization helps to guard against such hazardous diseases. In the past two decades, vaccines have shown a tremendous ability in preventing serious illnesses, and averted death in millions of cases. They have proved to be one of the most effective tools ever created to help babies live a healthy life. The article lists the immunization schedule for babies, in infancy and later. Read on to know about the timings of important vaccines.

Immunization Time Schedule

Mandatory Vaccines

Age	Disease	Vaccination
AT BIRTH	HEPATITIS B	HEP B VACCINE -I
AT BIRTH	POLIO	ORAL PV 0 DOSE
BIRTH TO 6 WEEKS	TUBERCULOSIS	BCG
4 -6 WEEKS	HEPATITIS B	HEP B VACCINE -II
6 WEEKS	DIPHTHERIA PERTUSIS TETANUS POLIO	DPT-I OPV -I
10 WEEKS	DIPHTHERIA PERTUSIS TETANUS POLIO HEPATITIS B	DPT-II OPV-II HEP B VACCINE III

Age	Disease	Vaccination
14 WEEKS	DIPHTHERIA PERTUSIS TETANUS POLIO	DPT-III OPV- III HEP B VACCINE IV
24 WEEKS	HEPATITIS B	HEP B VACCINE III
9 -12 MONTHS	POLIO MEASLES	OPV-IV MEASLES
15-18 MONTHS	MUMPS MEASELES RUBELLA	MMR
18 MONTHS	DIPHTHERIA PERTUSIS TETANUS POLIO	DPT –BOOSTER I OPV –V
24 MONTHS	TYPHOID	TYPHOID
4-5 YEARS	DIPHTHERIA PERTUSIS TETANUS POLIO	DPT BOOSTER – II OPV -VI

Other Vaccines

Age	Disease	Vaccination
6 WEEKS	H influenza B	HiB
10 WEEKS	H influenza B	HiB
14 WEEKS	H influenza B	HiB
18 MONTHS	H influenza B	HiB
24 MONTHS	HEPATITIS A	H A VACCINE-I
30 MONTHS	HEPATITIS A	H A VACCINE -II
12 MONTHS	CHICKENPOX	VARICELLA VACCINE
24 MONTHS	MENINGOCOCCAL A&C	MENINGOCOCCAL VACCINE
12 MONTHS	PNEUMOCOCCAL	PNEUMOCOCCAL VACCINE
12 MONTHS	INFLUENZA	INFLUENZA VACCINE
5 YEARS	TYPHOID	TYPHOID
5 YEARS	MENINGOCOCCAL A&C	MENINGOCOCCAL VACCINE
10 YEARS	TETANUS	TT

It is important to follow the immunization schedule accurately. If you miss an immunization date, you need to consult your doctor immediately to fix a new date. If the baby is very ill when immunization is due, it is advisable

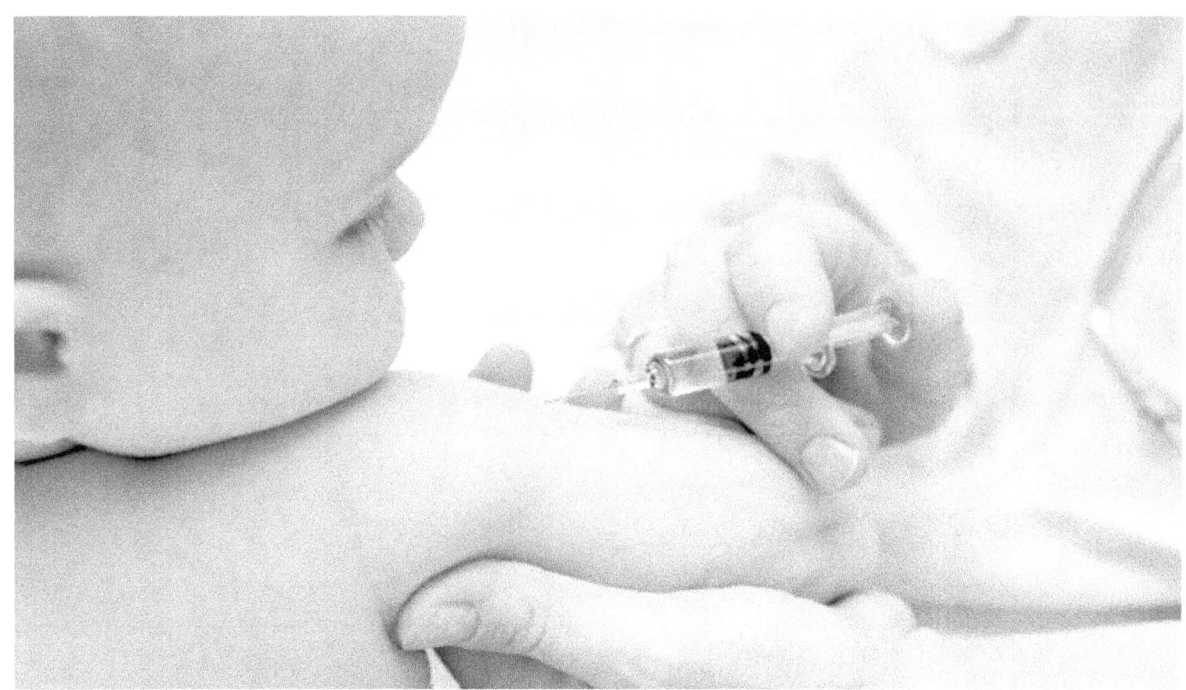
A child getting vaccinated

to consult the doctor/pediatrician and reschedule immunization. But if your baby has a slight cold or cough, then you can go ahead with vaccination. In case your baby has had an acute reaction to a dose of immunization, consult your doctor/pediatrician before you give him the booster dose.

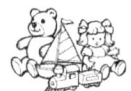

FAQs

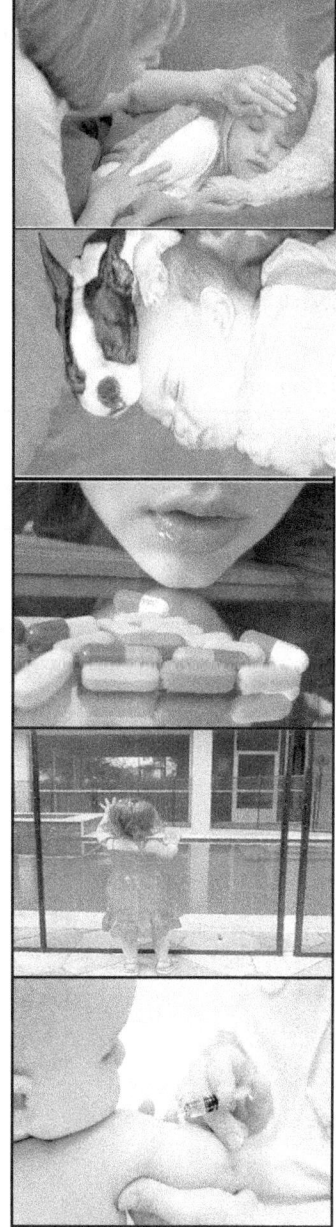

Q-1. My daughter is nine months old. Can I put the thermometer in her mouth to check her temperature?

Ans. Use a clinical thermometer to check her temperature. It is preferable to check the temperature by keeping it in the arm pit till your baby is at least 4-5 years old. When she can understand that she is not supposed to bite the thermometer, then put it inside her mouth. While placing the thermometer in the arm pit, make sure that the tip of the thermometer touches the skin and not the clothing.

Q-2. What should I keep in my first-aid kit?

Ans. A first-aid kit helps in giving immediate help to the victim before medical help reaches them. A first-aid kit should contain antiseptic lotion, sterile cotton and gauze, band aid, burnol. Some emergency drugs may be kept in the first-aid box as per doctor's recommendations.

Q-3. What should I do if I miss any dose of a vaccine for my daughter?

Ans. If you have missed any dose of a vaccine, then just start from the dose you missed and go ahead with rest of the vaccines in schedule. You do not have to repeat the whole cycle all over again.

Q-4. What are the general symptoms which tell me that my baby might be sick and I should consult a doctor?

Ans. Look for these signs in your baby and consult a doctor/pediatrician if you find any one of them in your baby:
- ➤ The baby has fever, cough and cold.
- ➤ The baby is sleeping more than usual.
- ➤ Baby is continuously crying and none of your efforts seem to placate the baby.
- ➤ Your baby is breathing faster with unusual sounds and appears uncomfortable while breathing.
- ➤ Your baby appears blue or very pale and feels cold to touch.
- ➤ The baby has not passed urine for more than 12 hours.
- ➤ The baby has not passed stool for past four days.
- ➤ The baby has diarrhea and vomiting.
- ➤ The baby is passing red/black stools.
- ➤ The baby is not taking the feed at all.

Q-5. My daughter received her BCG vaccination soon after birth, but she did not develop a scar even after three months. What should be done?

Ans. You need to repeat the vaccine before she is one year old. Keep in mind that BCG and Measles vaccines should not be given together. There should be a gap of at least one month between these two vaccines.

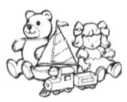

General Care

Appendix – I
Average Weight and Height of Boys and Girls at Different Ages

	Boys			Girls	
Age	Weight (Kg)	Height (cm)	Age	Weight (kg)	Height (cm)
Birth	3.0	50.0	Birth	2.9	48.5
6 months	7.2	66.0	6 months	6.6	64.2
1 year	9.5	75.0	1 year	9.0	72.5
2 year	11.5	85.5	2 year	11.0	84.0
3 year	13.5	94.0	3 year	13.0	93.0
4 year	15.4	100.0	4 year	15.0	99.0
5 year	17.2	106.5	5 year	16.5	105.5
6 year	19.0	112.5	6 year	18.0	111.5
7 year	21.0	118.0	7 year	19.8	117.0
8 year	22.0	123.0	8 year	22.0	122.0
9 year	25.4	128.0	9 year	25.3	127.8
10 year	28.0	133.4	10 year	28.7	133.6
11 year	31.2	139.0	11 year	32.4	140.0
12 year	35.0	144.5	12 year	36.5	147.0
13 year	40.0	150.5	13 year	40.5	152.8
14 year	45.2	157.0	14 year	44.5	156.0
15 year	51.0	163.0	15 year	47.8	157.0
16 year	56.0	168.5	16 year	50.0	157.8

Appendix – II
CDC Growth Charts

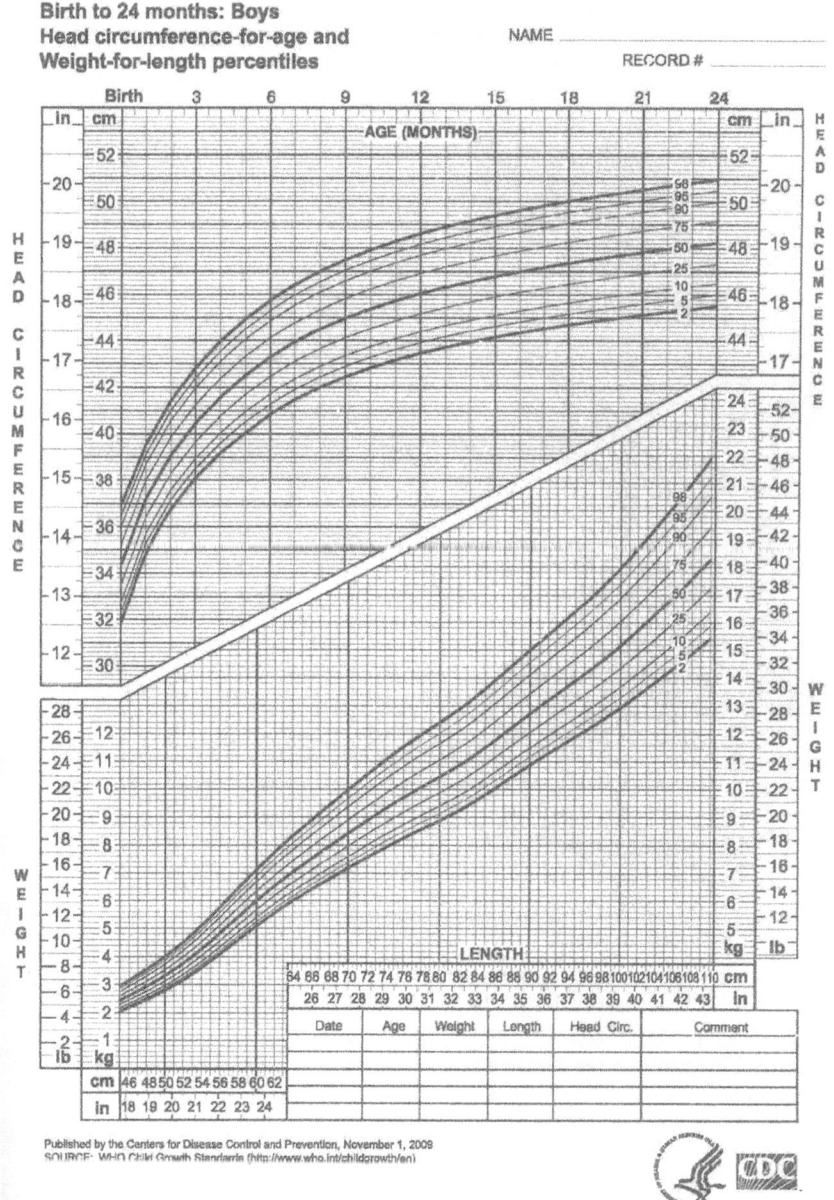

CDC Growth Charts

189

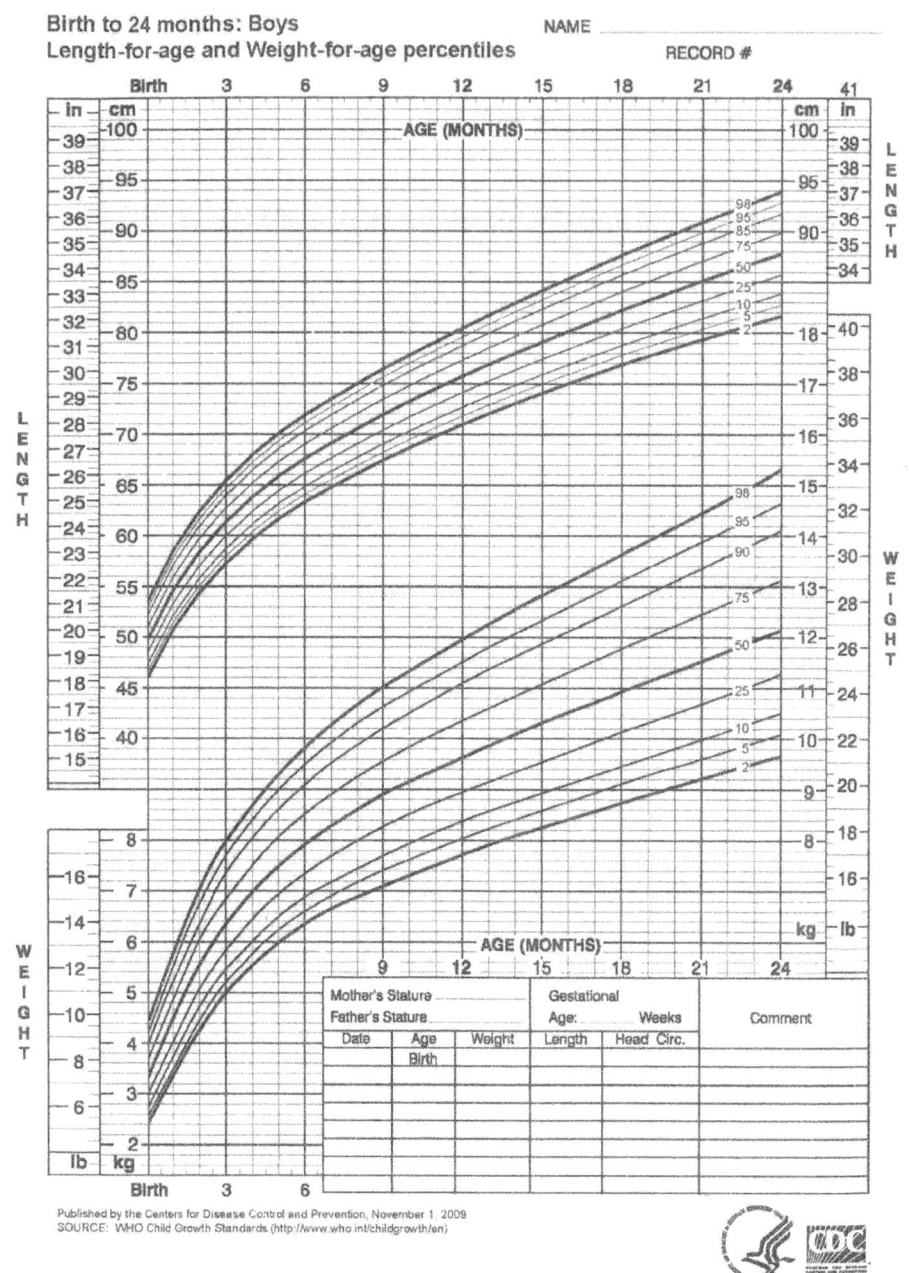

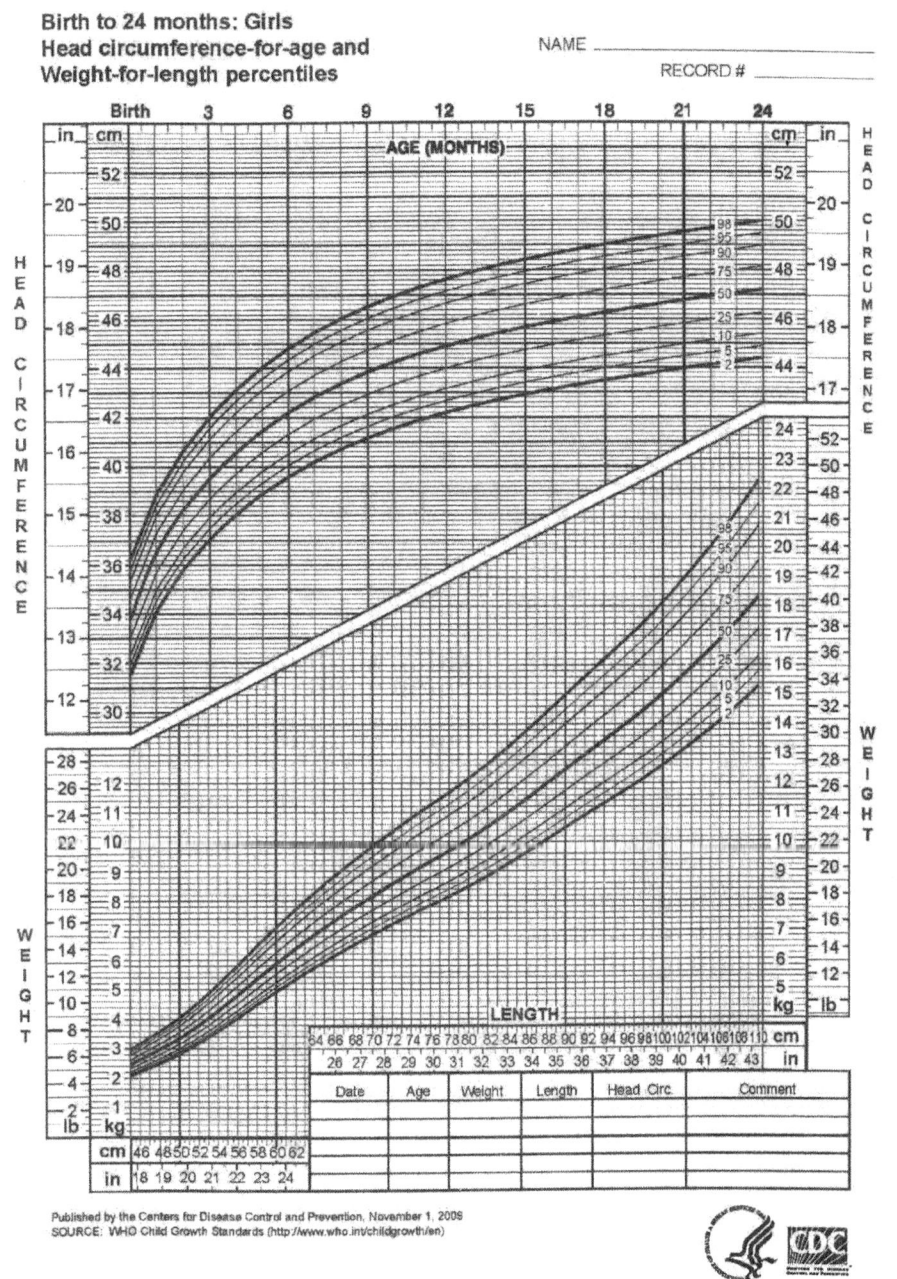

CDC Growth Charts

Birth to 24 months: Girls
Head circumference-for-age and
Weight-for-length percentiles

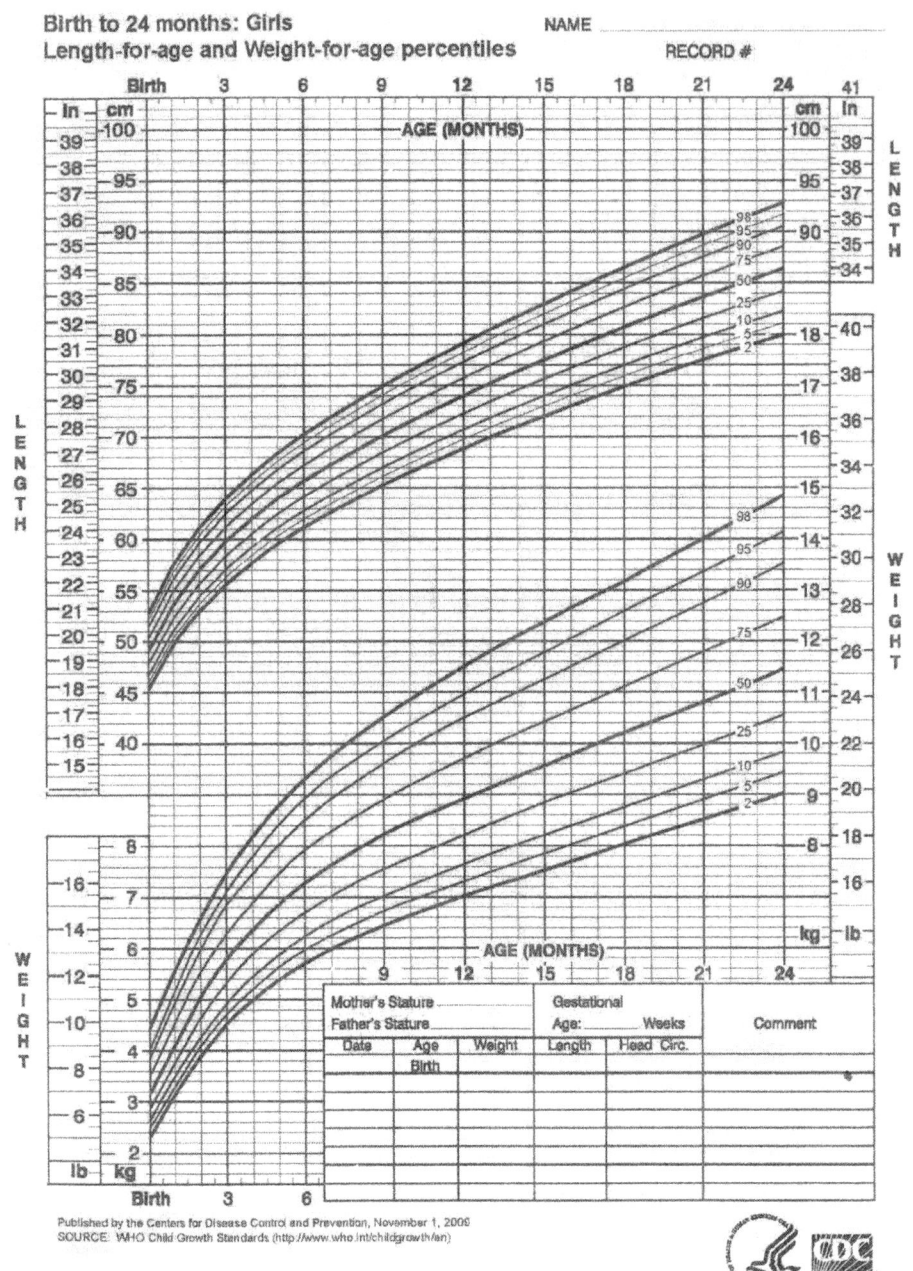

Appendix – III
Recipes of Common Weaning Foods

1. Suji Ki Kheer

Suji	25 gm
Sugar	10 gm
Milk	250 ml (¼ litre)

Method: Boil milk and add suji. Cook on a slow fire till it becomes semisolid. Add sugar. Cool and serve lukewarm to the baby.

2. Rice Kheer

Rice	10 gm
Sugar	10 gm
Milk	250 ml

Method: Wash rice after cleaning and picking it. Boil milk and add rice. Cook on a slow fire till it becomes semisolid. Add sugar. serve at lukewarm temperature.

3. Khichdi

Rice	50gm
Dehusked moong dal	25 gm
Spinach (optional)	50 gm
Oil	2 teaspoons
Salt	to taste

Method: Cook rice and dal together and mash. Boil spinach, mash and strain. Add the spinach puree, salt and heated oil to the rice-dal mixture and stir. Cool and serve lukewarm.

4. Porridge of Khichdi

Wheat dalia (Porridge)	50 gm
Moong dal or Green Gram	50 gm

Potato	in amounts desired
Any green vegetable	in amounts desired
Oil	1 teaspoon
Salt	to taste
Onion	1 small
Ginger	2 gm
Bay leaf and cardamom (optional)	1 each

Method: Clean and wash dalia and dal separately and cut vegetables. To boiling water add onion, ginger, bay leaf, cardamom and dalia. Cook until half-cooked. Then add dal and vegetables and cook until soft. Season with salt and oil.

5. Rice Upma

Rice	25 gm
Green gram dal	25 gm
Onion	1 large
Mustard	½ teaspoons
Groundnut oil	4 teaspoons
Salt	to taste
Water	2 cups

Method: Roast rice and dal and grind into granules. Cook green gram dal with ¾ cup water and mash. To hot oil, add mustard, onion and fry and then add water and salt. Add the rice granules and vegetables to the water and stir cook for 10 minutes and add the green gram dal paste. Drumstick leaves may also be used instead of vegetables.

Note: Suji Upma may also be made in the same way. Use suji in place of rice and dal.

6. Poha

Puffed rice (soaked)	50 gm
Onions	1 small
Potatoes or other vegetables	½ cup
Cumin and mustard seeds	¼ teaspoons
Mustard oil	1 teaspoons

Method: Saute onions and cumin and mustard seeds in oil. Add vegetables and cook till tender, adding minimum quantity of water. Finally add puffed and soaked rice, and cook for 2-3 minutes.

7. Ragi Adai-Sweet

Ragi flour	30 gm
Roasted Bengal gram dal	3 teaspoons
Jaggery	15 gm

Coconut scrapings	1 teaspoons
Oil (groundnut)	2 teaspoons
Water	3 teaspoons

Method: Dissolve jaggery in water. Add Bengal gram flour, ragi flour and coconut scrapings to the jaggery water to make thick dough. Prepare the adai on a greased iron pan or tawa.
Note: Ragi is good for the growth of babies

8. Apple Carrot Soup

Apple	1 small (deseeded)
Carrot	1 small
Cinnamon stick	1 cm stick
Salt to taste	

Method: Peel and dice the apple and carrot. Boil then in a pressure cooker with 2 cups of water. Add the cinnamon stick to the mixture. Open the cooker and remove the cinnamon stick. Blend the mixture in a blender till the required consistency. Heat and simmer the soup for five minutes. Serve hot.

9. Biscuit Custard

Milk	½ cup
Carrot	1 crushed
Sugar to taste	

Method: Methods bring the milk and sugar to a boil and add the crushed biscuit. Allow it to mix with the milk so that the milk thickens. Mix well so that the custard does not have any lumps.
Note: Instead of using refined cornflour to make custard, digestive biscuit makes this custard healthy.

10. Banana Smoothie

Banana	1 (peeled)
Milk	1 cup
Sugar to taste	

Method: Pour all ingredients in blender. Mix it for 30 seconds and serve cool.

Source: Selected Nutritious Recipes – 1983 National Institutes of Public Cooperation and Child Development, New Delhi.

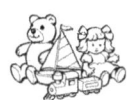

Children are like wet cement, whatever falls on them makes an impression — Haim Ginott

Parents often have a tendency to blame children for their failings — little realising that their own role in their personality development is of much greater significance than their offsprings'. Parents need to look within to see how they can be model parents and provide a healthy environment for proper mental, emotional and physical growth of their children. However protection or restrictiveness can spoil a child; permissiveness or indulgence can make him anti-social, rejection can work on his personality, why he takes to lying, stealing or mud-eating.

How to Shape Your Kids Better

Author: Hari Datt Sharma
Language: English
Type: Paperback
Pages: 124
Price: ₹ 96

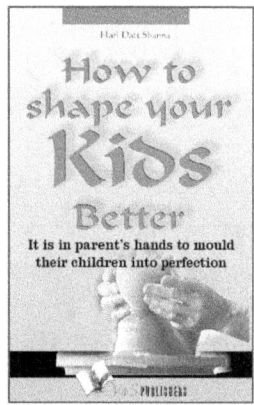

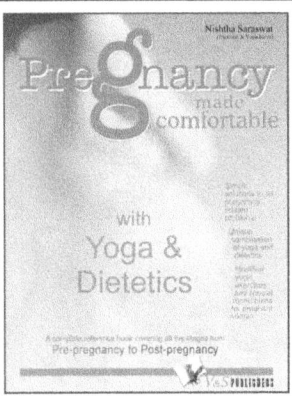

Pregnancy

Author: Nishtha Saraswat
Language: English
Type: Paperback
Pages: 129
Price: ₹ 150

This unique and must read book by Nishtha Saraswat is the only one of its kind that deals with pregnancy related problems with the help of unique combination of yoga and dietetics, two of the most relevant subjects in today's social context.

The effort has been put behind understanding various stages involved in pregnancy in a simple and easy to understand manner. The stress has been laid on providing practical solutions to the common problems faced by women before, during and after pregnancy. A combination of yogic exercises, meditation and special menu plans has been recommended keeping in mind the needs of Indian women.

The mother of two daughters, the author has used both her own experience and suggestions from peers to give valuable insights on bringing up a daughter in 21st century India. She has not only attempted to highlight the problems of bringing up a daughter today, but also tried to show how these can be tackled and how the best of our traditional values can be combined with current requirements to bring up a well-adjusted daughter.

Raising a Daughter in 21st Century India

Author: Rupa Chatterjee
Language: English
Type: Paperback
Pages: 136
Price: ₹ 120

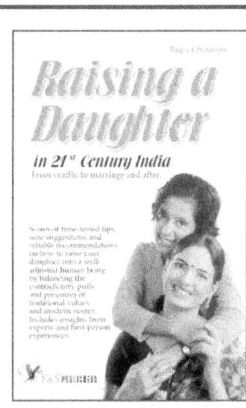

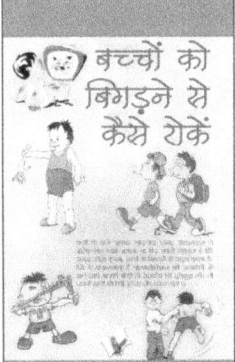

बच्चों को बिगड़ने से कैसे रोकें

लेखक: चुन्नीलाल सलूजा
भाषा: हिन्दी
टाइप: पेपर बैक
पृष्ठ: 152
मूल्य: ₹ 96

आज पश्चिम की स्वच्छंद और भोगवादी संस्कृति के कारण हमारा परिवेश ही बदल गया है। आनंद मनाने, योजनाओं में जीने और चकाचौंध-भरी दुनिया में सुध-बुध बिसार देने की होड़ मची है। ऐसी जीवन शैली से सर्वप्रथम बच्चे ही प्रभावित होते है, क्योंकि सीखने-समझने, परिपक्व बनने की कच्ची उम्र में ही उन्हें परलोक जैसा काल्पनिक संसार आकर्षित कर रहा होता है। राह संक्रमण काल भयावह है, जिससे बचना अवश्यंभावी है।

PARENTING

info@vspublishers.com • www.vspublishers.com

COOKING

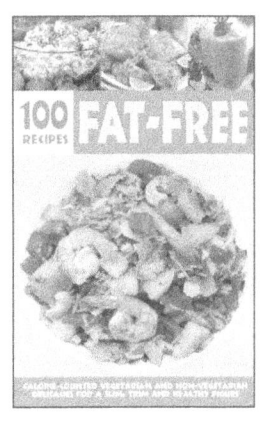

100 Recipes
FAT-FREE

Author: Elizabeth Jyothi Mathew
Language: English
Type: Paperback
Pages: 117
Price: ₹ 96

With fast food and junk foods being the order of the day, thanks to our rushed modern existence, staying healthy is of prime importance. More often than not, we forego some of the most delicious food in order to stay healthy. It is not necessary to give up culinary delicacies to maintain good health. This book shows just how.

The author discribes dishes that are nutritious, low in calories and high on taste. This book takes readers on a journey of culinary experimentation with different recipes that can be incorporated into a healthy lifestyle.

There is a famous saying, *"Cooking is one of the oldest arts and one which has rendered us the most important service in civic life."* It has, indeed, changed our lifestyle from the early man to the present man of the 21st century.

After an incredibly successful run for over two decades, the *New Modern Cookery Book* is now back in an all new avatar with about *150 mouth-watering recipes* from all over the country and across the globe.

New Modern Cookery Book

Author: Asha Rani Vohra
Language: English
Type: Paperback
Pages: 176
Price: ₹ 150

Also available in Hindi

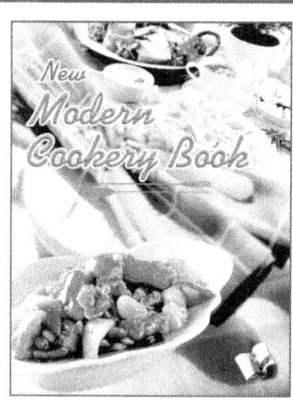

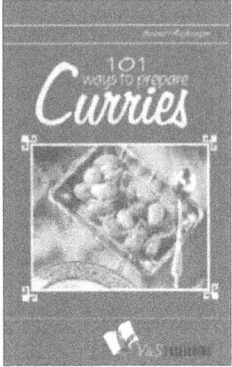

101 ways to prepare Curries

Author: Aroona Reejhsinghani
Language: English
Type: Paperback
Pages: 136
Price: ₹ 80

India is identified with its curries. Curries are vegetarian non-vegetarian preparations in rich gravies. Because of diversity and rich cultural legacy, India has an endless variety of curries, each better than the other.

In the book, *101 ways to prepare Curries*, author has included curries from across the country all of which have their unique and distinctive flavours. The recipes of these curries have been explained in easy-to-follow language to facilitate easy preparation; and can be enjoyed in every part of India.

व्यंजनों के बादशाह आलू की जगह अब पनीर ने ले ली है। लंच हो या डिनर, शाम की चाय हो या सुबह का नाश्ता, शादी–ब्याह हो या किटी–पार्टी अथवा बर्थ डे पार्टी, पनीर के व्यंजनों के बिना खाना आधा–अधूरा लगता है। बच्चे, स्त्री–पुरुष, बड़े–बूढ़े और बीमार सभी के लिए पनीर के ऐसे-ऐसे चटपटे, मसालेदार और स्वादिष्ट व्यंजन, प्रस्तुत पुस्तक में दिये गये हैं जो हर किसी को भरपूर तृप्ति देगा।

पनीर अपने आप में बेहद स्वादिष्ट भी है और पौष्टिक भी। तमाम तरह के भारतीय व्यंजनों में यह अपनी पहचान अलग रखता है।

101 व्यंजनों से सजा
पनीर खाना ख़ज़ाना

लेखक: चित्रा गर्ग
भाषा: हिन्दी
टाइप: पेपर बैक
पृष्ठ: 125
मूल्य: ₹ 96

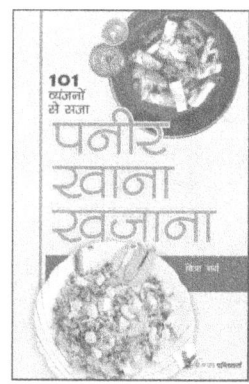

---

info@vspublishers.com • **www.vspublishers.com**

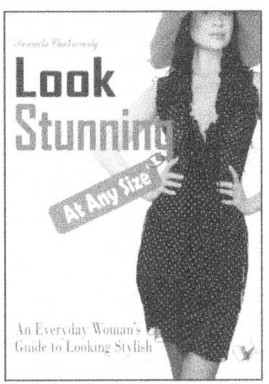

Look Stunning – At Any Size

Author: Parimita Chakravorty
Language: English
Type: Paperback
Pages: 172
Price: ₹ 495

The book has been written, keeping in mind the contemporary Indian woman, her needs, her lifestyle and demands of her personal and professional life. It has information specifically suited for Indian colour, tone, texture as well as sense of style. It intends to bring together a comprehensive overview about how to be presentable and confident with comfortable styling and dressing.

It has make-up suggestions, hairstyle suggestions, hair and beauty care suggestions for all. Everyone will find something useful in this book as it tries to cover most of the problem areas of today's woman. It is not about fashion but identifying one's innate style sense and the quest to look beautiful.

A seasoned housewife who is also a professional interior designer, is one such handy help that deals with the subject in a critical and comprehensive manner. Never before so many tips and suggestions, covering every aspect of the subject, have been put together in a single volume. From interior decoration, time management, cleaning of house and its security, maintaining of gadgets and household articles to household budget, etiquette for all occasions, first aid, travel and transfer, personal grooming, gardening, it goes on to cover tips on energy conservation and interpersonal relationships.

A must for all who wish to make their home a paradise.

Smart Housekeeping

Author: Rupa Chatterjee
Language: English
Type: Paperback
Pages: 252
Price: ₹ 150

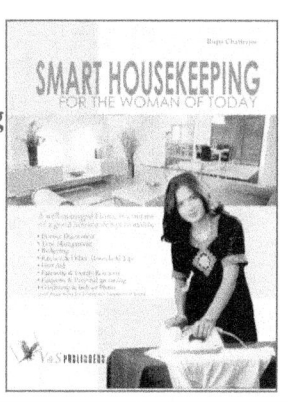

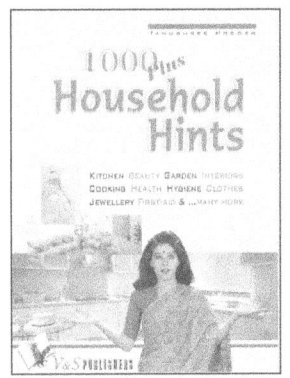

1000 Plus Household Hints

Author: Tanushree Pooder
Language: English
Type: Paperback
Pages: 192
Price: ₹ 150

The fast life of the present day does not permit learning through experience. The new millennium will find people busier with life, leaving little time for anyone to try out the 'trial and error' method of learning. Young women who are setting up their own homes, with little or no experience in running the different departments of the household, face a plethora of problems in their day-to-day work. With the break-up of the joint family system, there are no elderly members in the house to advise them about the solutions to these problems.

Sex being a taboo in our society, several misconceptions and myths have gained currency. Backed by suitable illustrations the book dispels several myths associated with it; as it makes for an informative, educative and enjoyable reading material. This book dissects the entire gamut of sexual artistry, with special references from celebrated sex manuals like Kamasutra and other proven texts on the subject.

All You wanted to know about SEX

Author: Hari Dutt Sharma
Language: English
Type: Paperback
Pages: 144
Price: ₹ 96

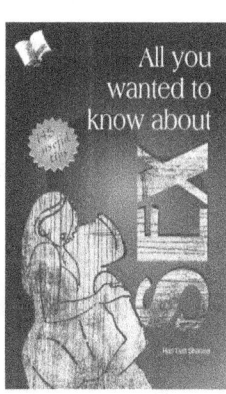

HOUSEKEEPING

info@vspublishers.com • www.vspublishers.com

www.ingramcontent.com/pod-product-compliance
Lightning Source LLC
Chambersburg PA
CBHW080550230426

43663CB00015B/2779